Updates in Pediatric Otolaryngology

Editors

SAMANTHA ANNE
JULINA ONGKASUWAN

OTOLARYNGOLOGIC CLINICS OF NORTH AMERICA

www.oto.theclinics.com

Consulting Editor
SUJANA S. CHANDRASEKHAR

October 2019 • Volume 52 • Number 5

ELSEVIER

1600 John F. Kennedy Boulevard • Suite 1800 • Philadelphia, Pennsylvania, 19103-2899

http://www.oto.theclinics.com

OTOLARYNGOLOGIC CLINICS OF NORTH AMERICA Volume 52, Number 5
October 2019 ISSN 0030-6665, ISBN-13: 978-0-323-70912-5

Editor: Jessica McCool
Developmental Editor: Laura Kavanaugh

Otolaryngologic Clinics of North America (ISSN 0030-6665) is published bimonthly by Elsevier, Inc., 360 Park Avenue South, New York, NY 10010-1710. Months of issue are February, April, June, August, October, and December. Business and Editorial Offices: 1600 John F. Kennedy Blvd., Suite 1800, Philadelphia, PA 19103-2899. Customer Service Office: 6277 Sea Harbor Drive, Orlando, FL 32887-4800. Periodicals postage paid at New York, NY and additional mailing offices. Subscription prices are $412.00 per year (US individuals), $889.00 per year (US institutions), $100.00 per year (US student/resident), $548.00 per year (Canadian individuals), $1127.00 per year (Canadian institutions), $564.00 per year (international individuals), $1127.00 per year (international institutions), $270.00 per year (international & Canadian student/resident). Foreign air speed delivery is included in all *Clinics*' subscription prices. All prices are subject to change without notice. **POSTMASTER:** Send address changes to *Otolaryngologic Clinics of North America*, Elsevier Health Sciences Division, Subscription Customer Service, 3251 Riverport Lane, Maryland Heights, MO 63043. **Telephone: 1-800-654-2452 (U.S. and Canada); 314-447-8871 (outside U.S. and Canada). Fax: 314-447-8029. E-mail: journalscustomerservice-usa@elsevier.com (for print support); journalsonlinesupport-usa@elsevier.com (for online support).**

Reprints. For copies of 100 or more of articles in this publication, please contact the Commercial Reprints Department, Elsevier Inc., 360 Park Avenue South, New York, NY 10010-1710. Tel.: 212-633-3874; Fax: 212-633-3820; E-mail: reprints@elsevier.com.

Otolaryngologic Clinics of North America is also published in Spanish by McGraw-Hill Interamericana Editores S.A., P.O. Box 5-237, 06500 Mexico D.F., Mexico.

Otolaryngologic Clinics of North America is covered in *MEDLINE/PubMed (Index Medicus), Current Contents/Clinical Medicine, Excerpta Medica, BIOSIS, Science Citation Index,* and *ISI/BIOMED.*

Contributors

CONSULTING EDITOR

SUJANA S. CHANDRASEKHAR, MD, FACS, FAAOHNS
Past President, American Academy of Otolaryngology–Head and Neck Surgery,
Secretary-Treasurer, American Otological Society, Partner, ENT & Allergy Associates,
LLP, Clinical Professor, Department of Otolaryngology–Head and Neck Surgery, Zucker
School of Medicine at Hofstra-Northwell, Hempstead, New York; Clinical Associate
Professor, Department of Otolaryngology–Head and Neck Surgery, Icahn School of
Medicine at Mount Sinai, New York, New York

EDITORS

SAMANTHA ANNE, MD, MS
Associate Professor of Surgery, Medical Director, Pediatric Ear and Hearing Disorders,
Department of Otolaryngology–Head and Neck Surgery, Otolaryngology, Head & Neck
Institute, Cleveland Clinic, Cleveland, Ohio

JULINA ONGKASUWAN, MD, FAAP, FACS
Associate Professor of Surgery, Adult and Pediatric Laryngology, Bobby R. Alford
Department of Otolaryngology–Head and Neck Surgery, Baylor College of Medicine,
Texas Children's Hospital, Houston, Texas

AUTHORS

SAMANTHA ANNE, MD, MS
Associate Professor of Surgery, Medical Director, Pediatric Ear and Hearing Disorders,
Department of Otolaryngology–Head and Neck Surgery, Otolaryngology, Head & Neck
Institute, Cleveland Clinic, Cleveland, Ohio

SWATHI APPACHI, MD
Otolaryngology Resident, Head & Neck Institute, Cleveland Clinic, Cleveland,
Ohio

CRISTINA M. BALDASSARI, MD, FAAP, FACS
Associate Professor, Departments of Otolaryngology–Head and Neck Surgery, and
Pediatric Sleep Medicine, Eastern Virginia Medical School, Children's Hospital of the
King's Daughters, Norfolk, Virginia

RYAN BELCHER, MD
Department of Otolaryngology, Pediatric Otolaryngology, Vanderbilt University Medical
Center, Nashville, Tennessee

MARGO McKENNA BENOIT, MD, FACS
Associate Professor, Department of Otolaryngology, University of Rochester Medical
Center, Rochester, New York

ANDREW E. BLUHER, MD
Department of Otolaryngology–Head and Neck Surgery, Eastern Virginia Medical School, Norfolk, Virginia

KAY W. CHANG, MD
Professor, Division of Pediatric Otolaryngology, Lucile Packard Children's Hospital at Stanford, Department of Otolaryngology, Stanford University School of Medicine, Palo Alto, California

DANIEL C. CHELIUS Jr, MD, FAAP, FACS
Department of Otolaryngology–Head and Neck Surgery, Assistant Professor, Baylor College of Medicine, Pediatric Thyroid Tumor Program, Pediatric Head and Neck Tumor Program, Texas Children's Hospital, Houston, Texas

DAVID CHI, MD
Chief, Division of Pediatric Otolaryngology, UPMC Children's Hospital of Pittsburgh, Pittsburgh, Pennsylvania

ROBERT CHUN, MD
Associate Professor of Otolaryngology, Medical College of Wisconsin, Milwaukee, Wisconsin

JOHN P. DAHL, MD, PhD, MBA
Attending Physician, Pediatric Otolaryngology, Seattle Children's Hospital, Assistant Professor, Department of Otolaryngology–Head and Neck Surgery, University of Washington School of Medicine, Seattle, Washington

KELLY DEAN, MD
Otolaryngology Resident, Department of Otolaryngology–Head and Neck Surgery, UNC Hospitals, The University of North Carolina at Chapel Hill, Chapel Hill, North Carolina

AMY L. DIMACHKIEH, MD
Department of Otolaryngology–Head and Neck Surgery, Assistant Professor, Baylor College of Medicine, Pediatric Thyroid Tumor Program, Pediatric Head and Neck Tumor Program, Texas Children's Hospital, Houston, Texas

AMELIA F. DRAKE, MD
ND Fischer Distinguished Professor of Otolaryngology, Department of Otolaryngology–Head and Neck Surgery, UNC Hospitals, Director, Craniofacial Center, The University of North Carolina at Chapel Hill, Chapel Hill, North Carolina

MANUELA FINA, MD
Assistant Professor, Department of Otolaryngology, Minneapolis, Minnesota; Staff Associate, HealthPartners Medical Group, St Paul, Minnesota

CHRISTIAN R. FRANCOM, MD
Department of Otolaryngology, University of Colorado School of Medicine, Children's Hospital Colorado, University of Colorado, Aurora, Colorado

ELLEN M. FRIEDMAN, MD, FACS, FAAP
Center for Professionalism, Office of the Provost, Baylor College of Medicine, Houston, Texas

GLENN E. GREEN, MD
Professor, Pediatric Otolaryngology, Department of Otolaryngology–Head and Neck Surgery, University of Michigan, Ann Arbor, Michigan

CATHERINE K. HART, MD, MS
Associate Professor, Pediatric Otolaryngology, Cincinnati Children's Hospital Medical Center, University of Cincinnati College of Medicine, Cincinnati, Ohio

BRANDON HOPKINS, MD
Pediatric Otolaryngology, Assistant Professor, Surgical Director, Pediatric Center for Airway Voice and Swallowing, Cleveland Clinic, Cleveland, Ohio

DAVID L. HORN, MD, MS
Associate Professor, Department of Otolaryngology–Head and Neck Surgery, Division of Pediatric Otolaryngology, University of Washington School of Medicine, Seattle, Washington

ANNE HSEU, MD
Boston Children's Hospital, Boston, Massachusetts

STACEY L. ISHMAN, MD, MPH
Professor, Divisions of Pediatric Otolaryngology–Head and Neck Surgery, and Pulmonary Medicine, Department of Otolaryngology–Head and Neck Surgery, Cincinnati Children's Hospital Medical Center, University of Cincinnati College of Medicine, Cincinnati, Ohio

ROMAINE F. JOHNSON, MD, MPH, FACS
Department of Otolaryngology– Head and Neck Surgery, The University of Texas Southwestern Medical Center, Dallas, Texas

KEN KAZAHAYA, MD, MBA, FACS
Associate Director, Division of Pediatric Otolaryngology, Associate Professor of Clinical Otolaryngology–Head and Neck Surgery, University of Pennsylvania, Co-Lead Surgeon, Pediatric Thyroid Center, Children's Hospital of Philadelphia, Philadelphia, Pennsylvania

KRISTA K. KIYOSAKI, MD
Division of Pediatric Otolaryngology, Lucile Packard Children's Hospital at Stanford, Department of Otolaryngology, Stanford University School of Medicine, Palo Alto, California

DANIEL J. LEE, MD
Director, Pediatric Otology and Neurotology, Associate Professor, Department of Otology and Laryngology, Harvard Medical School, Massachusetts Eye and Ear Infirmary, Boston, Massachusetts

VICTORIA S. LEE, MD
Department of Otolaryngology–Head and Neck Surgery, Johns Hopkins School of Medicine, Johns Hopkins Outpatient Center, Baltimore, Maryland

SANDRA Y. LIN, MD
Department of Otolaryngology–Head and Neck Surgery, Johns Hopkins School of Medicine, Johns Hopkins Outpatient Center, Baltimore, Maryland

C. CARRIE LIU, MD, MPH
Pediatric Otolaryngology–Head and Neck Surgery, Seattle Children's Hospital, Seattle, Washington

KIMBERLY LUU, MD
Division of Pediatric Otolaryngology, UPMC Children's Hospital of Pittsburgh, Pittsburgh, Pennsylvania

AMY MANNING, MD
Clinical Fellow, Pediatric Otolaryngology, Cincinnati Children's Hospital Medical Center, Cincinnati, Ohio

CINZIA L. MARCHICA, MD, FRCSC, MSc
Fellow, Pediatric Otolaryngology, Children's Healthcare of Atlanta, Emory University, Atlanta, Georgia

KIMBERLY A. MILLER, MD
Resident, Department of Otolaryngology, University of Minnesota, Minneapolis, Minnesota

JULINA ONGKASUWAN, MD, FAAP, FACS
Associate Professor of Surgery, Adult and Pediatric Laryngology, Bobby R. Alford Department of Otolaryngology–Head and Neck Surgery, Baylor College of Medicine, Texas Children's Hospital, Houston, Texas

JEREMY D. PRAGER, MD, MBA
Department of Otolaryngology, University of Colorado School of Medicine, Children's Hospital Colorado, Associate Professor, University of Colorado, Aurora, Colorado

NIKHILA RAOL, MD, MPH
Attending Physician, Pediatric Otolaryngology, Children's Healthcare of Atlanta, Assistant Professor, Department of Otolaryngology–Head and Neck Surgery, Emory University, Atlanta, Georgia

JEFFREY RASTATTER, MD
Associate Professor of Otolaryngology, Northwestern University, Chicago, Illinois

SOPHIE G. SHAY, MD
Assistant Professor of Otolaryngology, Medical College of Wisconsin, Milwaukee, Wisconsin

TAHER VALIKA, MD
Assistant Professor of Otolaryngology, Northwestern University, Chicago, Illinois

JONATHAN WALSH, MD
Assistant Professor, Department of Otolaryngology–Head and Neck Surgery, Johns Hopkins University, Baltimore, Maryland

DANIEL J. WEHRMANN, MD
Fellow, Pediatric Otolaryngology, Department of Otolaryngology–Head and Neck Surgery, University of Michigan, Ann Arbor, Michigan

CHRISTOPHER T. WOOTTEN, MD, MMHC
Department of Otolaryngology, Pediatric Otolaryngology, Associate Professor, Vanderbilt University Medical Center, Nashville, Tennessee

Contents

have allowed the otologic surgeon to improve surgical outcomes while minimizing intervention.

The article describes the unique benefits and challenges of transcanal (and transmastoid) endoscopic ear surgery (EES) for management of middle ear disease in children. It provides a rationale for EES in children and describes differences in anatomy between the pediatric and adult ear. The basic principles of EES, from operating room layout, choice of surgical instruments, and tips and pearls to avoid complications specific to the endoscope, are reviewed. Finally, techniques and outcomes in pediatric EES for tympanic membrane perforation, congenital cholesteatoma, and acquired cholesteatoma are summarized.

The work-up and management of sensorineural hearing loss in children has been an area of rapid evolution. With the availability of genetic and cytomegalovirus testing, the diagnostic process is continuously refined. Aural rehabilitation should be provided to children in a timely manner. At present, the main surgical options for the treatment of sensorineural hearing loss are bone conduction sound processors and cochlear implants. Investigations into modalities such as auditory brainstem implants are ongoing. With further technological and medical advancements, the evaluation and management of pediatric sensorineural hearing loss will undoubtedly continue to change.

Food allergy and allergic rhinitis are childhood diseases with special relevance to the pediatric otolaryngologist. Much of the diagnosis of food allergy can be made on history alone; strict avoidance is the mainstay treatment. Skin prick testing and serum-specific IgE testing play a stronger role in allergic rhinitis diagnosis. If pharmacotherapy fails, allergen immunotherapy is an option. Currently, there is intense investigation on diagnostic tests, novel treatments, and prevention strategies that could dramatically affect the way these diseases are identified and managed. This article summarizes the epidemiology, pathophysiology, diagnosis, and management of food allergy and allergic rhinitis.

Although there have been many advances in new tools and procedures for endonasal sinus surgery in children, the management and care for pediatric chronic rhinosinusitis has remained relatively unchanged. However, there have been advances in skull base surgery and tumor removal and new knowledge about perioperative concerns in children. This article discusses the role and risks of endoscopic sinus surgery, the use of balloon sinuplasty in children, management of complicated rhinosinusitis, and advances in skull base tumors and choanal atresia repair.

Andrew E. Bluher, Stacey L. Ishman, and Cristina M. Baldassari

 Video content accompanies this article at http://www.oto.theclinics. com.

Pediatric obstructive sleep apnea (OSA) affects 2% to 4% of American children, and is associated with metabolic, cardiovascular, and neurocognitive sequelae. The primary treatment for pediatric OSA is adenotonsillectomy. Children with obesity, craniofacial syndromes, and severe baseline OSA are at risk for persistent disease. Evaluation of persistent OSA should focus on identifying the causes of upper airway obstruction. Interventions should be tailored to address the patient's symptomatology, sites of obstruction, and preference for surgical versus medical management. Further research is needed to identify management protocols that result in improved outcomes for children with persistent OSA.

Brandon Hopkins, Kelly Dean, Swathi Appachi, and Amelia F. Drake

Craniofacial interventions are common and the surgical options continue to grow. The issues encountered include micrognathia, macroglossia, midface hypoplasia, hearing loss, facial nerve palsy, hemifacial microsomia, and microtia. In addition, a unifying theme is complex upper airway obstruction. Throughout a child's life the focus of interventions may change from airway management to speech, hearing, and language optimization, and finally to decannulation and procedures aimed at social integration and self-esteem. Otolaryngologists play an important role is this arena and provide high-quality care while continuing to expand what can be done for our patients.

Amy Manning, Daniel J. Wehrmann, Catherine K. Hart, and Glenn E. Green

The management of pediatric airway stenosis has evolved considerably over time. At the outset, dilation was the mainstay of management. In the 1900s, open surgery in the form of cricoid expansion procedures or resection procedures was the primary treatment with subsequent development of the slide tracheoplasty. Now in the twenty-first century, advances in endoscopic management, balloon dilation, and stenting, along with the advent of external scaffolds and tissue replacement continue to advance pediatric airway surgery.

Christopher T. Wootten, Ryan Belcher, Christian R. Francom, and Jeremy D. Prager

The early efforts of pediatric airway surgeons, gastroenterologists, and pulmonologists to optimize surgical outcomes involved evaluating multiple organ systems for diseases negatively affecting surgery. This resulted in coordinated clinics with multiple services, ancillary testing, and endoscopic procedures, known as aerodigestive programs. These programs have nationally increased the value of care, with multidisciplinary experts delivering organized and efficient care to children with complex needs. This article describes the origin and value of aerodigestive programs within the modern health care landscape, serving as a primer for providers and administrators investigating how to facilitate aerodigestive or similar programs.

Pediatric dysphonia is common; however, not all vocal fold pathology in children is due to nodules. Laryngeal stroboscopy (transoral or transnasal) often is essential for the diagnosis of other not-nodule lesions. As in adults, multidisciplinary care with a speech language pathologist helps with patient buy-in for therapy. Breathy dysphonia due to glottic incompetence may be related to vocal fold movement impairment (VFMI) or posterior glottic insufficiency. There are several medialization procedures available for children with VFMI due to recurrent laryngeal nerve injury.

This article summarizes the current management of pediatric thyroid disease, with an emphasis on surgical management. Medical and surgical approaches to hyperthyroidism are reviewed as well as pathways for evaluation of nodules and malignancy. Differences between pediatric and adult thyroid management are highlighted.

Professionalism, quality, and safety have become essential components of pediatric otolaryngology. Professionalism, as defined by Osler, refers to the long tradition of physicians carrying out the noble cause of providing health care to patients and families. The importance of professionalism cannot be overstated and now is widely understood to be a core competency of every practicing physician. The attention to quality and safety is also a central tenet of current surgical practice. Quality is doing the right thing at the right time for the right persons. Safety is providing care to patients that is free from undue harm.

OTOLARYNGOLOGIC CLINICS
OF NORTH AMERICA

SERIES OF RELATED INTEREST

Facial Plastic Surgery Clinics
Available at: https://www.facialplastic.theclinics.com/

THE CLINICS ARE AVAILABLE ONLINE!
Access your subscription at:
www.theclinics.com

Erratum

An error was made in the June 2019 issue of *Otolaryngologic Clinics* (Volume 52, Issue 3) in the Preface, written by guest editors Melissa A. Pynnonen and Cecelia E. Schmalbach (pgs. xv–xvi).

References were made to Appendix I and Appendix II within the Preface; however, no appendices were included in the print or online versions of the issue.

The print and online versions of the Preface have now been corrected to include these appendices.

Otolaryngol Clin N Am 52 (2019) xiii
https://doi.org/10.1016/j.otc.2019.07.002
oto.theclinics.com

Foreword

Not Just Smaller Ears, Noses, Throats, and Necks

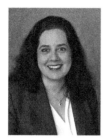

Sujana S. Chandrasekhar, MD, FACS, FAAOHNS
Consulting Editor

On the first day of my clinical rotation in Pediatrics as a third-year medical student, I was handed the Harriet Lane Handbook and told, with some ferocity, that "children are not just little adults." Similarly, otolaryngologic problems in children are not just smaller versions of those problems in adults. Although otolaryngologists have always cared for children, and the fundamental nature of their specialty is conducive to treating diseases in children (otitis media, upper respiratory infections, and so forth), Dr Sylvan Stool pointed out the necessity of developing the discipline of pediatric otolaryngology and how it helps all otolaryngologists treat these patients. In his article written for the centennial year of the American Academy of Otolaryngology–Head and Neck Surgery, he details the thought processes that have culminated in focused scientific attention to pediatric otolaryngologic disorders.[1] He points out that the first edition of Bluestone and Stool's textbook *Pediatric Otolaryngology* had 89 chapters. The fifth edition, published in 2014, has nearly double that number.

Drs Anne and Ongkasuwan have achieved a remarkable feat. They have assembled, in just 14 separate articles, this single issue of *Otolaryngologic Clinics of North America* devoted to Updates in Pediatric Otolaryngology. The reader of this issue will be thoroughly briefed on the state-of-the-art, with each article being written by experts. Every single article is worth a close read. Here are some highlights:

What is often considered the most "routine" of all operations, tonsillectomy, is consistently in the news, particularly because it is almost exclusively performed in children. Indications change, pain management changes, but, despite major advances in patient safety, the mortality of tonsillectomy of 1 in 10,000 in 1965[2] was still between 1 in 10,000 and 1 in 35,000 in 2010.[3] Dr Raol's article regarding what's new in tubes,

Otolaryngol Clin N Am 52 (2019) xv–xvii
https://doi.org/10.1016/j.otc.2019.07.001
oto.theclinics.com

tonsils, and adenoids touches on all of the factors that minimize risk and maximize outcome for these commonly performed procedures.

Ear surgery in children ranges from chronic otitis media procedures to implantable auditory devices. Minimally invasive methodologies including endoscopic ear surgery, and the ability of implants to afford high quality of life options are explained in 3 important articles.

The 'snot-nosed kid' can have several problems, each of which must be assessed and treated correctly. The articles on allergy and endonasal sinus surgery delineate this. Sleep apnea in children is much more than just big tonsils. Craniofacial anomalies can now be addressed more directly and less invasively. The articles about these topics offer pearls to the practicing otolaryngologist, for assessment, counseling, and intervention.

Pediatric airway management has evolved very quickly, with advances in not only pediatric otolaryngology but also pediatric anesthesiology as well. The articles on airway surgery, pediatric voice, and holistic management of aerodigestive issues are thorough and insightful. Tongue-tie has become a great concern to parents of newborns who may be having feeding/suckling issues. Management of less than severe ankyloglossia requires the otolaryngologist to understand the nuances of this issue, and when and how best to intervene, and, of course, when intervention is not indicated. The article by Dr Benoit on this is highly educational.

Thyroid disease in children is clearly a much different issue than that in adults. Ramifications include physical and mental retardation as well as hearing loss. Much like that old Harriet Lane Handbook, the article on this topic is required reading.

All of the articles mentioned above provide information to enhance quality and safety in pediatric otolaryngology. Drs Johnson and Friedman tie that into the role of professionalism in this field. Respectful communication between members of the health care team, the patient, and the family members is clearly shown to effect better outcomes.

Again, I commend Drs Anne and Ongkasuwan, the guest editors of this issue of *Otolaryngologic Clinics of North America*. They have provided a wealth of important information from which all otolaryngologists and their patients can benefit. I hope you enjoy reading it as much as I did.

Sujana S. Chandrasekhar, MD, FACS, FAAOHNS
Past President, American Academy of Otolaryngology-Head and Neck Surgery
Secretary-Treasurer, American Otological Society
Partner, ENT & Allergy Associates, LLP
Clinical Professor, Department of Otolaryngology–Head and Neck Surgery
Zucker School of Medicine at Hofstra-Northwell
Hempstead, NY, USA

Clinical Associate Professor, Department of Otolaryngology–Head and Neck Surgery
Icahn School of Medicine at Mount Sinai
New York, NY, USA

ENT & Allergy Associates, LLP
18 East 48th Street, 2nd Floor
New York, NY 10017, USA

E-mail address:
ssc@nyotology.com

REFERENCES

1. Stool SE. A brief history of pediatric otolaryngology. Otolaryngol Head Neck Surg 1996;115(4):278–82.
2. Tonsillectomy mortality. JAMA 1965;194(7):824. https://doi.org/10.1001/jama. 1965.03090200132029.
3. Oron Y, Marom T, Russo E, et al. Don't overlook the complications of tonsillectomy. J Fam Pract 2010;59(10):E4–9.

Preface

Updates in Pediatric Otolaryngology

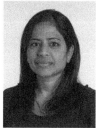 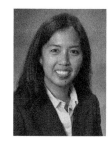

Samantha Anne, MD, MS   Julina Ongkasuwan, MD, FAAP, FACS
Editors

Pediatric Otolaryngology as a field has gone through incredible advancement over the past 40 years since its inception as a discipline of medicine. This *Otolaryngologic Clinics of North America* issue reviews these various developments. In otology, the authors present innovations in the use of otoendoscopes and in the evaluation of sensorineural hearing loss. In rhinology, new technology, such as balloon dilation, and transnasal approaches to the skull base are discussed. Contemporary management with multidisciplinary care of complex aerodigestive disorders, craniofacial disorders, and thyroid disorders is presented. In addition, management options for pediatric voice disorders, refractive obstructive sleep apnea, and ankyloglossia are presented.

Otolaryngol Clin N Am 52 (2019) xix–xx
https://doi.org/10.1016/j.otc.2019.06.011
0030-6665/19/© 2019 Published by Elsevier Inc.

As the field continues to evolve, it is hoped that these innovations and updates will serve as breeding ground for new ideas and improvements.

Samantha Anne, MD, MS
Section of Pediatric Otolaryngology
Head & Neck Institute
Cleveland Clinic
9500 Euclid Avenue A71
Cleveland, OH 44195, USA

Julina Ongkasuwan, MD, FAAP, FACS
Adult and Pediatric Laryngology
Bobby R. Alford Department of
Otolaryngology Head and Neck Surgery
Baylor College of Medicine
Texas Children's Hospital
6701 Fannin, Suite 640
Houston, TX 77030, USA

E-mail addresses:
annes@ccf.org (S. Anne)
julinao@bcm.edu (J. Ongkasuwan)

What's New with Tubes, Tonsils, and Adenoids?

Cinzia L. Marchica, MD, FRCSC, MSc[a,b], John P. Dahl, MD, PhD, MBA[c,d], Nikhila Raol, MD, MPH[a,b,*]

KEYWORDS

- Tympanostomy tubes • Otitis • Otitis media with effusion • Tonsillectomy
- Adenoidectomy • Sleep apnea • Recurrent tonsillitis

KEY POINTS

- Understand the current indications for tympanostomy tube placement.
- Evaluate the role for adenoidectomy in the context of middle ear effusion.
- Understand the current indications for tonsillectomy.
- Review current clinical practice guidelines for the various professional organizations on these topics.

INTRODUCTION

Otolaryngology procedures, including tympanostomy tube insertion, adenoidectomy, and tonsillectomy, are among the most common procedures performed in children. Evidence-based recommendations are constantly being updated regarding the indication for the surgical management of common pediatric conditions such as otitis media, recurrent tonsillitis, and sleep disordered breathing. Appropriate knowledge regarding the disease entities, as well as clinical practice and treatment guidelines, is essential for providing evidence-based care.

Current Concepts and Guidelines in Acute Otitis Media, Otitis Media with Effusion, and Tympanostomy Tube Insertion

Otitis media is one of the most prevalent conditions seen in childhood,[1,2] accounting for a high proportion of primary care office visits.[3] It encapsulates different disease

Disclosures: Dr. Raol receives funding from American Society of Pediatric Otolaryngology Career Development Award. Rest of the authors do not have any disclosures.
[a] Pediatric Otolaryngology, Children's Healthcare of Atlanta, USA; [b] Department of Otolaryngology Head and Neck Surgery, Emory University, 2015 Uppergate Dr., Atlanta, GA 30322, USA; [c] Pediatric Otolaryngology, Seattle Children's Hospital, 4800 Sand Point Way NE, Seattle, WA 98105, USA; [d] Department of Otolaryngology Head & Neck Surgery, University of Washington School of Medicine, Seattle, WA, USA
* Corresponding author. Department of Otolaryngology Head and Neck Surgery, Emory University, 2015 Uppergate Dr., Atlanta, GA 30322.
E-mail address: nikhila.p.raol@emory.edu

Otolaryngol Clin N Am 52 (2019) 779–794
https://doi.org/10.1016/j.otc.2019.05.002
0030-6665/19/© 2019 Elsevier Inc. All rights reserved.

oto.theclinics.com

entities, including acute otitis media (AOM), defined as the rapid onset of signs and symptoms of inflammation of the middle ear, and otitis media with effusion (OME), the presence of fluid in the middle ear without signs or symptoms of acute ear infection.[2,4] Recurrent AOM (rAOM) refers to 3 or more well-documented and separate AOM episodes in the past 6 months or at least 4 AOM episodes in the past 12 months with at least 1 in the past 6 months[4,5]. Chronic otitis media with effusion (COME) is defined as OME persisting for greater than or equal to 3 months from the date of onset (if known) or from the date of diagnosis (if onset is unknown)[2,4]

Acute Otitis Media

AOM has an average incidence of 10.8 new episodes per 100 individuals yearly.[6,7] A decline in this incidence has been seen in developed countries because of vaccines as well as the adoption of clinical practice guidelines (CPGs) providing strict diagnostic criteria and indications for antibiotic use.

The American Academy of Pediatrics (AAP) 2013 guidelines on the diagnosis and management of AOM[8] stated that in order to diagnose AOM a middle ear effusion (MEE) with tympanic membrane (TM) bulging as well as recent onset of otalgia or intense TM erythema must be present. AOM severity is defined by the presence of 1 or more of the following[8]:

- Moderate or severe otalgia
- Otalgia greater than or equal to 48 hours
- Temperature greater than or equal to 39°C (102.2°F)

Risk factors

Both environmental and genetic factors are thought to be associated with AOM, including exposure to tobacco smoke, pacifier use, supine bottle feeding, day care attendance, and low socioeconomic status.[7] Pneumococcal and influenza vaccination are recommended by the AAP CPG, which have been shown decreased frequency of AOM and the risk of developing a serious systemic complication. Breastfeeding in the first 6 months of life is also recommended, because it has been shown to reduce episodes of AOM/rAOM.[8,9] Lifestyle changes, such as supine bottle feeding, pacifier use, and child care attendance, potentially reduce AOM incidence or recurrence. However, there are insufficient data for the AAP to set forth a guideline/recommendation.[8]

Management

Analgesia in acute otitis media

Pain is the most common symptom associated with AOM, therefore a clear role exists for pain management as an adjunct in the treatment algorithm. A strong recommendation for good pain control has been made by the AAP, with acetaminophen/ibuprofen recommended for mild to moderate pain and narcotic analgesia for moderate to severe pain (used with caution because of the risk of respiratory depression and altered mental status). The incorporation of parent/caregiver preference should also be taken into consideration when selecting appropriate analgesia options. Topical analgesics applied to the TM may show potential but short-lived benefit, with limited studies clearly showing their effectiveness.[7,8,10]

Antibiotics in acute otitis media

A more judicious use of antibiotics in AOM has occurred in part because of guidelines regarding their indications. These indications include:

- Bilateral or unilateral AOM in children greater than 6 months old with severe signs or symptoms (severe otalgia, temperature>39°C [102.2°F])
- Bilateral AOM in children less than 2 years old without signs or symptoms of severe disease
  - Mild otalgia (<48 hours)
  - Temperature less than 39°C (102.2°F)
- AOM with otorrhea

First-line antibiotic therapy in patients with uncomplicated AOM is high-dose amoxicillin (80–90 mg/kg/d) as long as the patient has not received amoxicillin in the past 30 days or has purulent conjunctivitis. If a penicillin allergy exists, the AAP recommends the use of any of the following: cefdinir, cefuroxime, cefpodoxime, or ceftriaxone. Second-line agents, such as amoxicillin-clavulanate, are recommended when the patient has received amoxicillin in the last 30 days, has purulent conjunctivitis, or has failed first-line therapy within 48 to 72 hours (severe otalgia, temperature>39°C).[8]

With regard to treatment duration, the AAP recommends a 10-day course for children less than 2 years old or those with severe symptoms. A 7-day course is acceptable for children between 2 and 5 years of age with mild or moderate AOM. In addition, a 5-day to 7-day course of antibiotic has been proposed for those children greater than or equal to 6 years old with mild to moderate symptoms.[8] A recently published noninferiority study evaluating antibiotic duration in children 6 to 23 months old showed that a 5-day treatment course was inferior to the 10-day treatment when evaluating symptom score and clinical signs. However, the investigators commented that this difference is small and questioned its clinical significance.[11] Hospital admission with intravenous antibiotics is reserved for refractory disease and the presence of complications of AOM, including mastoiditis, sigmoid sinus thrombosis, and cerebral abscess.

Systemic corticosteroids
Based on a Cochrane Review evaluating the role for systemic corticosteroids in improving treatment outcomes for AOM, their role remains uncertain because of the low quality of current studies in the literature.[12]

Myringotomy with tympanostomy tube insertion
A Cochrane Review evaluating the effectiveness of tympanostomy tube (TT) insertion in rAOM identified only 5 randomized control studies, all published before the institution of the pneumococcal vaccine. According to this review, the placement of TTs for rAOM in children showed an average decrease of 1.5 AOM episodes at 6 months compared with active monitoring and placebo medication; however, this difference was 0.55 AOM episodes at 12 months. Their effectiveness compared with antibiotics was uncertain. These studies were regarded to provide low-quality to very-low-quality evidence, and therefore need to be interpreted with caution.[13]

Otitis Media with Effusion

OME is common among the pediatric population, affecting 90% of children before 5 years of age. It can occur as a result of eustachian tube dysfunction, during an upper respiratory tract infection, or following the inflammatory process of AOM.[14–16] Although OME resolves spontaneously in most cases, up to 40% of patients have repeated episodes, with 10% of them lasting more than a year.[15,16] The prevalence of OME has also been shown to be higher in the Down syndrome and cleft palate population of children.[17,18]

MEE present for more than 3 months has been associated with decreased hearing levels, balance disorders, worse quality of life, and poor school performance.[4,19] With the potential impact of OME on the development of children, minimizing variations in treatment practices has been the objective of the American Academy of Otolaryngology–Head and Neck Surgery (AAO-HNS) CPG.[15] The current guidelines target patients aged 2 to 12 years. They also include and define children who are considered at risk of developmental difficulties, such as children with physical, sensory, or cognitive delays or disorders.[4] This at-risk group of children includes those with autism-spectrum disorder, children with blindness or hearing loss irrespective of OME, syndromic children, and those with cleft palate or developmental delay.[4,15]

Per the AAO-HNS CPG, there is a strong recommendation for clinicians to document the presence of MEE with pneumatic otoscopy when diagnosing OME. In addition, children presenting with hearing loss, otalgia, or both should be evaluated with pneumatic otoscopy to rule out OME.[15] Despite this, in a survey sampling providers within the San Antonio military health system, only 67.3% had pneumatic otoscopes, with only 38.5% of those actually using them for diagnostic purposes.[1] Diagnosing the presence of long-standing OME is imperative because of its effect on hearing and speech development, as well as its effect on the TM with potential development of retraction pockets and eventual formation of cholesteatoma.[20]

If diagnosis is still uncertain after pneumatic otoscopy, or attempt thereof, tympanometry should be obtained (strong recommendation).[15] This advice is similarly endorsed by the international consensus (ICON) on management of OME.[20] As with the TT guidelines discussed later, at-risk children need to be identified by the provider and should be evaluated for the presence of OME. This evaluation should be repeated at 12 to 18 months of age (recommendation), in contrast with healthy children who need not be screened regularly for OME if otherwise asymptomatic. However, if healthy children do present with OME, watchful waiting for a period of 3 months from diagnosis of OME is strongly recommended given the natural history of self-resolution of OME. Usually, up to 90% of cases of OME self-resolve in the span of 3 months.[15]

The current guidelines also discuss the recommendations against intranasal or systemic steroids, antibiotics,[21] antihistamines, or decongestants in the treatment of OME because of lack of evidence showing their effectiveness compared with placebo.[15,22,23] However, patients with concomitant allergic rhinitis may benefit from intranasal steroids, which can decrease the inflammatory component likely contributing to the presence of OME.[24] Note that although an association between allergy and OME has been postulated, evidence for direct causation is lacking in the literature. As for other nonsurgical options, the ICON panelists have agreed that autoinsufflation may partially restore eustachian tube function, leading to clearance of the MEE; however, additional studies are required to clearly show its effectiveness.[20]

Tympanostomy Tube Insertion

In 2012, the AAO-HNS published the CPG on TT insertion in children between 6 months and 12 years of age.[4] TTs are the most common elective surgery performed in the United States, with 6.8% of children having TT insertion by age 3 years.[4,25] The main reasons for TT insertion are the presence of MEE and recurrent/persistent ear infections. The presence of fluid in the middle ear is common in children after upper respiratory tract infections. Their increased risk of developing the former is partly explained by their immature immune systems, as well as poor ventilator function of the eustachian tube caused in part by a more horizontal position.[26] Therefore, the

AAO-HNS guidelines state that OME present for a period of less than 3 months does not qualify as an indication for TT placement. The exception to this includes the at-risk children previously defined.

An observational surveillance interval of 3 to 6 months should be established in children with OME in order to identify one of the following courses of the disease:

1. OME resolves
2. Hearing loss is detected
3. Abnormalities in the structure of the TM or middle ear are suspected or observed

This surveillance period allows reassessment of surgical intervention, helps avoid complications, and permits continual family counseling. Because of the high-volume nature of pediatric otolaryngology practices with the possibility of loss to follow-up for these patients, pediatricians should be made aware of these recommendations as well so that one of the disease courses listed earlier is ensured by either provider.

A valuable and recommended component of the evaluation of chronic OME is an age-appropriate hearing evaluation of children who are otherwise candidates for TT placement. Establishing hearing levels helps to document baseline hearing thresholds, identifies presence of concomitant sensorineural component, and aids in the clinical decisions regarding the need for surgery.

Indications for TT placement as per AAO-HNS guidelines include the following:

- Bilateral OME present greater than or equal to 3 months with documented hearing loss
- Unilateral or bilateral OME greater than or equal to 3 months with symptoms, including ear discomfort, vestibular problems, behavioral issues (including poor school performance), as well as decreased quality of life measures
- rAOM and unilateral or bilateral MEE at time of evaluation
- At-risk children with unilateral or bilateral OME that is thought to have a low probability of resolving spontaneously, or the presence of OME for greater than or equal to 3 months

The AAO-HNS[15] and ICON[20] OME guidelines also document a distinction between children less than 4 years of age and those aged 4 years and older. When TT insertion is recommended for children less than 4 years of age, adenoidectomy should not be concurrently performed unless a clear indication for this surgical procedure exists, such as chronic adenoiditis or nasal obstruction caused by adenoid hypertrophy. This guideline is in contrast with children more than 4 years of age, whereby TT insertion, adenoidectomy, or both are recommended for the treatment of OME.[15] These recommendations were the product of a systematic review with meta-analysis evaluating the effect of concurrent adenoidectomy on repeated TT placement, rAOM, OME, as well as otorrhea. When the data were stratified by age, adenoidectomy showed a protective effect in children more than 4 years old.[27] This finding is an important distinction from prior guidelines[28] as well as AAP guidelines[8] that recommended adenoidectomy when repeat surgery for OME was needed. Limited evidence has been published to support the previous recommendation, and thus was it modified in the most recent guideline.

Studies have shown a positive effect of TT insertion on reducing the prevalence of MEE long term,[29] improving hearing,[4,29,30] and positively affecting quality of life.[31] These effects may be enhanced in children at risk of having developmental difficulties.[32] In a meta-analysis evaluating individual patient data from 7 randomized control trials, patients with high infection load or older children with greater than 25 decibels hearing level (dB HL) loss with MEE present for more than 12 weeks benefitted from TT placement.[32] Studies have shown a 32% decreased prevalence of MEE after TT insertion in patients with COME with an improvement in hearing levels by 5 to 12 dB HL.[32,33]

In the context of rAOM, if the child does not have any MEE at the time of assessment, TT should not be performed. This recommendation is based on randomized controlled trials evaluating the natural history of the disease and showing that TT in children without MEE does not decrease the incidence of AOM.[4,19] Note that this specific criterion is omitted in the AAP CPG,[8] which may lead to some confusion among primary care providers and patients' families. However, the AAO-HNS guidelines do specify exceptions to this, which include children with a history of a severe or persistent episode of AOM; presence of immunosuppression; or the presence of a complication of AOM, such as mastoiditis, meningitis, or facial nerve paralysis. TT may also be an option for children who have allergies or intolerances to multiple antibiotics.[4]

Various ventilation tubes exist on the market and the choice of tube type must be made in the context of the child's clinical context and individualized treatment strategy. TTs, such as Paparella tubes, can extrude within a 6-month to 12-month period compared with Armstrong tubes, which extrude usually within a 9-month to 14-month period. In addition, TTs are considered long-term tubes lasting up to 2 years.[20,34]

Perioperative education and family counseling are imperative in the care of these patients and allow caregivers to understand the nature and course of the disease, postsurgical expectations, as well as identifying any complications. One of the more common, but usually transient, complications of TT insertion is tube otorrhea, seen in up to 26% of children with TTs.[35] It is recommended that, in otherwise uncomplicated tube otorrhea, otic eardrops alone be prescribed.[4] The local drug levels of otic drops are 1000 times higher than with the same oral antibiotic.[20] These otic preparations are efficacious against ear pathogens, such as *Pseudomonas aeruginosa* and methicillin-resistant *Staphylococcus aureus*, allowing the use of systemic antibiotics to be limited in immunosuppressed children or in cases of acute complications, including cellulitis of adjacent skin or concurrent bacterial infections of the sinuses or pharynx.

Other reported complications of TTs are tube blockage (7%), early tube extrusion (4%), granulation tissue (4%), and rarely displacement of the TT into the middle ear (0.5%).[35] Myringosclerosis and the associated minimal effects on hearing can be among the long-term sequelae of TT presence.

Water precautions in children with TT are not routinely encouraged unless there is presence of otalgia with water exposure, swimming in lake water, deep sea diving, or presence of tube otorrhea.[4] A Cochrane Review discussing water precautions in TTs identified 2 randomized-controlled trials that met inclusion criteria for evaluating the effectiveness of water precautions on TT otorrhea.[36] The first study investigated 201 children and showed a 0.36 reduction in the number of otorrhea episodes per year (95% confidence interval [CI], −0.45 to −0.27). Additional results showed no differences in hearing or tube extrusion. The second study evaluated 212 patients and did not find any significant difference between those patients who observed water precautions and those who did not.

Trends in Tonsillectomy and Adenoidectomy

Adenotonsillectomy is the second most common procedure performed by otolaryngologists in patients less than 15 years old after the insertion of TT.[37,38] Although tonsillectomy was frequently performed for recurrent infection in the past, the primary indication for this procedure is now obstructive sleep disordered breathing.[38,39]

Indications

When evaluating recurrent tonsillitis as an indication for tonsillectomy, the recent 2019 update to the AAO-HNS CPG[38] on tonsillectomy now strongly recommends watchful waiting for those children who have a history of less than 7 infections in the past year, less than 5 infections per year for the past 2 years, or less than 3 episodes per year in the past 3 years. A positive episode is defined as the presence of sore throat with greater than or equal to 1 of the following: temperature greater than 38.3°C, cervical adenopathy, tonsillar exudates, or positive group A beta-hemolytic streptococcus (GABHS) test, which must be well documented in the medical record. This definition is based on literature describing limited benefits of tonsillectomy if performed in children with mild disease. Once patients fulfill these so-called Paradise criteria,[40] physicians can consider tonsillectomy as a treatment option.

The current literature shows a moderate reduction in severity and frequency of throat infections up to a year after tonsillectomy.[38,41] In addition, the favorable natural history of disease is reflected by seeing similar outcomes for surgery versus watchful waiting over time. In contrast, a past history of more than 1 peritonsillar abscess, rheumatic heart disease/fever, Lemierre syndrome, or severe pharyngotonsillitis episodes requiring hospitalizations may not need to achieve the frequency criteria to be reasonably considered for tonsillectomy. Other modifying factors that need to be taken into consideration when patients do not meet frequency criteria include periodic fever, aphthous stomatitis, pharyngitis, and adenitis (PFAPA) and multiple allergies/intolerance to medications. The current guidelines have not made any recommendations regarding pediatric autoimmune neuropsychiatric disorders associated with streptococcal infections (PANDAS) because of lack of evidence in the literature.[42] Therefore, a shared decision-making approach should be considered.

Many studies have questioned whether removing the tonsils, which are producers of the 5 immunoglobulin isotypes, would have any effect on children's immunity. There is a population-based cohort study evaluating the effect of adenoidectomy, tonsillectomy, or both on the risk of acquiring allergic, infectious, or respiratory diseases long term in the Danish population. Data obtained from the Denmark national health registry were used. The investigators concluded that adenoidectomy and tonsillectomy were associated with a 2-fold to 3-fold increased risk of developing upper respiratory tract diseases, questioning the long-term effects of such surgical procedures.[43] However, the study has inherent flaws. First, baseline characteristics of cohort and control groups are likely significantly different. In addition, there is a lack of information regarding the indications for surgery.[44] Thus, currently, there is no significant clinical impact shown in the published literature.[38]

In addition, there are various other indications that have been discussed in the literature for undergoing tonsillectomy, although they have been inadequately studied to be included in the AAO-HNS CPG. These indications include chronic tonsillitis, cryptic tonsils, chronic carriers of group A β-hemolytic *Streptococcus*, malocclusion, halitosis, and febrile seizures. If the patient shows more than 1 of these entities, shared decision making is necessary.[38]

Obstructive sleep disordered breathing (oSDB) is characterized by a spectrum of sleep disturbances from snoring to sleep apnea and occurs in approximately 12% of children.[45,46] Tonsillar and adenoid hypertrophy act as an anatomic overcrowding of the nasopharynx and oropharynx and are leading factors contributing to obstructive symptoms during sleep.[45,46] oSDB is now the leading indication for adenotonsillectomy. Note that the size of either tonsil or adenoids alone does not directly correlate with the severity of the oSDB but, taken together, show higher correlations.[38,47–49] Other variables that influence oSDB severity include craniofacial development and overall muscle tone.[38]

Table 1
Effects of tonsillectomy on symptoms associated with obstructive sleep disordered breathing

Symptoms in Children with oSDB	Effects Described After Tonsillectomy
Behavioral disturbances	Significantly improved[a]
Attention-deficit disorder	Improved
Neurocognitive disturbances (including depression, memory difficulties)	Significantly improved[a]
Secondary enuresis	Resolved or improved
Failure to thrive	Height, weight, and growth increased significantly
Overall quality of life	Significantly improved[a]
Asthma exacerbations	Asthma outcomes improved[b]

[a] Effects seen up to 2 years following tonsillectomy.
[b] Asthma exacerbations, respiratory medication use, emergency room visits, overall symptoms.

There are a multitude of symptoms commonly observed in children with oSDB that have been shown to either significantly improve or resolve following tonsillectomy (**Table 1**). Physicians should seek out this information and comorbid conditions from the medical history.

A polysomnogram (PSG) is recommended before surgical treatment of children less than 2 years old or if they show the following comorbidities:

- Obesity (body mass index [BMI] greater than or equal to 95th percentile)
- Craniofacial abnormalities
- Down syndrome
- Neuromuscular disorders
- Sickle cell disease
- Mucopolysaccharidoses

A PSG is considered the gold standard for diagnosing obstructive sleep apnea (OSA) and aids in clinical decision making in these children who, at baseline, show increased risk of surgical and anesthetic complications. The PSG helps define central versus obstructive events, as well as the severity of the apneas, in order to guide preoperative and postoperative consultations, evaluations, and admission planning. Physicians should advocate a PSG in cases in which the need for tonsillectomy is unclear because of discordance between history and physical examination.[38]

Table 2
Comparison of American Academy of Otolaryngology–Head and Neck Surgery and American Academy of Sleep Medicine clinical practice guidelines on indications for polysomnography

Guideline	AAO-HNS	AASM	AAP
PSG indications	<2 y of age, obesity, trisomy 21, craniofacial disorder, sickle cell disease, mucopolysaccharidoses, neuromuscular diseases, uncertain diagnosis	*All* patients undergoing tonsillectomy for oSDB	Snoring on a regular basis and any signs or symptoms of OSA
If PSG not readily available	Portable monitoring home system can be considered	Refer to otolaryngologist or sleep medicine specialist	—

PSG indications vary between the currently published AAO-HNS CPG and the American Academy of Sleep Medicine (AASM) CPG. Key differences are shown in **Table 2**. Abnormal PSG results in children are considered when the apnea-hypopnea index (AHI) is greater than 1 and/or pulse oximetry is less than 92%.[38,50] Ranges for increasing severity of OSA vary in the literature but most studies define them as follows:

- Mild OSA = AHI 1 to 4.9
- Moderate OSA = AHI 5 to 9.9
- Severe OSA = AHI greater than or equal to 10

For OSA documented on PSG, tonsillectomy should be recommended in order to reduce morbidity associated with untreated OSA. This recommendation is consistent among the 3 academic bodies, AAO-HNS, AAP, and AASM. Despite this recommendation, access to PSG may be difficult to obtain because of differing resources as well as insurance coverage. Physicians thus often decide to forgo the PSG or request a portable monitoring device in otherwise healthy children with a strong history and physical examination consistent with sleep disordered breathing, unless parents request a confirmatory diagnosis.[46]

Surgical treatment is the mainstay for OSA and was evaluated against watchful waiting in the Childhood Adenotonsillectomy Trial (CHAT).[51] This study showed that, in the school-aged population, tonsillectomy reduced symptoms and improved polysomnography results as well as quality-of-life measures.[51] Note that baseline values were similar between groups for the primary outcome of the developmental neuropsychological assessment for attention and executive functioning scores. In addition, the watchful waiting group had a normalization in their PSG findings in 46% versus 79% in the tonsillectomy group.[51] For patients with mild OSA, a limited number of studies have shown oral montelukast and nasal steroids to be effective alternatives to surgery, although the duration of treatment needed with these medications is unclear.[52,53]

In at-risk populations, such as children with obesity or trisomy 21, evidence shows that tonsillectomy is often not curative, although an improvement in AHI is frequently seen.[54] For example, up to 76% of obese children show persistent OSA after undergoing tonsillectomy, although AHI may show improvement.[54] It is thus important to counsel parents accordingly. Risk factors associated with persistent OSA are shown in **Box 1**. It is imperative to understand the multitude of factors playing a role in the development of oSDB in order to help guide long-term management in patients with persistent OSA.

Box 1
Risk factors associated with persistent obstructive sleep apnea

Obesity

Age greater than 7 years

Down syndrome

Craniofacial

Asthma

Metabolic disorders

Neuromuscular

Perioperative antibiotics
There is a strong recommendation against the use of perioperative antibiotics in the setting of tonsillectomy. Based on the results of a Cochrane systematic review, antibiotic use did not show significant reductions in pain/use of pain medication, bleeding rates, or time to normal activity.[55] Certain exclusions to this are tonsillectomy in the setting of palate surgery; tonsil biopsy; unilateral tonsillectomy for carcinoma; or those patients requiring prophylactic antibiotics for medical conditions, including heart murmurs or implants.[55]

Indications for steroids
In children undergoing tonsillectomy, the current AAO-HNS guidelines[38] continue to strongly recommend a single intraoperative intravenous dose of dexamethasone. Various studies have shown significant improvement in postoperative nausea and vomiting, pain, and time to normal diet following this procedure.[56] The most commonly used dose for dexamethasone is 0.5 mg/kg, although other doses have been shown to result in positive effects.

Postoperative complications
Although tonsillectomy is a surgical procedure that has been shown to have positive effects on both recurrent infections as well as oSDB, it is associated with a degree of morbidity. Postoperative hemorrhage has been quoted to be 0.2% to 2.2% for primary bleeding occurring less than 24 hours from surgery and from 0.1% to 3% for bleeding occurring greater than 24 hours postsurgery.[57] Factors influencing the risk of posttonsillectomy hemorrhage (PTH) are shown in **Box 2**.[58] Other complications may include respiratory compromise, injury to soft tissues and surrounding vascular structures, vomiting, dehydration, and pain.

Pain control
Pain management is an important aspect in the postoperative care of tonsillectomy patients. Pain is considered an important cause of the morbidity associated with this procedure, leading to a downward spiral of decreased oral intake, dehydration, and readmission. Nonpharmacologic options for pain management include drinking, eating, chewing gum, cold application, minimizing noise, and distraction with games.[38,59,60] These options should supplement pharmacologic treatments.

Pharmacologic treatments are divided into nonopioid and opioid options. The AAO-HNS strongly recommends the use of ibuprofen, acetaminophen, or a combination of the two in the treatment of posttonsillectomy pain. The use of nonsteroidal antiinflammatory drugs (NSAIDs), such as ibuprofen, has been shown to decrease postoperative

---

Box 2
Factors influencing posttonsillectomy hemorrhage: national prospective tonsillectomy audit

Increasing age

Male sex

History of recurrent acute tonsillitis

Previous peritonsillar abscess, including Quincy tonsillectomy

Data from The Royal College of Surgeons of England. National prospective tonsillectomy audit: final report of an audit carried out in England and Northern Ireland between July 2003 and September 2004. Available at: https://www.rcseng.ac.uk/library-and-publications/rcs-publications/docs/tonsillectomy-audit/.

narcotic medication use, nausea, and vomiting without increasing the incidence of adverse events such as bleeding.[61,62] A study by Mudd and colleagues[63] evaluated the association of ibuprofen use with the severity of PTH being surgically managed. Their retrospective cohort study found a 3.3% incidence of surgically managed PTH, with 6.8% of those patients receiving blood transfusions. Although ibuprofen was not associated with increased risk of surgically managed PTH, ibuprofen use increased transfusion risk 3-fold.

Ketorolac has also been evaluated as a potential analgesic for posttonsillectomy pain but continues to remain controversial. A systematic review and meta-analysis of the literature evaluating the risk of PTH with ketorolac showed no association of relative risk (RR) of bleeding with its use in children less than 18 years old undergoing tonsillectomy (RR, 1.39; 95% CI, 0.84–2.30; P<.20).[64] This finding is also corroborated by a Cochrane Review evaluating the use of ketorolac versus other NSAIDs.[65]

With regard to opioid analgesics, there is a strong recommendation against using any codeine, or medication containing codeine, in children after tonsillectomy because of the risk of severe respiratory depression in children who are ultrarapid metabolizers. Oxycodone and morphine can be used with caution for posttonsillectomy pain management, although physicians should consider lower dosages, particularly for patients with OSA.[38]

Surgical techniques Various surgical techniques exist for the removal of tonsillar tissue. These techniques include cold dissection, electrocautery dissection, coblation, radiofrequency ablation, and harmonic scalpel. Frequencies of PTH show inconsistent results between these techniques, with no clear difference in rates based on technique.[38] In addition, tonsillotomy, also referred to as intracapsular tonsillectomy, and complete tonsillectomy are often compared in order to identify the method with the best postsurgical results and minimal postoperative risks.

A recent retrospective cohort study by Sakki and colleagues,[66] evaluating the changing trends in tonsillectomy techniques at a single institution, showed a reoperation rate of 1.5% in their cohort of 1781 children less than 16 years old undergoing tonsillotomy. More than 50% of these patients were less than 3 years old.[66] This study also showed a decreased number of postoperative hemorrhages with tonsillotomy compared with the cold-knife tonsillectomy technique (0.6% vs 6.3%, P<.05, respectively). Similar findings were seen in a review of 86 studies by Windfuhr and colleagues,[67] which showed repeat surgery being necessary in 1.6% of the original 5877 tonsillotomy cases.

With regard to surgical techniques, including coblation, cold steel, or hot electrocautery, there are insufficient data in the literature to evaluate whether a significant difference is seen with regard to postoperative pain or bleeding between these various techniques. A recent Cochrane Review evaluating coblation versus other techniques concluded that data are limited and low quality; thus, adequate conclusions could not be drawn regarding the superiority of one technique to the others.[68] The current CPG on tonsillectomy also comments on the variability of various studies on this topic.[38]

Postoperative admission criteria

The current CPGs from the AAO-HNS recommend the following admission criteria posttonsillectomy: (1) documented severe OSA (AHI $\geq$10, oxygen saturation of <80%, or both), (2) significant comorbidities, and/or (3) age less than 3 years.[38] The largest study included is the analysis by Amoils and colleagues[69] (2016), which showed that risks for adverse events, including airway complications, were greater in younger patients. Notably, this risk was greatest in the 2-month to 11-month age group, and decreased with age, with lower risks were seen after 3 years of age. Weight less

Table 3
Population of children benefitting from inpatient admission posttonsillectomy

Severe OSA (AHI ≥10 and/or O_2<80%)	Obesity (BMI >95%)
Age <3 y	Cardiac comorbidities
Weight <14 kg	Neuromuscular disorders
Down syndrome	Failure to thrive
Craniofacial anomalies	Behavioral factors predicting for poor oral intake

than 14 kg has also been associated with increased perioperative respiratory complications.[70] In addition, various factors have been associated with escalation of care requiring pediatric intensive care unit admission, including younger age, higher AHI, increased total time in the recovery room or oxygen needed for longer in the immediate postoperative period, neurologic comorbidities, and gastrostomy tube presence.[71,72]

In a recent retrospective review by Evans and colleagues[73] (2019), this age criterion was reevaluated using 2 cohorts of posttonsillectomy patients; one comprising patients 24 to 35 months old and a second comprising patients 36 to 42 months old. No significant differences in readmission rates, emergency room visits, or complication rates were seen between the older and younger groups. **Table 3** lists the various indications for impatient admission posttonsillectomy suggested in the literature.

SUMMARY

CPGs for the most common medical conditions (ie, AOM, COME, oSDB, and recurrent tonsillitis) and surgical procedures (ie, TTs, adenotonsillectomy) being performed in pediatric otolaryngology are designed to decrease variability in an evidence-based manner. Although seemingly simple procedures, TTs, as well as adenotonsillectomy, have been shown to have significantly positive effects on children's overall health and quality of life, when performed in the context of recommended indications. It is important to understand these indications and the body of research that supports these recommendations, in order to appropriately counsel patients and caregivers regarding appropriate management. Evidence gaps do remain, despite the abundance of published research, and thus shared decision making is required in particular situations.

REFERENCES

1. Harvey M, Bowe SN, Laury AM. Clinical practice guidelines: whose practice are we guiding? Otolaryngol Head Neck Surg 2016;155(3):373–5.
2. Rosenfeld RM, Shin JJ, Schwartz SR, et al. Clinical practice guideline: otitis media with effusion executive summary (Update). Otolaryngol Head Neck Surg 2016;154(2):201–14.
3. Forrest CB, Fiks AG, Bailey LC, et al. Improving adherence to otitis media guidelines with clinical decision support and physician feedback. Pediatrics 2013; 131(4):e1071–81.
4. Rosenfeld RM, Schwartz SR, Pynnonen MA, et al. Clinical practice guideline: tympanostomy tubes in children–executive summary. Otolaryngol Head Neck Surg 2013;149(1):8–16.
5. Casselbrant ML, Kaleida PH, Rockette HE, et al. Efficacy of antimicrobial prophylaxis and of tympanostomy tube insertion for prevention of recurrent acute otitis media: results of a randomized clinical trial. Pediatr Infect Dis J 1992;11(4): 278–86.

6. Monasta L, Ronfani L, Marchetti F, et al. Burden of disease caused by otitis media: systematic review and global estimates. PLoS One 2012;7(4):e36226.
7. Schilder AG, Chonmaitree T, Cripps AW, et al. Otitis media. Nat Rev Dis Primers 2016;2:16063.
8. Lieberthal AS, Carroll AE, Chonmaitree T, et al. The diagnosis and management of acute otitis media. Pediatrics 2013;131(3):e964–99.
9. Duncan B, Ey J, Holberg CJ, et al. Exclusive breast-feeding for at least 4 months protects against otitis media. Pediatrics 1993;91(5):867–72.
10. Foxlee R, Johansson A, Wejfalk J, et al. Topical analgesia for acute otitis media. Cochrane Database Syst Rev 2006;(3):CD005657.
11. Venekamp RP, Schilder AGM. Clinical failure is more common in young children with acute otitis media who receive a short course of antibiotics compared with standard duration. Evid Based Med 2017;22(3):100.
12. Ranakusuma RW, Pitoyo Y, Safitri ED, et al. Systemic corticosteroids for acute otitis media in children. Cochrane Database Syst Rev 2018;(3):CD012289.
13. Venekamp RP, Mick P, Schilder AG, et al. Grommets (ventilation tubes) for recurrent acute otitis media in children. Cochrane Database Syst Rev 2018;(5):CD012017.
14. Paradise JL, Rockette HE, Colborn DK, et al. Otitis media in 2253 Pittsburgh-area infants: prevalence and risk factors during the first two years of life. Pediatrics 1997;99(3):318–33.
15. Rosenfeld RM, Shin JJ, Schwartz SR, et al. Clinical practice guideline: otitis media with effusion (Update). Otolaryngol Head Neck Surg 2016;154(1 Suppl):S1–41.
16. Tos M. Epidemiology and natural history of secretory otitis. Am J Otol 1984;5(6):459–62.
17. Flynn T, Moller C, Jonsson R, et al. The high prevalence of otitis media with effusion in children with cleft lip and palate as compared to children without clefts. Int J Pediatr Otorhinolaryngol 2009;73(10):1441–6.
18. Maris M, Wojciechowski M, Van de Heyning P, et al. A cross-sectional analysis of otitis media with effusion in children with Down syndrome. Eur J Pediatr 2014;173(10):1319–25.
19. Rosenfeld RM, Kay D. Natural history of untreated otitis media. Laryngoscope 2003;113(10):1645–57.
20. Simon F, Haggard M, Rosenfeld RM, et al. International consensus (ICON) on management of otitis media with effusion in children. Eur Ann Otorhinolaryngol Head Neck Dis 2018;135(1S):S33–9.
21. Venekamp RP, Burton MJ, van Dongen TM, et al. Antibiotics for otitis media with effusion in children. Cochrane Database Syst Rev 2016;(6):CD009163.
22. Hussein A, Fathy H, Amin SM, et al. Oral steroids alone or followed by intranasal steroids versus watchful waiting in the management of otitis media with effusion. J Laryngol Otol 2017;131(10):907–13.
23. Simpson SA, Lewis R, van der Voort J, et al. Oral or topical nasal steroids for hearing loss associated with otitis media with effusion in children. Cochrane Database Syst Rev 2011;(5):CD001935.
24. Lack G, Caulfield H, Penagos M. The link between otitis media with effusion and allergy: a potential role for intranasal corticosteroids. Pediatr Allergy Immunol 2011;22(3):258–66.
25. Kogan MD, Overpeck MD, Hoffman HJ, et al. Factors associated with tympanostomy tube insertion among preschool-aged children in the United States. Am J Public Health 2000;90(2):245–50.

26. Bluestone CD, Swarts JD. Human evolutionary history: consequences for the pathogenesis of otitis media. Otolaryngol Head Neck Surg 2010;143(6):739–44.
27. Mikals SJ, Brigger MT. Adenoidectomy as an adjuvant to primary tympanostomy tube placement: a systematic review and meta-analysis. JAMA Otolaryngol Head Neck Surg 2014;140(2):95–101.
28. Rosenfeld RM, Culpepper L, Doyle KJ, et al. Clinical practice guideline: otitis media with effusion. Otolaryngol Head Neck Surg 2004;130(5 Suppl):S95–118.
29. Berkman ND, Wallace IF, Steiner MJ, et al. Otitis media with effusion: comparative effectiveness of treatments 2013. Rockville (MD).
30. Hellstrom S, Groth A, Jorgensen F, et al. Ventilation tube treatment: a systematic review of the literature. Otolaryngol Head Neck Surg 2011;145(3):383–95.
31. Rosenfeld RM, Bhaya MH, Bower CM, et al. Impact of tympanostomy tubes on child quality of life. Arch Otolaryngol Head Neck Surg 2000;126(5):585–92.
32. Rovers MM, Black N, Browning GG, et al. Grommets in otitis media with effusion: an individual patient data meta-analysis. Arch Dis Child 2005;90(5):480–5.
33. Browning GG, Rovers MM, Williamson I, et al. Grommets (ventilation tubes) for hearing loss associated with otitis media with effusion in children. Cochrane Database Syst Rev 2010;10:CD001801.
34. Soderman AC, Knutsson J, Priwin C, et al. A randomized study of four different types of tympanostomy ventilation tubes - One-year follow-up. Int J Pediatr Otorhinolaryngol 2016;89:159–63.
35. Kay DJ, Nelson M, Rosenfeld RM. Meta-analysis of tympanostomy tube sequelae. Otolaryngol Head Neck Surg 2001;124(4):374–80.
36. Moualed D, Masterson L, Kumar S, et al. Water precautions for prevention of infection in children with ventilation tubes (grommets). Cochrane Database Syst Rev 2016;(1):CD010375.
37. Hall MJ, Schwartzman A, Zhang J, et al. Ambulatory surgery data from hospitals and ambulatory surgery centers: United States, 2010. Natl Health Stat Report 2017;(102):1–15.
38. Mitchell RB, Archer SM, Ishman SL, et al. Clinical practice guideline: tonsillectomy in children (Update). Otolaryngol Head Neck Surg 2019;160(1_suppl):S1–42.
39. Parker NP, Walner DL. Trends in the indications for pediatric tonsillectomy or adenotonsillectomy. Int J Pediatr Otorhinolaryngol 2011;75(2):282–5.
40. Paradise JL, Bluestone CD, Bachman RZ, et al. Efficacy of tonsillectomy for recurrent throat infection in severely affected children. Results of parallel randomized and nonrandomized clinical trials. N Engl J Med 1984;310(11):674–83.
41. Morad A, Sathe NA, Francis DO, et al. Tonsillectomy versus watchful waiting for recurrent throat infection: a systematic review. Pediatrics 2017;139(2) [pii: e20163490].
42. Farhood Z, Ong AA, Discolo CM. PANDAS: a systematic review of treatment options. Int J Pediatr Otorhinolaryngol 2016;89:149–53.
43. Byars SG, Stearns SC, Boomsma JJ. Association of long-term risk of respiratory, allergic, and infectious diseases with removal of adenoids and tonsils in childhood. JAMA Otolaryngol Head Neck Surg 2018;144(7):594–603.
44. Kitipornchai L, Mackay SG. Limitations to the association of risk of airway disease with removal of adenoids and tonsils in children. JAMA Otolaryngol Head Neck Surg 2018. [Epub ahead of print]. https://doi.org/10.1001/jamaoto.2018.2447.
45. Ali NJ, Pitson DJ, Stradling JR. Snoring, sleep disturbance, and behaviour in 4-5 year olds. Arch Dis Child 1993;68(3):360–6.

46. Roland PS, Rosenfeld RM, Brooks LJ, et al. Clinical practice guideline: polysomnography for sleep-disordered breathing prior to tonsillectomy in children. Otolaryngol Head Neck Surg 2011;145(1 Suppl):S1–15.

47. Arens R, McDonough JM, Corbin AM, et al. Upper airway size analysis by magnetic resonance imaging of children with obstructive sleep apnea syndrome. Am J Respir Crit Care Med 2003;167(1):65–70.

48. Arens R, McDonough JM, Costarino AT, et al. Magnetic resonance imaging of the upper airway structure of children with obstructive sleep apnea syndrome. Am J Respir Crit Care Med 2001;164(4):698–703.

49. Howard NS, Brietzke SE. Pediatric tonsil size: objective vs subjective measurements correlated to overnight polysomnogram. Otolaryngol Head Neck Surg 2009;140(5):675–81.

50. Traeger N, Schultz B, Pollock AN, et al. Polysomnographic values in children 2-9 years old: additional data and review of the literature. Pediatr Pulmonol 2005; 40(1):22–30.

51. Marcus CL, Moore RH, Rosen CL, et al. A randomized trial of adenotonsillectomy for childhood sleep apnea. N Engl J Med 2013;368(25):2366–76.

52. Kheirandish-Gozal L, Bhattacharjee R, Bandla HPR, et al. Antiinflammatory therapy outcomes for mild OSA in children. Chest 2014;146(1):88–95.

53. Kheirandish-Gozal L, Gozal D. Intranasal budesonide treatment for children with mild obstructive sleep apnea syndrome. Pediatrics 2008;122(1):e149–55.

54. Andersen IG, Holm JC, Homoe P. Obstructive sleep apnea in obese children and adolescents, treatment methods and outcome of treatment - a systematic review. Int J Pediatr Otorhinolaryngol 2016;87:190–7.

55. Dhiwakar M, Clement WA, Supriya M, et al. Antibiotics to reduce post-tonsillectomy morbidity. Cochrane Database Syst Rev 2012;(12):CD005607.

56. Steward DL, Grisel J, Meinzen-Derr J. Steroids for improving recovery following tonsillectomy in children. Cochrane Database Syst Rev 2011;(8):CD003997.

57. Windfuhr JP, Chen YS, Remmert S. Hemorrhage following tonsillectomy and adenoidectomy in 15,218 patients. Otolaryngol Head Neck Surg 2005;132(2): 281–6.

58. National prospective tonsillectomy audit: final report of an audit carried out in England and Northern Ireland between July 2003 and September 2004. Available at: https://www.rcseng.ac.uk/library-and-publications/college-publications/docs/tonsillectomy-audit/.

59. Dorkham MC, Chalkiadis GA, von Ungern Sternberg BS, et al. Effective postoperative pain management in children after ambulatory surgery, with a focus on tonsillectomy: barriers and possible solutions. Paediatr Anaesth 2014;24(3): 239–48.

60. Sutters KA, Isaacson G. Posttonsillectomy pain in children. Am J Nurs 2014; 114(2):36–42 [quiz 43].

61. Moss JR, Watcha MF, Bendel LP, et al. A multicenter, randomized, double-blind placebo-controlled, single dose trial of the safety and efficacy of intravenous ibuprofen for treatment of pain in pediatric patients undergoing tonsillectomy. Paediatr Anaesth 2014;24(5):483–9.

62. Riggin L, Ramakrishna J, Sommer DD, et al. A 2013 updated systematic review & meta-analysis of 36 randomized controlled trials; no apparent effects of non steroidal anti-inflammatory agents on the risk of bleeding after tonsillectomy. Clin Otolaryngol 2013;38(2):115–29.

63. Mudd PA, Thottathil P, Giordano T, et al. Association between ibuprofen use and severity of surgically managed posttonsillectomy hemorrhage. JAMA Otolaryngol Head Neck Surg 2017;143(7):712–7.

64. Chan DK, Parikh SR. Perioperative ketorolac increases post-tonsillectomy hemorrhage in adults but not children. Laryngoscope 2014;124(8):1789–93.

65. Lewis SR, Nicholson A, Cardwell ME, et al. Nonsteroidal anti-inflammatory drugs and perioperative bleeding in paediatric tonsillectomy. Cochrane Database Syst Rev 2013;(7):CD003591.

66. Sakki A, Makinen LK, Roine RP, et al. Changing trends in pediatric tonsil surgery. Int J Pediatr Otorhinolaryngol 2018;118:84–9.

67. Windfuhr JP, Savva K, Dahm JD, et al. Tonsillotomy: facts and fiction. Eur Arch Otorhinolaryngol 2015;272(4):949–69.

68. Pynnonen M, Brinkmeier JV, Thorne MC, et al. Coblation versus other surgical techniques for tonsillectomy. Cochrane Database Syst Rev 2017;(8):CD004619.

69. Amoils M, Chang KW, Saynina O, et al. Postoperative complications in pediatric tonsillectomy and adenoidectomy in ambulatory vs inpatient settings. JAMA Otolaryngol Head Neck Surg 2016;142(4):344–50.

70. Baijal RG, Bidani SA, Minard CG, et al. Perioperative respiratory complications following awake and deep extubation in children undergoing adenotonsillectomy. Paediatr Anaesth 2015;25(4):392–9.

71. Arambula AM, Xie DX, Whigham AS. Respiratory events after adenotonsillectomy requiring escalated admission status in children with obstructive sleep apnea. Int J Pediatr Otorhinolaryngol 2018;107:31–6.

72. Lavin JM, Smith C, Harris ZL, et al. Critical care resources utilized in high-risk adenotonsillectomy patients. Laryngoscope 2019;129(5):1229–34.

73. Evans SS, Cho DY, Richman J, et al. Revisiting age-related admission following tonsillectomy in the pediatric population. Laryngoscope 2019. [Epub ahead of print]. https://doi.org/10.1002/lary.27795.

Ankyloglossia and Other Oral Ties

Jonathan Walsh, MD[a], Margo McKenna Benoit, MD[b],*

KEYWORDS

• Ankyloglossia • Tongue-tie • Lip-tie • Frenulectomy • Frenotomy

KEY POINTS

- Ankyloglossia, or tongue-tie, has become a topic of great interest and some controversy over the past 20 to 30 years, as rates of breastfeeding initiation have increased.
- Tongue-tie can result in various degrees of difficulty with breastfeeding, oral hygiene, speech, and dentition.
- Diagnosis must include a functional assessment of tongue mobility, in addition to the physical appearance of the frenulum.
- Procedures to address ankyloglossia and other oral ties are commonly accepted as safe; however, serious complications such as severe bleeding, infection, and worsening glossoptosis have been reported.
- There is little evidence to date supporting surgical intervention for maxillary, mandibular, or other oral ties.

INTRODUCTION

The lingual frenulum is formed during the fourth week of gestation as the 2 lateral lingual swellings move medially to fuse with the tuberculum impar, forming the anterior two-thirds of the tongue. The tongue then separates from the floor of mouth to form the lingual sulcus. Failure of release results in varying degrees of ankyloglossia, or tongue-tie, in which a fibrous band in the midline tethers the tongue to the alveolar ridge or floor of mouth. Ankyloglossia can be asymptomatic or may have a wide array of consequences, including difficulty with breastfeeding, oral hygiene, dental development, speech, and other social factors. Treatment often involves division of the band to provide better tongue mobility. Although this is generally accepted to be a minor and safe procedure, there is considerable debate about when and how to intervene. In addition, several case reports have documented serious and potentially

Disclosure Statement: The authors have nothing to disclose.
[a] Department of Otolaryngology–Head and Neck Surgery, Johns Hopkins University, 601 North Caroline Street, 6th Floor, Baltimore, MD 21287, USA; [b] Department of Otolaryngology, University of Rochester Medical Center, 601 Elmwood Avenue, Box 629, Rochester, NY 14642, USA
* Corresponding author.
E-mail address: Margo_Benoit@urmc.rochester.edu

life-threatening complications associated with frenotomy. In addition to anterior and posterior lingual ties, there is growing interest in clinical practice and in the literature on how best to evaluate and manage upper lip-tie (ULT) and other oral ties. Within the multidisciplinary community of providers interested in ankyloglossia, there exists a need for a solid understanding of the available literature and best practice recommendations to make discerning diagnostic and treatment decisions for patients. This article presents an evidence-based approach to ankyloglossia and other oral ties.

HISTORY AND EPIDEMIOLOGY

Ankyloglossia, commonly known as tongue-tie, is an anatomic variant of tongue anatomy that has been recognized for centuries. Some of the first references to a disorder of the tongue being tethered to the floor of mouth appear in days of Aristotle in the third century BC, and the operative technique of dividing a tongue-tie was first described in the seventh century AD. In the middle ages, debate first arose between midwives, who used a long fingernail to perform the procedure, and surgeons, who were allowed to use instruments. In medieval times up and through the early 1900s, tongue-ties were released routinely. In fact, the instruments necessary to clip a tongue-tie appeared in circumcision trays because both procedures were commonly performed before a newborn was sent home from the hospital.[1,2] Around 1950, the culture in the United States changed with the introduction of baby formula and rates of breastfeeding fell dramatically. By the 1960s and 1970s, ankyloglossia was considered to be an outdated topic, and many pediatricians denied that tongue-tie existed or that it caused a problem with feeding in newborns.[3] The natural childbirth movement in the 1970s brought renewed interest in breastfeeding as a first choice for infants, and with this change came increasing recognition of tongue-tie as a potential road block to successful breastfeeding. A few case reports and observational studies appeared, proposing a link between ankyloglossia and breastfeeding difficulty. In the past 20 years, ankyloglossia has become a controversial topic in medicine, with many strong opinions held by a diverse group of providers, including pediatricians, neonatologists, feeding and speech therapists, lactation consultants, dentists, and otolaryngologists.[4]

Walsh and colleagues,[5] in a study of the KIDS database, reported an increase in the diagnosis of tongue-tie by 834% from 1997 to 2012 and a similar increase in the number of frenotomy procedures performed over that same time period. Similar epidemiologic studies in Australia and Canada have shown a marked increase in ankyloglossia diagnosis and frenotomy rates.[6,7] Along with this increase in clinical interest has come an increase in published literature on the topic of ankyloglossia.[8] As is the case for any rapid change in medicine, high-quality research has often lagged behind the explosion of clinical interest, leaving clinicians with little guidance regarding the best approach for diagnosis and treatment, and generating heated controversy in the medical community.[9,10]

The incidence of tongue-tie in the general population is estimated between 0.02% and 12%. These rates are variable, at least in part, because no consensus exists on the best way to diagnose tongue-tie.[11] Using the Coryllos classification (see later discussion), Haham and colleagues[12] evaluated 200 newborns within 3 days of birth, and found that all but 1 baby had "an observable or palpable lingual frenulum" that was Coryllos class 1 (frenulum attached to the tip of tongue) through 4 (frenulum attaches at the base of tongue). The investigators found no correlation between Coryllos type and presence of breastfeeding difficulty. Two studies using the Hazelbaker tool reported an incidence and prevalence ranging from 4.2% to 12.8%.[13,14] Other studies attempting to estimate the incidence and prevalence of tongue-tie in babies have used varying methods for diagnosis, including "when the lingual frenulum attaches close to the tongue tip," "when the frenum extends to the papillary surface of the tongue," and "when the frenum caused a fissure in the tongue during movement."[11,12] Characterization of posterior tongue-tie has proven even more difficult and controversial. Descriptions of posterior tongue-tie include the presence of a "thick, fibrous cord posterior to the ventral tongue mucosa...obscured by the 'mucosal curtain'"[15] or "when the lingual frenulum was not very prominent on inspection but was thought to be tight on manual palpation or was found to be abnormally prominent, short, thick or fibrous cord-like with the use of the grooved director."[16] In an observational study, up to 59% of healthy newborns fit these criteria.[17] The true incidence of posterior tongue-tie is unknown.[18] The natural history and outcomes for patients with tongue-tie also have not been established.[19] An online Web-based survey conducted by Jin and colleagues[19] found that professional opinions about tongue-tie varied greatly based on profession and geography. One recent study looked at Website quality and trends for ankyloglossia, and found that, although overall the quality of Websites is good, many of the published Websites available to patients and the community are opinion pieces without clear sources and with inherent bias toward performing frenotomy for tongue-tie.[20] Potentially in response to the marked increase in the diagnosis and treatment of tongue-tie, some centers have put safeguards in place to minimize unnecessary procedures in newborns thought to have tongue-tie.[21]

As understanding of ankyloglossia and other oral ties evolves, the epidemiology of this disorder will continue to change as well (**Fig. 1**).

GENETICS

Multiple studies consistently demonstrate male-to-female ratios from 1.1:1 to 3:1.[14,22–34] These findings would suggest X-linked or autosomal dominant inheritance. This understanding is complicated by distinctions between sporadic and familial cases of ankyloglossia.[35] Most cases of ankyloglossia are thought to be sporadic and have a higher male predilection than the familial cases. Environmental or teratogen causes of ankyloglossia have been reported as well.[36] Additional heterogeneity is seen with differing ankyloglossia grading types. O'Callahan and colleagues[37] reported that the male predominance decreased from 68% for Coryllos types 1 and 2, to 59% for type 3, and to 46% for type 4 ankyloglossia. Similar trends were noted by Haham and colleagues.[12]

An X-linked cause is supported by the X-linked cleft palate syndrome.[22,38] This syndrome is caused by TBX22 gene mutation, a T-box gene involved in early vertebrate development. In addition to this association, in isolated ankyloglossia cases, a Finnish familial cohort demonstrated autosomal dominant inheritance with no TBX22 mutations.[23,24] Another pedigree study of 149 Korean subjects with isolated ankyloglossia was most suggestive of X-linked inheritance.[39] A mouse model of LGR5 knockout, a G protein–coupled receptor, has also been demonstrated to be a candidate gene for ankyloglossia in mice.[25] The mice have high mortality but do consistently have ankyloglossia. No studies have demonstrated LGR5 mutations in humans with ankyloglossia.

An autosomal dominant inheritance has been suggested through pedigree studies of families with inherited ankyloglossia.[35] Studies that evaluate multiple generations of familial ankyloglossia follow an autosomal dominant with incomplete penetrance pattern rather than X-linked.[23,26,35,39] In these situations, both TBX22 and LGR5 were excluded as potential candidates.

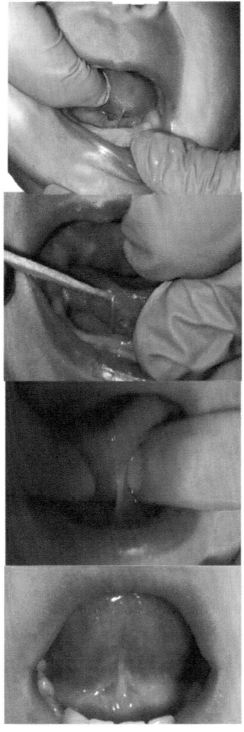

Fig. 1. Coryllos Lingual Frenulum Classification. Top to bottom: type 1 attaches to tip of tongue, type 2 attaches 2-4 mm from tongue tip, type 3 attaches to mid-tongue, type 4 attaches with a posterior attachment.

With these findings in mind, the embryologic development of the tongue is still an evolving story. The described inheritance patterns found in ankyloglossia are consistent with significant genetic heterogeneity with no clear single gene locus currently known.

PRESENTATION AND IMPACT

Tongue-tie in infants and children can have wide-ranging effects, depending on the age of the child and the degree and pattern of tongue-tie. The domain in which this has been studied most is the effect of tongue-tie on breastfeeding in infants. Effective breastfeeding requires formation of an adequate seal between the baby's oral cavity and the mother's nipple, which allows creation of an intraoral vacuum, and a coordinated peristaltic mechanism. Tongue position is important for all of these steps.[3,40] Some of this positioning and suckling can be observed directly, paying special attention to the depth of the baby's latch, adequate positioning, sucking motion, and coordination. Ultrasound studies have also been helpful in characterizing the mechanism of breastfeeding, including the intraoral positioning and motions of the tongue.[41]

For babies noted to have tethering of the tongue, some characteristic presentation features have been widely recognized, whereas others are still being debated. Consensus in the literature and from clinical experience suggests that babies with limited tongue mobility due to ankyloglossia can have a shallow latch and poor oral seal around the nipple. This can result in maternal nipple pain, which is sometimes severe enough to cause early cessation of breastfeeding. Nipple trauma such as cracking, bleeding, and ulceration can also occur, leading to plugged milk ducts and mastitis in severe cases. Puapornpong and colleagues[42] studied nipple pain specifically in 1649 postpartum breastfeeding women. They found that moderate to severe tongue-tie was the primary reason for nipple pain in 122 women and that frenotomy was effective in relieving this pain. Ankyloglossia also makes the transfer of milk less efficient, which can lead to a decrease in milk supply, poor infant weight gain, prolonged feedings, and failure to thrive. The intermittent loss of the oral nipple seal also leads to a clicking sound and aerophagia, which some investigators have hypothesized may contribute to symptomatic reflux in infants.[43,44] The psychosocial wellbeing of both mother and child can be affected by a short lingual frenulum, in particular for mothers who are unable to continue breastfeeding. Wong and colleagues[45] looked at online forum discussions among breastfeeding women and found that many threads contained language related to maternal distress, including fear, anger, frustration, and depressed mood.

Tethering of the tongue from ankyloglossia also raises concerns about oral hygiene, dental health, and orthognathic development. Tongue mobility is essential for sweeping the oral cavity and cleaning the teeth after feedings, to remove residual food debris that could contribute to caries. An association between a tight lingual frenulum and increased dental caries is thought to be due to restrictions in the ability of the tongue to adequately reach and clean all of the teeth on a regular basis. In addition to dental caries, some studies have implicated the lingual frenulum in contributing to problems with normal occlusion and craniofacial development.[46–48] This is based on the premise that alterations in tongue mobility, sucking motion, and coordination can alter the developmental balance of the stomatognathic system, leading to changes in the shape of the dental arches and malocclusion.[48] Specifically, 2 studies have reported an association between a short lingual frenulum and class III occlusion.[46,47] In the absence of larger prospective studies, establishing a causal link is more challenging.

There is evidence in the literature that ankyloglossia can also have an impact on speech articulation disorders. Messner and Lalakea[49] conducted a prospective study evaluating speech articulation in 30 children before and after frenuloplasty. There were documented articulation errors thought to be due to tongue-tie in 15 out of 21 subjects, 9 of whom improved following frenuloplasty. In addition to improvement on speech pathology reports, the parents' perception of speech intelligibility also improved significantly. Dollberg and colleagues[50] looked at speech intelligibility in children 4 to 8 years old who had difficulty with tongue-tie as infants. Half of these infants had been treated with frenulectomy and half with observation. The investigators found that intelligibility was not different between children with untreated tongue-tie versus those with treated tongue-tie. There was no comparison with a control group without tongue-tie. A study evaluating speech outcomes for subjects older than the age of 3 years undergoing frenulum Z-plasty found that a 4-flap frenulum Z-plasty resulted in greater improvements in articulation compared with a horizontal-to-vertical Z-plasty.[51] Although some studies lend support to the idea that tethering of the tongue affects speech articulation in some children with ankyloglossia, and that releasing the frenulum has the potential to create objective and subjective improvements in speech intelligibility, the evidence is limited and sometimes contradictory. A comprehensive review by Webb and colleagues[52] concluded that the quality of evidence regarding speech outcomes is low and definite conclusions cannot be drawn. Most clinicians advise against performing frenotomy or frenuloplasty in a newborn infant for an indication of concerns about speech disorders in the future because there is currently no reliable way to predict which of these babies will go on to have speech problems.

Ankyloglossia most often presents in isolated fashion in familial reports, but it can also appear in syndromic form, such as in Ehlers Danlos and oro-facio-digital syndrome.[53–55] Male-to-male transmission in some families supports an autosomal dominant inheritance pattern, with incomplete penetrance.[26,35] Other genes implicated in ankyloglossia show an X-linked pattern, as with mutations in TBX22, also associated with cleft palate.[38] The lingual frenulum was also reported to be abnormal as part of the spectrum of birth defects associated with congenital Zika syndrome, either as an absent lingual frenulum[56] or as a posteriorly positioned frenulum.[57]

There several other functional and social considerations related to ankyloglossia that may need to be considered. School-aged children may be more bothered by limitations in tongue elevation and protrusion that can lead to difficulty participating in social events, including licking an ice cream cone and kissing in teens.[4] Some students have reported difficulty playing wind instruments due to poor tongue positioning. Adolescents can also struggle wearing orthodontic and dental appliances because the lingual frenulum interferes with comfortable insertion. Although these concerns are often not mentioned in the scientific literature, they are heard commonly in providers' offices and can be primary reasons for older children and their families to seek treatment of release of the lingual frenum.

DIAGNOSTICS

Universally agreed on classification and consistent diagnostic algorithms are lacking for the diagnosis of ankyloglossia. The severe form of ankyloglossia is readily apparent, it is for mild to moderate ankyloglossia that confusion arises. Diagnosis not only uses patient and maternal symptoms but also requires a thorough oral cavity structural and functional examination. A brief visual inspection of the tongue is inadequate for diagnosis. Current understanding of ankyloglossia and its impact on breastfeeding necessitates anatomic and functional grading.

With regard to diagnostic examination, the initial examination can be performed in infants lying supine with their head toward the examiner. The mouth and lips are examined, the resting tongue position is noted, and tongue and suck reflexes are elicited. Craniofacial appearance is noted along with jaw size and position, nasal airway, and retrognathia. The tongue is then elevated with fingers or a grooved retractor. The authors find that a grooved retractor may alter the tongue appearance and the frenulum may be missed or overestimated depending on tongue and retractor position. Attachment location on the tongue and alveolus, frenulum length, and thickness is evaluated. After anatomic assessment, a gloved finger is used to illicit a suck reflex. The latch functions, such as cupping, lift, peristalsis, suction, and snap back, can then be evaluated. Additional assessment can be made with a breastfeeding or bottle feeding trial.

Most grading systems for anatomic criteria use the point of tongue attachment, length of the frenulum, or tongue protrusion.[49,58–60] The Coryllos classification has 4 types of frenulum based on the point of attachment and is the most widely used.[58] Similar to Coryllos system, the Kotlow grading systems measure the free tongue length from the tip of the tongue to the frenulum attachment.[59,60] The frenulum length, as measured from origin to insertion, interincisal distance, or tongue protrusion, are not often practical in infants or impossible to obtain owing to lack of erupted dentition.[61–64] Functional anatomy classifications include the Hazelbaker Assessment Tool for Lingual Frenulum Function (HATLFF) and the Bristol Tongue Assessment Tool (BTAT).[65,66] The HATLFF is a 12-item scale with 10 points for frenulum appearance and 14 points for tongue function. A score of 24 has normal function and normal anatomy. According to the scale, frenotomy is necessary for symptomatic ankyloglossia if the appearance score is less than 8 or the function score is less than 11. For perfect function scores regardless of appearance, frenotomy is not recommended. By allowing for functional assessment, it enables inclusion of posterior ankyloglossia, which may be missed in attachment-only scales. Routine use of the HATLFF can be difficult because assessment is complex and it requires an in-depth understanding of function and anatomy.[27,67] The BTAT was developed to incorporate much of the benefits of the HATLFF but to make it more portable and teachable. The scale has 4 items to grade tongue tip appearance, alveolar attachment location, tongue lift, and tongue protrusion. It was found to correlate well with HATLFF findings.[66] However, it does not fully address functional assessment. More recent studies have incorporated breastfeeding ultrasound to examine latch and tongue position, as well as milk intake.[28] Breastfeeding ultrasound is a promising tool can assist with functional assessment but is not specific to ankyloglossia.

In summary, current best practice should include an objective standardized anatomic and functional assessment of tongue appearance and mobility, as well as latch, regardless of grading system used.

TREATMENT

There are a variety of intervention options for breastfeeding difficulty in infants. These include changes in breastfeeding technique or positioning, or assisting devices such as nipple shields. Other complementary medical treatments have included craniosacral therapy, orofacial myofunctional therapy, chiropractic care, and naturopathy. Many of these same treatment options have been used to improve breastfeeding in the setting of suspected ankyloglossia. There are no high-quality outcome studies to inform providers on the efficacy of these techniques.

Other than lactation consultant expertise and assistance, the primary treatment of ankyloglossia in infants is frenotomy, which involves surgical division of the lingual frenum. Additional surgical techniques such as frenulectomy, or removal of the frenulum; frenotomy with myotomy; and frenulum Z-plasty have been described.[51,61,68–70] Despite these additional surgical options, frenotomy is sufficient in most infants. Shared decision-making about treatment options, with involvement of the family, is encouraged (**Fig. 2**).

The frenotomy technique isolates the frenulum with a grooved retractor. The frenulum is divided through the fibroelastic tissues of the frenum but not into the muscle, with scissors. Hemostasis is typically achieved with digital pressure, gauze with oxymetazoline, silver nitrate, or (rarely) suturing. Other common techniques follow the same principles but use carbon dioxide, diode, erbium: yttrium aluminium garnet

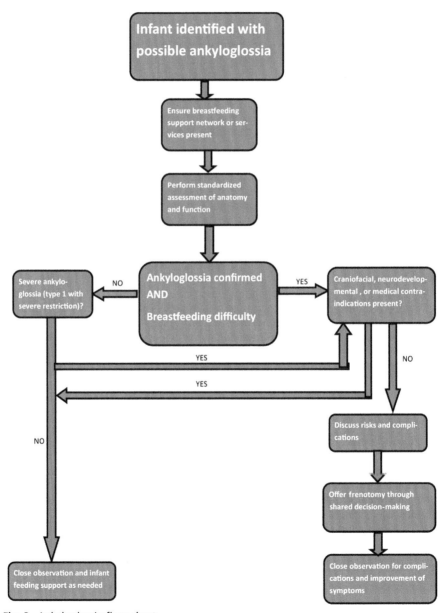

Fig. 2. Ankyloglossia flow chart.

(YAG), or neodymium-doped (Nd):YAG lasers, or electrocautery.[60,68,71–73] There are no comparative trials of scissor versus laser techniques for frenotomy in infants; however, in animal models of oral injury, cold surgical techniques have quicker healing,[74,75] possibly due to reduced thermal injury to the frenum and surrounding tissues. One study of adult labial frenotomy showed slight benefit of diode laser,[76] with an added benefit of concurrent hemostasis.

With regard to topical anesthesia, a randomized clinical trial concluded that topical anesthesia options are ineffective and need not be used.[77] An additional risk of topical anesthetic agents is methemoglobinemia. Common topical amide and ether anesthetics such as benzocaine have been implicated, and children younger the age of 2 years are at particular risk.[78] Instead of topical anesthesia, a 24% sucrose solution given orally before the procedure, accompanied by postprocedure nutritive or nonnutritive sucking, can help reduce discomfort.[79]

OUTCOMES

As previously discussed, a variety of dental, speech, feeding, and sleep-related outcomes are attributed to untreated ankyloglossia. Unfortunately, the ability to predict the natural history of untreated ankyloglossia is limited owing to the wide range of published ages of presentation, literature bias toward treatment, wide variation of symptom severity, and difficulty determining causation from retrospective association studies. Two systematic reviews recently analyzed the published studies regarding the impact of surgical treatment of ankyloglossia on breastfeeding and nonbreastfeeding issues. These reports noted improvement in breastfeeding and nipple pain as assessed by maternal report, but the overall strength and quality of evidence in support of frenotomy is low.[80,81] Outside of surgical complications, surgical frenotomy outcomes are consistently positive. Most outcomes are prospective cohort or retrospective studies. Of the few published randomized controlled trials (RCTs), most of the control subjects had crossover to frenotomy as part of the study designs. Two RCTs evaluated immediate results only because most control subjects had frenotomy shortly after sham procedure.[82,83] Three other RCTs had almost entire crossover of the control arms to the treatment groups during the course of the study.[84–86]

It is the inherent bias and heterogeneity within the literature that makes comprehensive assessment of frenotomy outcomes difficult. What is clear from the body of evidence is that some infants will indeed benefit from frenotomy and others who have multifactorial causes of feeding difficulty may have minimal or no benefit from the procedure. The positive predictive value of preoperative diagnosis is limited compared with rising frenotomy treatment.[5] The need for revision treatment of recurrent symptoms has not been studied directly, but rates for revision have been reported between 2.6% and 6.5%.[87,88] For posterior tongue-tie, the revision rates can be as high as 21%.[16]

Expected treatment outcomes change by the type of ankyloglossia, that is, anterior or posterior ankyloglossia, and presence of associated findings, such as ULT. A recent Web-based postintervention maternal report study found 100% improvement in latching difficulties for type 1 and type 2 classic ankyloglossia, and 49% improvement for type 4 posterior ankyloglossia. For maternal pain, there was 79% improvement in type 1 and 2, and 63% improvement in type 4.[37] The maternal breast's transition to breastfeeding or the experience of the mother may also play a role beyond the presence of ankyloglossia.[17] First-time mothers seem to be more likely to have an infant who is diagnosed with ankyloglossia and are also less likely determine if frenotomy had been performed based on breastfeeding efficacy.[5,85]

Despite these limitations, treatment outcome measures, such as the Breastfeeding Self-Efficacy Scale (BSES), the Infant Breastfeeding Assessment Tool (IBFAT), and the Latch, Audible swallowing, Type of nipple, Comfort, Hold (LATCH) tool have generally shown improvements in retrospective studies, but controlled studies are limited.[80]

There are insufficient data to determine the association of ankyloglossia with issues other than breastfeeding.[51,82] Therefore, the effect of frenotomy on speech, malocclusion, mandibular incisor irregularity, gingival recession, mandibular growth, and tongue mobility in older children is primarily described only in retrospective or cohort studies. Because tongue mobility can be restricted in ankyloglossia, the restricted mobility may affect speech articulation.[89] Messner and Lalakea[49] described the improvement of speech articulation issues in a cohort of children with frenotomy. The improvement or prevention of dental and craniofacial abnormalities is controversial, with benefits shown only in small retrospective case series.[55]

POTENTIAL COMPLICATIONS

Frenotomy is considered to be a safe procedure in almost all cases. The most common risks include infection and minor bleeding at the site, pain and discomfort, and a risk of injury to the salivary ducts that are located near the frenulum. Other considerations that should be discussed with patients and family members during informed consent include the possibility of no improvement or the need for additional revision surgical procedures in the future. Pain and discomfort associated with the procedure are often concerns because topical anesthetic agents are contraindicated in children younger than the age of 2 years, who are at higher risk of methemoglobinemia (www. fda.gov/Drugs/DrugSafety/ucm608265.htm). Postprocedure pain from extensive dissection or cautery in the floor of mouth can lead to oral aversion in severe cases. Most research studies that have been done on tongue-tie report no complications occurring in their cohort of subjects,[82,84,85] thus lending weight to the idea that frenotomy is, in most cases, without significant morbidity.

Despite this common understanding among providers and the public about the relative safety of frenotomy, there have been case reports of very serious complications occurring after frenotomy. As the diagnosis and treatment of tongue-tie have increased in the past 20 years (see previous discussion), these cautionary reports began to appear in the literature. One of the earliest of such case reports was published by Isaiah and Pereira[90] in 2013, regarding a 2-year-old boy who underwent outpatient frenotomy under general anesthesia with scissor technique and presented on postoperative day 2 with fever, tongue swelling, and drooling. Intraoral examination revealed an infected sublingual hematoma. This patient was treated with local evacuation and debridement, intravenous steroids, and antibiotics, and he made a full recovery.

Another case report included 2 patients with Pierre Robin sequence who presented with feeding difficulty and a short lingual frenulum.[91] Both patients developed increasing respiratory symptoms after frenotomy, presumed to be due to worsening of glossoptosis after the anterior attachments of the tongue to the floor of mouth had been released. Both patients had significant daytime symptoms of cyanosis and increased work of breathing with feeds, and both had severe obstructive sleep apnea noted on overnight polysomnogram. Surgical management of glossoptosis (tongue–lip adhesion in 1 patient and mandibular distraction osteogenesis in the other) was effective in improving respiratory symptoms; however, both patients eventually required feeding tube insertion for inadequate oral intake.

In 2017, Tracy and colleagues[92] described 2 pediatric patients who experienced heavy intraoral bleeding leading to hypovolemic shock. Both patients were older than 1 year of age and underwent frenotomy under anesthesia or sedation, and both presented hours to days after the procedure with significant intraoral bleeding requiring transfusion in both cases and cardiopulmonary resuscitation in 1 case.

These reports highlight the risk of airway compromise with any complication arising in the floor of mouth. Otolaryngologists are particularly sensitive to airway compromise from infection or hematoma in the floor of mouth, but other practitioners who also perform frenotomy may not be as attuned to this possibility and may not be comfortable or facile in managing the airway in these rare circumstances. All providers treating tongue-tie need to be aware that such serious complications can occur so that patients receive timely identification and treatment.

MAXILLARY AND OTHER ORAL TIES

Along with the increased interest in lingual ties, there has been a recent increase in clinical concern about labial ties, including the maxillary and mandibular midline frena, as well as lateral oral ties. To date, the literature on the anatomic significance and potential impact of these ties is sparse. Cadaver studies have demonstrated that these frena are composed of dense collagenous connective tissue, often at the reflections or interface of musculature in the area.[93,94] Observational studies have shown a wide variety of morphologic variation, with some investigators advising caution about interpreting these normal variants as pathologic.[95] Many potential issues have been purported to be due to tight maxillary and mandibular labial ties, including formation of a midline diastema between the teeth, increased caries and periodontal disease, gingival recession, difficulty in wearing dentures or retainers, difficulty with lip mobility, and possible esthetic or psychological consequences.[93,94]

The midline maxillary labial frenum, which can form an ULT, has recently been implicated in breastfeeding difficulty due to inability to properly flange the upper lip to obtain a proper latch. Because of the controversy surrounding the identification, diagnosis, and impact of an ULT, recent studies have attempted to characterize the normal anatomy of the maxillary labial frenum in newborns.[96,97] Santa Maria and colleagues[97] studied 100 healthy newborns and developed the Stanford Classification System, which had higher interrater and intrarater reliability than prior studies. Up to 11% of these babies had a class 3 upper lip frenulum that attached along the inferior margin of the alveolar papilla or onto the palate. The authors point out that the natural history of this structure is not known, and performing procedures to release it without adequate evidence that it is impactful may not be advisable.

Clinical research on tongue-tie may also include subsets of subjects with both tongue-tie and ULT. Pransky and colleagues[98] reported that, in a group of 618 infants with breastfeeding difficulty, 2% had an isolated ULT, 6% had concurrent ULT and anterior ankyloglossia, and 5% had concurrent ULT and posterior ankyloglossia. With treatment of these ties, more than 85% to 100% reported improvement in breastfeeding. Of those with isolated ULT, 100% reported improvement in breastfeeding after release. Benoiton and colleagues[99] also reported on a mixed group of subjects with tongue-tie and ULT and found that, for isolated ULT, 2 out of 3 subjects reported improvement, and, for combined posterior tongue-tie and ULT, 9 out of 10 subjects eventually reported improvement in breastfeeding. Finally, in 2017, Ghaheri and colleagues[44] reported a statistically significant improvement on the BSES following release of both tongue-tie and ULT in a cohort of 178 infants. Results from these studies are difficult to interpret due to various methodological limitations, including a lack of control group, assessment of procedures performed in combination, and subjective outcome measures. More evidence will be needed before division of ULT or other oral ties can be recommended for breastfeeding difficulty.

SUMMARY

Ankyloglossia is a complex multidisciplinary issue, with interplay and impact on a mother–infant dyad, and with many providers from different backgrounds involved in evaluation and treatment. Knowledge about the genetics and epidemiology of this group of disorders continues to evolve. To date, there is high-quality evidence from randomized prospective trials that division of an anterior tongue-tie is helpful in improving breastfeeding in some dyads. Although evidence is emerging on posterior tongue-tie and other oral ties, these studies are often limited by a lack of consensus on diagnosis, indications for treatment, and validated outcomes. As understanding improves, all disciplines will need to work toward cohesive treatment recommendations based on high-quality evidence.

REFERENCES

1. Knox I. Tongue tie and frenotomy in the breastfeeding newborn. Neoreviews 2010;11:e513–9.
2. Obladen M. Much ado about nothing: two millennia of controversy on tongue-tie. Neonatology 2010;97:83–9.
3. Hall DMB, Renfrew MJ. Tongue tie. Arch Dis Child 2005;90:1217–8.
4. Messner AH, Lalakea ML. Ankyloglossia: controversies in management. Int J Pediatr Otorhinolaryngol 2000;54(2–3):123–31.
5. Walsh J, Links A, Boss E, et al. Ankyloglossia and lingual frenotomy: national trends in inpatient diagnosis and management in the United States, 1997-2012. Otolaryngol Head Neck Surg 2017;156(4):735–40.
6. Lisonek M, Liu S, Dzakpasu S, et al. Changes in the incidence and surgical treatment of ankyloglossia in Canada. Paediatr Child Health 2017;22(7):382–6.
7. Kapoor V, Douglas PS, Hill PS, et al. Frenotomy for tongue-tie in Australian children, 2006-2016: an increasing problem. Med J Aust 2018;208(2):88–9.
8. Bin-Nun A, Kasirer YM, Mimouni FB. A dramatic increase in tongue tie-related articles: a 67 years systematic review. Breastfeed Med 2017;12(7):410–4.
9. Douglas PS. Conclusions of Ghaheri's Study that laser surgery for posterior tongue and lip ties improves breastfeeding are not substantiated. Breastfeed Med 2017;12:180–1.
10. Ghaheri BA, Cole M. Response to Douglas Re: "Conclusions of Ghaheri's Study that laser surgery for posterior tongue and lip ties improves breastfeeding are not substantiated. Breastfeed Med 2017;12:182–3.
11. Segal LM, Stephenson R, Dawes M, et al. Prevalence, diagnosis, and treatment of ankyloglossia: methodologic review. Can Fam Physician 2007;53(6):1027–33.
12. Haham A, Marom R, Mangel L, et al. Prevalence of breastfeeding difficulties in newborns with a lingual frenulum: a prospective cohort series. Breastfeed Med 2014;9(9):438–41.
13. Ballard JL, Auer CE, Khoury JC. Ankyloglossia: assessment, incidence, and effect of frenuloplasty on the breastfeeding dyad. Pediatrics 2002;110(5):e63.
14. Ricke LA, Baker NJ, Madlon-Kay DJ, et al. Newborn tongue-tie: prevalence and effect on breast-feeding. J Am Board Fam Pract 2005;18(1):1–7.
15. Chu MW, Bloom DC. Posterior ankyloglossia: a case report. Int J Pediatr Otorhinolaryngol 2009;73(6):881–3.

16. Hong P, Lago D, Seargeant J, et al. Defining ankyloglossia: a case series of anterior and posterior tongue ties. Int J Pediatr Otorhinolaryngol 2010;74(9):1003–6.

17. Walker RD, Messing S, Rosen-Carole C, et al. Defining tip-frenulum length for ankyloglossia and its impact on breastfeeding: a prospective cohort study. Breastfeed Med 2018;13(3):204–10.

18. Douglas PS. Rethinking "posterior" tongue-tie. Breastfeed Med 2013;8(6):503–6.

19. Jin RR, Sutcliffe A, Vento M, et al. What does the world think of ankyloglossia? Acta Paediatr 2018;107(10):1733–8.

20. Aaronson NL, Castaño JE, Simons JP, et al. Quality, readability, and trends for websites on ankyloglossia. Ann Otol Rhinol Laryngol 2018;127(7):439–44.

21. Dixon B, Gray J, Elliot N, et al. A multifaceted programme to reduce the rate of tongue-tie release surgery in newborn infants: observational study. Int J Pediatr Otorhinolaryngol 2018;113:156–63.

22. Gorski SM, Adams KJ, Birch PH, et al. Linkage analysis of X-linked cleft palate and ankyloglossia in Manitoba Mennonite and British Columbia Native kindreds. Hum Genet 1994;94(2):141–8.

23. Klockars T. Familial ankyloglossia (tongue-tie). Int J Pediatr Otorhinolaryngol 2007;71(8):1321–4.

24. Klockars T, Kyttanen S, Ellonen P. TBX22 and tongue-tie. Cleft Palate Craniofac J 2012;49(3):378–9.

25. Morita H, Mazerbourg S, Bouley DM, et al. Neonatal lethality of LGR5 null mice is associated with ankyloglossia and gastrointestinal distension. Mol Cell Biol 2004;24(22):9736–43.

26. Lenormand A, Khonsari R, Corre P, et al. Familial autosomal dominant severe ankyloglossia with tooth abnormalities. Am J Med Genet A 2018;176(7):1614–7.

27. Madlon-Kay DJ, Ricke LA, Baker NJ, et al. Case series of 148 tongue-tied newborn babies evaluated with the assessment tool for lingual frenulum function. Midwifery 2008;24(3):353–7.

28. Douglas P, Geddes D. Practice-based interpretation of ultrasound studies leads the way to more effective clinical support and less pharmaceutical and surgical intervention for breastfeeding infants. Midwifery 2018;58:145–55.

29. Jorgenson RJ, Shapiro SD, Salinas CF, et al. Intraoral findings and anomalies in neonates. Pediatrics 1982;69(5):577–82.

30. Garcia Pola MJ, González García M, García Martín JM, et al. A study of pathology associated with short lingual frenum. ASDC J Dent Child 2002;69(1):59–62, 12.

31. Sedano HO. Congenital oral anomalies in Argentinian children. Community Dent Oral Epidemiol 1975;3(2):61–3.

32. Salem G, Holm SA, Fattah R, et al. Developmental oral anomalies among schoolchildren in Gizan region, Saudi Arabia. Community Dent Oral Epidemiol 1987;15(3):150–1.

33. Voros-Balog T, Vincze N, Banoczy J. Prevalence of tongue lesions in Hungarian children. Oral Dis 2003;9(2):84–7.

34. Messner AH, Lalakea ML, Aby J, et al. Ankyloglossia: incidence and associated feeding difficulties. Arch Otolaryngol Head Neck Surg 2000;126(1):36–9.

35. Klockars T, Pitkaranta A. Inheritance of ankyloglossia (tongue-tie). Clin Genet 2009;75(1):98–9.

36. Harris EF, Friend GW, Tolley EA. Enhanced prevalence of ankyloglossia with maternal cocaine use. Cleft Palate Craniofac J 1992;29(1):72–6.

37. O'Callahan C, Macary S, Clemente S. The effects of office-based frenotomy for anterior and posterior ankyloglossia on breastfeeding. Int J Pediatr Otorhinolaryngol 2013;77(5):827–32.

38. Braybrook C, Doudney K, Marçano AC, et al. The T-box transcription factor gene TBX22 is mutated in X-linked cleft palate and ankyloglossia. Nat Genet 2001; 29(2):179–83.
39. Han SH, Kim MC, Choi YS, et al. A study on the genetic inheritance of ankyloglossia based on pedigree analysis. Arch Plast Surg 2012;39(4):329–32.
40. Patel J, Anthonappa RP, King NM. All tied up! influences of oral frenulae on breastfeeding and their recommended management strategies. J Clin Pediatr Dent 2018;42(6):407–13.
41. Geddes DT, Langton DB, Gollow I, et al. Frenulotomy for breastfeeding infants with ankyloglossia: effect on milk removal and sucking mechanism as imaged by ultrasound. Pediatrics 2008;122(1):e188–94.
42. Puapornpong P, Paritakul P, Suksamarnwong M, et al. Nipple pain incidence, the predisposing factors, the recovery period after care management, and the exclusive breastfeeding outcome. Breastfeed Med 2017;12:169–73.
43. Kotlow LA. The influence of the maxillary frenum on the development and pattern of dental caries on anterior teeth in breastfeeding infants: prevention, diagnosis, and treatment. J Hum Lact 2010;26(3):304–8.
44. Ghaheri BA, Cole M, Fausel SC, et al. Breastfeeding improvement following tongue-tie and lip-tie release: a prospective cohort study. Laryngoscope 2017; 127(5):1217–23.
45. Wong K, Patel P, Cohen MB, et al. Breastfeeding infants with ankyloglossia: insight into mothers' experiences. Breastfeed Med 2017;12:86–90.
46. Jang GJ, Lee SL, Kim HM. [Breast feeding rates and factors influencing breast feeding practice in late preterm infants: comparison with preterm born at less than 34 weeks of gestational age]. J Korean Acad Nurs 2012;42(2):181–9.
47. Meenakshi S, Jagannathan N. Assessment of lingual frenulum lengths in skeletal malocclusion. J Clin Diagn Res 2014;8(3):202–4.
48. Pompeia LE, Ilinsky RS, Ortolani CLF, et al. Ankyloglossia and its influence on growth and development of the stomatognathic system. Rev Paul Pediatr 2017; 35(2):216–21.
49. Messner AH, Lalakea ML. The effect of ankyloglossia on speech in children. Otolaryngol Head Neck Surg 2002;127(6):539–45.
50. Dollberg S, Manor Y, Makai E, et al. Evaluation of speech intelligibility in children with tongue-tie. Acta Paediatr 2011;100(9):e125–7.
51. Heller J, Gabbay J, O'Hara C, et al. Improved ankyloglossia correction with four-flap Z-frenuloplasty. Ann Plast Surg 2005;54(6):623–8.
52. Webb AN, Hao W, Hong P. The effect of tongue-tie division on breastfeeding and speech articulation: a systematic review. Int J Pediatr Otorhinolaryngol 2013; 77(5):635–46.
53. Devasya A, Sarpangala M. Familial ankyloglossia -a rare report of three cases in a family. J Clin Diagn Res 2017;11(2):ZJ03–4
54. Mintz SM, Siegel MA, Seider PJ. An overview of oral frena and their association with multiple syndromic and nonsyndromic conditions. Oral Surg Oral Med Oral Pathol Oral Radiol Endod 2005;99(3):321–4.
55. Suter VG, Bornstein MM. Ankyloglossia: facts and myths in diagnosis and treatment. J Periodontol 2009;80(8):1204–19.
56. Del Campo M, Feitosa IM, Ribeiro EM, et al. The phenotypic spectrum of congenital Zika syndrome. Am J Med Genet A 2017;173(4):841–57.
57. Fonteles CSR, Marques Ribeiro E, Sales Aragão Santos M, et al. Lingual frenulum phenotypes in Brazilian infants with congenital Zika syndrome. Cleft Palate Craniofac J 2018;55(10):1391–8.

58. Breastfeeding, A.A.o.P.S.o.. Congenital tongue-tie and its impact on breastfeeding 2004. Available at: https://urldefense.proofpoint.com/v2/url?u=http-3A__www.lunalactation.com_Ankyloglossia-5FAAPnewsletter.pdf&d=DwIFAg&c=4sF48jRmVAe_CH-k9mXYXEGfSnM3bY53YSKuLUQRxhA&r=xA2HPRJy1uN8376uKwD33sQTRrSRYfMjp9TI71yIeL8&m=f-py4WBjNhKe58-8Xxm4cFfycl70Z-2t0fX2zufQ5TE&s=sw6dtLPnRKe0hpR0YtZHeVYSlBYI4ZB9ovFCiWsUx6U&e=. Accessed July 7, 2019.

59. Kotlow LA. Ankyloglossia (tongue-tie): a diagnostic and treatment quandary. Quintessence Int 1999;30(4):259–62.

60. Kotlow L. Diagnosis and treatment of ankyloglossia and tied maxillary fraenum in infants using Er:YAG and 1064 diode lasers. Eur Arch Paediatr Dent 2011;12(2):106–12.

61. Lalakea ML, Messner AH. Ankyloglossia: does it matter? Pediatr Clin North Am 2003;50(2):381–97.

62. Williams WN, Waldron CM. Assessment of lingual function when ankyloglossia (tongue-tie) is suspected. J Am Dent Assoc 1985;110(3):353–6.

63. Notestine GE. The importance of the identification of ankyloglossia (short lingual frenulum) as a cause of breastfeeding problems. J Hum Lact 1990;6(3):113–5.

64. Ruffoli R, Giambelluca MA, Scavuzzo MC, et al. Ankyloglossia: a morphofunctional investigation in children. Oral Dis 2005;11(3):170–4.

65. Hazelbaker AK. Tongue-tie morphogenesis, impact, assessment and treatment. Columbus (OH): Aidan & Eva Press; 2010.

66. Ingram J, Johnson D, Copeland M, et al. The development of a tongue assessment tool to assist with tongue-tie identification. Arch Dis Child Fetal Neonatal Ed 2015;100(4):F344–8.

67. Ngerncham S, Laohapensang M, Wongvisutdhi T, et al. Lingual frenulum and effect on breastfeeding in Thai newborn infants. Paediatr Int Child Health 2013;33(2):86–90.

68. Junqueira MA, Cunha NN, Costa e Silva LL, et al. Surgical techniques for the treatment of ankyloglossia in children: a case series. J Appl Oral Sci 2014;22(3):241–8.

69. Choi YS, Lim JS, Han KT, et al. Ankyloglossia correction: Z-plasty combined with genioglossus myotomy. J Craniofac Surg 2011;22(6):2238–40.

70. Horton CE, Crawford HH, Adamson JE, et al. Tongue-tie. Cleft Palate J 1969;6:8–23.

71. Aras MH, Göregen M, Güngörmüş M, et al. Comparison of diode laser and Er:YAG lasers in the treatment of ankyloglossia. Photomed Laser Surg 2010;28(2):173–7.

72. Tuli A, Singh A. Monopolar diathermy used for correction of ankyloglossia. J Indian Soc Pedod Prev Dent 2010;28(2):130–3.

73. Chiniforush N, Ghadimi S, Yarahmadi N, et al. Treatment of ankyloglossia with carbon dioxide (CO_2) laser in a pediatric patient. J Lasers Med Sci 2013;4(1):53–5.

74. Morosolli AR, Veeck EB, Niccoli-Filho W, et al. Healing process after surgical treatment with scalpel, electrocautery and laser radiation: histomorphologic and histomorphometric analysis. Lasers Med Sci 2010;25(1):93–100.

75. D'Arcangelo C, Di Nardo Di Maio F, Prosperi GD, et al. A preliminary study of healing of diode laser versus scalpel incisions in rat oral tissue: a comparison of clinical, histological, and immunohistochemical results. Oral Surg Oral Med Oral Pathol Oral Radiol Endod 2007;103:764–73.

76. Gandhi D, Gandhi P. Comparison of healing period after frenectomy using scalpel, electrocautery and diode laser. Br J Med Med Res 2017;21(12):1–9.

77. Shavit I, Peri-Front Y, Rosen-Walther A, et al. A randomized trial to evaluate the effect of two topical anesthetics on pain response during frenotomy in young infants. Pain Med 2017;18(2):356–62.

78. Avarello JT, Gupta A, Silverman RA. Post-frenotomy methemoglobinemia associated with mepivacaine use in a 3 day old. Emergency Med 2013;3(1):1–3.

79. Stevens B, Yamada J, Ohlsson A, et al. Sucrose for analgesia in newborn infants undergoing painful procedures. Cochrane Database Syst Rev 2016;(7):CD001069.

80. Francis DO, Krishnaswami S, McPheeters M. Treatment of ankyloglossia and breastfeeding outcomes: a systematic review. Pediatrics 2015;135(6):e1458–66.

81. Chinnadurai S, Francis DO, Epstein RA, et al. Treatment of ankyloglossia for reasons other than breastfeeding: a systematic review. Pediatrics 2015;135(6):e1467–74.

82. Dollberg S, Botzer E, Grunis E, et al. Immediate nipple pain relief after frenotomy in breast-fed infants with ankyloglossia: a randomized, prospective study. J Pediatr Surg 2006;41(9):1598–600.

83. Berry J, Griffiths M, Westcott C. A double-blind, randomized, controlled trial of tongue-tie division and its immediate effect on breastfeeding. Breastfeed Med 2012;7(3):189–93.

84. Hogan M, Westcott C, Griffiths M. Randomized, controlled trial of division of tongue-tie in infants with feeding problems. J Paediatr Child Health 2005;41(5–6):246–50.

85. Buryk M, Bloom D, Shope T. Efficacy of neonatal release of ankyloglossia: a randomized trial. Pediatrics 2011;128(2):280–8.

86. Emond A, Ingram J, Johnson D, et al. Randomised controlled trial of early frenotomy in breastfed infants with mild-moderate tongue-tie. Arch Dis Child Fetal Neonatal Ed 2014;99(3):F189–95.

87. Argiris K, Vasani S, Wong G, et al. Audit of tongue-tie division in neonates with breastfeeding difficulties: how we do it. Clin Otolaryngol 2011;36(3):256–60.

88. Steehler MW, Steehler MK, Harley EH. A retrospective review of frenotomy in neonates and infants with feeding difficulties. Int J Pediatr Otorhinolaryngol 2012;76(9):1236–40.

89. Lalakea ML, Messner AH. Ankyloglossia: the adolescent and adult perspective. Otolaryngol Head Neck Surg 2003;128(5):746–52.

90. Isaiah A, Pereira KD. Infected sublingual hematoma: a rare complication of frenulectomy. Ear Nose Throat J 2013;92(7):296–7.

91. Genther DJ, Skinner ML, Bailey PJ, et al. Airway obstruction after lingual frenulectomy in two infants with Pierre-Robin sequence. Int J Pediatr Otorhinolaryngol 2015;79(9):1592–4.

92. Tracy LF, Gomez G, Overton LJ, et al. Hypovolemic shock after labial and lingual frenulectomy: a report of two cases. Int J Pediatr Otorhinolaryngol 2017;100:223–4.

93. Gartner LP, Schein D. The superior labial frenum: a histologic observation. Quintessence Int 1991;22(6):443–5.

94. Iwanaga J, Takeuchi N, Oskouian RJ, et al. Clinical anatomy of the frenulum of the oral vestibule. Cureus 2017;9(6):e1410.

95. Dasgupta P, Kamath G, Hs S, et al. Morphological variations of median maxillary labial frenum: a clinical study. J Stomatol Oral Maxillofac Surg 2017;118(6):337–41.

96. Kotlow LA. Diagnosing and understanding the maxillary lip-tie (superior labial, the maxillary labial frenum) as it relates to breastfeeding. J Hum Lact 2013;29(4):458–64.

97. Santa Maria C, Aby J, Truong MT, et al. The superior labial frenulum in newborns: what is normal? Glob Pediatr Health 2017;4. 2333794X17718896.
98. Pransky SM, Lago D, Hong P. Breastfeeding difficulties and oral cavity anomalies: the influence of posterior ankyloglossia and upper-lip ties. Int J Pediatr Otorhinolaryngol 2015;79(10):1714–7.
99. Benoiton L, Morgan M, Baguley K. Management of posterior ankyloglossia and upper lip ties in a tertiary otolaryngology outpatient clinic. Int J Pediatr Otorhinolaryngol 2016;88:13–6.

Updates in Pediatric Cholesteatoma

Minimizing Intervention While Maximizing Outcomes

Kimberly Luu, MD[a], David Chi, MD[a], Krista K. Kiyosaki, MD[b],
Kay W. Chang, MD[b],*

KEYWORDS

- Cholesteatoma • Otitis media with effusion • Mastoidectomy
- Eustachian tube dysfunction • Diffusion weighted MRI • Ossiculoplasty • Endoscopy

KEY POINTS

- Diffusion-weighted MRI has been shown to be both sensitive and specific for detecting cholesteatoma in the temporal bone.
- As surgical trends move toward minimally invasive surgery, we approach the use of canal wall down procedures cautiously.
- Single stage ossiculoplasty can provide equivalent hearing outcomes when compared with staged reconstruction.
- Endoscopic ear surgery has been validated as a valuable technique in cholesteatoma surgery.

INTRODUCTION

Otologic disease in the pediatric patient can pose a challenge to the otolaryngologist. The pediatric patient has a shorter, more horizontal, less rigid eustachian tubes that places them at high risk of middle ear disease, such as chronic otitis media with effusion and cholesteatoma. Small anatomy, a challenging examination, and more aggressive disease make these pathologies difficult to diagnose and treat. Recent advances in pediatric otology have given the pediatric otolaryngologist new tools for diagnosis and management. These advances are outlined in this article.

Disclosure Statement: The authors have nothing to disclose.
[a] Division of Pediatric Otolaryngology, UPMC Children's Hospital of Pittsburgh, Pittsburgh, PA 15224, USA; [b] Division of Pediatric Otolaryngology, Lucile Packard Children's Hospital at Stanford, Department of Otolaryngology, Stanford University School of Medicine, Palo Alto, CA 94304, USA
* Corresponding author. 801 Welch Road, Palo Alto, CA 94304, USA
E-mail address: kaychang@stanford.edu

Otolaryngol Clin N Am 52 (2019) 813–823
https://doi.org/10.1016/j.otc.2019.05.003
0030-6665/19/© 2019 Elsevier Inc. All rights reserved.

SURVEILLANCE: DIFFUSION-WEIGHTED MRI

The rates of recurrent and residual disease after tympanomastoidectomy for cholesteatoma can be as high as 57%.[1] Residual disease can grow in areas not easily assessed by otoscopy in the clinic. Thin cut computed tomography scans of the temporal bone are unable to distinguish between soft tissue types and has been shown to have a sensitivity of 43% and specificity of 48% for detecting cholesteatoma.[2] Given the high recurrence rates and challenges with clinical surveillance a second look surgery, 6 to 24 months is the standard of care for diagnosing recurrent or residual disease. The risk to the hearing and vestibular systems as well as to the facial nerve are significant considerations each time a patient undergoes otologic surgery. In the last decade, the development of diffusion-weighted (DW) MRI has provided a noninvasive surveillance alternative for the middle ear and mastoid. Imaging can provide a low-risk alternative to additional surgery. DWI does not require exposure to radiation and can therefore be especially beneficial in the pediatric population (**Fig. 1**).

DWI is a form of MRI based on measuring the motion of water molecules within tissue. Diffusion is the Brownian motion (errative and random movement) of molecules driven by thermal energy.[3] In the human body, different tissues have characteristic diffusion properties. Extracellular compartments exhibit relatively free diffusion, whereas intracellular compartments demonstrate restricted diffusion.[4] The cellular composition of each type of human tissue thus has predictable diffusion properties and variation from these properties can be an indication of pathology.[5] Diffusion is qualitatively evaluated on trace images and quantitatively evaluated by a calculated parameter called the apparent difficult coefficient (ADC). Tissue with restricted diffusion are bright on trace image and hypointense on the ADC map.

There is promising research for the use of DWI in a number of clinical specialties, including the peripheral nervous system, acute brain ischemia, and tumor detection, particularly in the brain, breast, hepatobiliary, thoracic, and head and neck.[6,7]

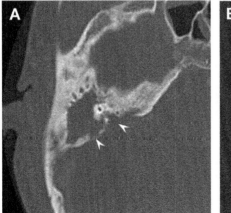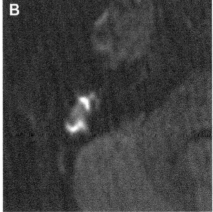

Fig. 1. Congenital cholesteatoma. Axial computed tomography scan through the right epitympanum (*A*) demonstrates complete opacification of the antrum and epitympanum with expansion of the aditus and erosion of the posterior petrous apex (*arrowheads*). The corresponding DW MR image (*B*) shows restricted diffusion (increased signal) within the cholesteatoma.

DIFFUSION-WEIGHTED IMAGING FOR CHOLESTEATOMA DETECTION

A large number of studies have reported on the usefulness of DW MRI for the detection of primary, recurrent, or residual cholesteatoma.[8–10] The majority of studies investigating this question have a prospective design. The number of subjects in each study is small, with the largest reported cohort of fewer than 100 patients.[8] Three systematic reviews have been published in an attempt to aggregate the data. Jindal and colleagues[9] published the first systematic review of 16 studies. Egmond and colleagues[10] and Muzaffar and colleagues[11] added to this literature with systematic reviews and meta-analysis of another 7 and 27 articles, respectively. The studies included in these reviews provide evidence on the usefulness of DW MRI for the detection of cholesteatoma and the difference between different MRI protocols, particularly echoplanar imaging (EPI) and non-EPI scans.

Usefulness is uniformly described by calculations of sensitivity, specificity, positive predictive value, and negative predictive value, with these values being clear and consistently reported. **Table 1** outlines the value ranges for each of these calculations as noted in Edmonds' systematic review. In general, studies report a high sensitivity, specificity, positive predictive value, and negative predictive value. Cholesteatomas missed on DWI but found in surgery range in size from 2 to 5 mm.[10]

DISEASE VARIATION

A number of disease factors influence the reported effectiveness of DW MRI at detecting cholesteatoma. Primary disease can occur in small retraction pockets that are difficult to detect on imaging and can have a higher rate of false-negative results.[7] Patients with canal wall down (CWD) surgeries are able to undergo surveillance in the office, thus imaging is likely more beneficial for patients who have received a canal wall up (CWU) mastoidectomy. The literature reports a large range in time between the imaging and confirmatory surgery, from 0 to 527 days. A long lag time between MRI and surgery could lead to small cholesteatomas being missed on scan and impacting sensitivity calculations.[10] Finally, patients with low likelihood of residual disease with negative MRIs are unlikely to consent for a second look procedure, resulting in selection bias and overestimation of positive predictive value.

IMAGING VARIATION

There is wide variation in the MRI techniques used among published studies that evaluate its effectiveness in cholesteatoma detection. Images are acquired and processed using different protocols depending on the manufacturer of the machine and the MR sequences used by that company. Common sequences seen in literature are

Table 1
Sensitivity, specificity, positive predictive value, and negative predictive value of cholesteatoma detection with DW MRI

Calculation	All Cases (%)[9]	Primary Cases (%)	Residual/ Recurrence (%)
Sensitivity	43–92	83–100	80–82
Specificity	58–100	50–100	90–100
Positive predictive value	50–100	85–100	96–100
Negative predictive value	64–100	50–100	64–85

half-Fourier-acquired single-shot turbo spin echo and periodically rotated overlapping parallel lines with enhanced reconstruction.[12]

The slice thickness of MRI images vary from 2.0 to 5.5 mm, which is a significant range when considering pathology in the middle ear that can be 2 mm or less. MRI is specifically proficient at providing detailed images of soft tissue, but inferior to other imaging techniques for bone. In the majority of study protocols, patients under surveillance for recurrent or residual cholesteatoma also underwent computed tomography scanning as part of the surveillance for cholesteatoma. A computed tomography scan can provide additional information, such as bony erosion and better resolution of the location and characteristics of soft tissue densities, which could alter the pretest probability when interpreting a DW MRI.

ECHOPLANAR IMAGING VERSUS NON-ECHOPLANAR IMAGING

The most important variation of DW MRI when used for cholesteatoma is EPI or non-EPI. In the early 1990s, the development of EPI DW MRI allowed DW technology to be clinically relevant by addressing issues such as imaging speed and motion artifact owing to respiration.[13] The introduction of non-EPI DW MRI further reduced artifact resulting in improved image quality and resolution. This improved resolution theoretically allows the detection of smaller lesions, which is especially important in the small area of concern in temporal bone imaging.

Jindal and colleagues[9] specifically compared the usefulness of non-EPI and EPI DW MRIs for the detection of cholesteatomas. They concluded that non-EPI DW MRI was able to detect smaller lesions with better spatial resolution and less artifact than EPI DW MRI. Muzaffar and colleagues[11] similarly concluded a statistically significant sensitivity of non-EPI DW MRI in detecting residual or recurrent cholesteatoma when compared with EPI DW MRI. Their pooled data showed superiority in non-EPI DW MRI in specificity and improvement in positive predictive value, and negative predictive value that was not statistically significant.[12]

TECHNICAL CHALLENGES OF DIFFUSION-WEIGHTED MRI

There are a number of technical challenges that remain with DW MRI. DWI is susceptible to various artifacts such as T2 shine through, T2 blackout, blurring, and distortion.[14] T2 shine through occurs when there is a prolonged T2 decay time in tissues that results in a high signal on DWI, which can be mistaken for the presence of cholesteatoma. T2 blackout occurs when there is a low signal owing to a lack of water protons. This blackout can be mistaken for restricted diffusion leading to a false-negative result. The DWI should be correlated with a low signal on T2-weighted fat-saturated images to confirm this effect. Finally, ADC values can vary from image to image even when using the same MRI machine and protocol. Variation results from a number of factors that include error in ADC calculations, artifacts, and distortions that are not currently mitigated by a consistent solution.[15]

In summary, DW MRI is an imaging technique using the diffusion properties of water molecules across different tissues in the human body. Restricted diffusion has been shown to be both sensitive and specific for detecting cholesteatoma in temporal bone MRI. There are 2 main categories of DW MRIs: EPI and non-EPI, with non-EPI showing superiority at detecting pathology. DW MRI can provide information on anatomic areas not easily seen on otoscopy, providing an adjunct to second-look surgery in surveillance of patients after cholesteatoma resection.

SURGICAL TECHNIQUES

Advances in the surgical management of cholesteatoma are also important in both initial management and surveillance of disease. Variables in surgical technique including CWU versus CWD surgery and the use of endoscopes impact surgical outcomes and should be considered while planning the management of cholesteatoma.

CANAL WALL UP VERSUS CANAL WALL DOWN SURGERY

The primary goals of cholesteatoma surgery are to eliminate disease and preserve or restore hearing. The indications and usefulness of CWU versus CWD tympanomastoidectomy in the pediatric population remains uncertain. As surgical trends move toward minimally invasive surgery, we approach the use of CWD procedures cautiously.

A CWU tympanomastoidectomy exposes the mastoid and middle ear, but maintains the superior and posterior portions of the bony external auditory canal. In CWD surgery, this bone is removed down to the vertical facial ridge. This creates an open mastoid, which requires regular debridement in the clinic and requires lifelong water precautions. These procedures become especially challenging in children, who are often difficult to examine and manipulate in clinic. Furthermore, they often have a more pneumatized mastoid, which leads to larger cavities.[16] Because CWD is a more extensive procedure, healing times are often longer than after CWU.

The argument for a CWD procedure is the lower recidivism rate and avoidance of a second look surgery. With CWD, the disease process has been exteriorized and there is no risk posed by any recurrence. Children are thought to be at twice the risk of recurrence compared with adults.[17] Despite the elimination of this risk, some argue that, owing to new bony growth in kids, mastoid revision surgery is sometimes still required after CWD surgery.[18] Several studies have demonstrated successful management of children after CWU procedures with recidivism rates ranging from 8% to 53%.[19–26] Further studies have shown that the rates of recurrence or residual disease between CWU and CWD procedures are equivocal.[27–29]

With CWU surgery, there are a wider variety of hearing rehabilitation options. Furthermore, many studies have shown CWU results in significantly better audiometric outcomes.[24,25,27] Tos and Lau[29] initially published on their results with 740 patients with a mean follow-up of 9.3 years and showed a significantly greater improvement in air bone gap in CWU versus CWD surgery. Since then, several large reviews have validated these findings. A review of 420 patients by Osborn and colleagues[30] found that the mean pure-tone average for CWU was 30 dB compared with 45 dB in CWD patients, which was independent of preoperative hearing levels. Similarly, in Schraff and Strasnick's study[28] of 278 cases, the average air bone gap improvement in patients after reconstruction was +10.8 dB in the CWU versus +3.7 dB in the CWD group.

In some cases, CWD surgery cannot be avoided owing to the extent of disease, location, and structures involved. However, otologic surgeons continue to innovate new techniques to minimize intervention and maximize outcome. One such alternative is obliteration of the mastoid cavity after CWD surgery. This maneuver allows for access to the epitympanum while eliminating the problem of an open mastoid. Those who advocate for this hybrid technique have shown that is safe and effective compared with traditional techniques.[19,20] Gantz and colleagues[31] reported successful outcomes with removing the posterior canal wall with a microsaggital saw with reconstruction during closure, a technique originally described by Mercke.[32] Godinho and colleagues[21] also demonstrated the usefulness of their technique using a canal wall window, which is a slit in the posterior canal wall as opposed to a full CWD approach. Moreover, as our technology progresses and we gain better visualization of difficult to access anatomic regions, we predict the role of CWD surgery further diminishing in the pediatric cholesteatoma population.

ENDOSCOPIC EAR SURGERY IN PEDIATRIC CHOLESTEATOMA SURGERY

In the early 1990s, Poe and colleagues[33] first described the use of endoscopes for middle ear exploration. This was followed by Tarabichi's work describing the endoscopic management of cholesteatoma.[34] As with any innovative technology, surgeons have been slow to adopt endoscopic ear surgery (EES) into regular practice. However, the development of smaller diameter endoscopes with high-definition capabilities have allowed for an expanded field of view and improved resolution compared with microscopic ear surgery (MES).[35,36] Furthermore, angled endoscopes allow surgeons significantly more visualization of recessed spaces like the facial recess, sinus tympani, and epitympanum.[35–37]

The challenge of pediatric cholesteatoma surgery is managing the increased rates of recidivism owing to more aggressive disease, while using conservative mastoid-preserving procedures. Endoscopes in cholesteatoma surgery may be used as an adjunct to traditional MES for intraoperative inspection of residual disease. Studies have shown endoscopically visible residual cholesteatoma rates of 16% to 38% after patients were thought to be microscopically free of disease.[38–42] With the advent of microscopic and curved instrumentation, the endoscope can also be effectively used in dissection (with or without the use of the microscope). Many studies have validated the safety and efficacy of EES compared with MES for pediatric cholesteatoma surgery.[42–47] A recent systematic review in pediatric patients by Han and colleagues[43] showed a significantly lower residual and recurrence rate in EES versus MES. Other outcomes such as the success of tympanoplasty graft and audiological outcomes were equivocal between the 2 techniques.[43,45–47] Marchioni and colleagues[48] examined the complications associated with EES and found that there were no major intraoperative complications and minor complications were low and comparable with traditional MES.

Beyond decreased recidivism rates, EES provides the potential for minimizing intervention and morbidity. A traditional microscopic view is limited by the narrowest portion of the ear canal, thus a postauricular incision and parallel channel through the mastoid is often required to visualize the attic. However, an endoscopic transcanal approach obviates the need for a postauricular incision. Although children have a smaller external auditory canal, Ito and colleagues[49] demonstrated that transcanal EES could be successfully performed in pediatric patients with canals as small as 3.2 mm in diameter. Studies have shown that EES leads to increased rates of ossicular chain preservation, which may be beneficial in hearing outcomes.[50,51] Others have demonstrated that EES is mastoid and mucosal sparing without compromise to functional outcomes.[52–54] In his 10-year retrospective review, Sajjadi reported that the incorporation of EES significantly reduced the need to perform a mastoidectomy during second look procedures.[38] Minimizing surgical morbidity with EES also leads to better postoperative pain and faster healing times.[55,56] Moreover, the decreased rates of residual cholesteatoma with the use of endoscopes may decrease the need for second look surgery in select patients. Sarcu and Isaacson[39] reviewed their practice with this strategy of selective second look surgery for children with high-risk disease and found a low rate (7%) of residual disease.

EES has been validated as a valuable technique in cholesteatoma surgery. Whereas MES offers the benefits of depth perception and 2-handed surgery, technological advances in instrumentation will continue to augment EES. The incorporation of single handpiece instruments like the flexible fiber CO_2 laser[57] and ultrasonic bone curette[58] have already broadened the indications for EES. As the EES toolbox expands, we anticipate a growing usefulness of EES in cholesteatoma management.

HEARING RECONSTRUCTION: SINGLE STAGE OSSCICULOPLASTY

The timing of ossicular reconstruction has long been debated. In the 1990s the House Institute advocated for delaying ossicular chain reconstruction (OCR) until the neotympanic membrane had healed and the inflammation in the middle ear was resolved.[59] This process was motivated by the assumption of better hearing results and lower risk of recurrent or residual disease. Sheehy, a prominent otologist, argued that the goal of the first stage should be to eradicate disease, create a healthy middle ear space, and intact tympanic membrane. A staged procedure, 6 to 24 months later, would ensure disease resolution and be a more appropriate time for OCR.[60]

Alternatively, Tos[61] argued that a single stage tympanomastoidectomy with OCR was cost effective with little risk to the patient. Crowson and colleagues[62] reported significantly decreased overall costs when comparing patients undergoing single stage and second look procedures, namely, $23,529 versus $41,411, respectively. The additional quality of life benefit of having immediate hearing rehabilitation should prompt clinicians to revisit the traditional assumption of better hearing outcomes with staged OCR.

In general, hearing outcomes in single stage procedures have been shown to be comparable with those from staged procedures.[63] However, there are a number of other hearing outcome prognostic factors that confound this conclusion.

There are 2 main types of operations performed for cholesteatoma, CWU and CWD. A number of studies have found that when compared with CWU surgeries, a CWD procedure is the strongest prognostic factor for poorer postoperative hearing.[64] A second look is not anticipated after a CWD mastoidectomy so tympanoplasty and ossiculoplasty are all performed in 1 stage. The reason for worse postoperative hearing is likely from the status of the mastoid rather than a single stage reconstruction.[27]

The status of the ossicular chain is an important factor to consider when deciding on staging OCR. Patients with severe disease should be considered more carefully. In a study where patients were stratified by the absence or presence of a stapes superstructure, staged procedure improved the postoperative the air–bone gap, leading the authors to conclude staging OCR may be advantageous in severe disease.[65] Patients with minimal disease have a lesser likelihood of recurrence that can even be followed with surveillance with diffusion-weighted MRI. This population may be particularly amenable to single stage reconstruction. If a reconstructed patient requires an additional operation, however, there is the additional risk of dislodging the prosthesis, resulting in worsening hearing.

A number of studies have investigated the significance of inflamed middle ear mucosa for hearing outcomes. Some studies have reported a weak association of inflamed mucosa with worse hearing outcomes, with ossicular chain and canal wall status being much stronger prognostic factors.[38,39,66] In contrast, other studies have found no association between inflamed middle ear mucosa and poorer hearing results.[67,68] However, these results could be biased because surgeons tend to not perform an OCR in the most severe cholesteatoma cases with the most inflammation. If all ears were reconstructed, regardless of the disease, the results may show poorer hearing for ears with inflamed mucosa.[69]

The timing of OCR in chronic ear surgery has been long debated. Single stage reconstruction can produce comparable hearing results with lower health care costs and benefits of hearing between surgical stages. Factors such as inflamed middle ear mucosa and disease severity should be considered when deciding on the timing of reconstruction.

SUMMARY

Innovation in pediatric otology has driven diagnosis and management of cholesteatoma to become less invasive while maintaining effectiveness. DW MRI differentiates disease from the surrounding soft tissue to an accuracy of 2 to 4 mm, providing surgeons a good alternative to a second look surgery for surveillance. Studies demonstrating eradication of disease with CWU surgery leads to less invasive surgery and allows for a wider range of hearing rehabilitation. Otoendoscopy is a growing technology that provides visualization of previously difficult to see areas and has become an integral addition to the surgeons' armamentarium. Finally, evidence of good outcomes with single stage ossiculoplasty again provides comparable benefit while lowering costs and intervention to the patient. These advances have moved the management of pediatric cholesteatoma toward improved surgical outcomes with minimized intervention.

REFERENCES

1. Rosenfeld R, Moura R, Bluestone C. Predictors of residual-recurrent cholesteatoma in children. Arch Otolaryngol Head Neck Surg 1992;118(4):384–91.
2. Tierney P, Pracy P, Blaney S, et al. An assessment of the value of the preoperative computed tomography scans prior to otoendoscopic 'second look' in intact canal wall mastoid surgery. Clin Otolaryngol Allied Sci 1999;24:274–6.
3. Jones D. Diffusion MRI: theory, methods, and applications. Oxford (USA): Oxford University Press; 2010.
4. Chilla G, Tan C, Xu C, et al. Diffusion weighted magnetic resonance imaging and its recent trend—a survey. Quant Imaging Med Surg 2015;5(3):407–22.
5. Baliyan V, Das C, Sharma G, et al. Diffusion weighted imaging: technique and applications. World J Radiol 2016;8(9):785–98.
6. Schouten C, de Graaf P, Alberts F, et al. Response evaluation after chemoradiotherapy for advanced nodal disease in head and neck cancer using diffusion-weighted MRI and 18F-FDG-PET-CT. Oral Oncol 2015;51:541–7.
7. Varoquaux A, Rager O, Dulguerov P, et al. Diffusion-weighted and PET/MR Imaging after radiation therapy for malignant head and neck tumors. Radiographics 2015;35:1502–27.
8. Akkari M, Gabrillargues J, Saroul N, et al. Contribution of magnetic resonance imaging to the diagnosis of middle ear cholesteatoma. analysis of a series of 97 cases. Eur Ann Otorhinolaryngol Head Neck Dis 2014;131:153–8.
9. Jindal M, Riskalla A, Jiang D, et al. A systematic review of diffusion-weighted magnetic resonance imaging in the assessment of postoperative cholesteatoma. Otol Neurotol 2011;32:1243–9.
10. Egmond S, Stegeman I, Grolman W, et al. A systematic review of non-echo planar diffusion-weighted magnetic resonance imaging for detection of primary and postoperative cholesteatoma. Otolaryngol Head Neck Surg 2016;154(2):233–40.
11. Muzaffar J, Colley S, Coulson C. Diffusion-weighted magnetic resonance imaging for residual and recurrent cholesteatoma: a systematic review and meta-analysis. Clin Otolaryngol 2017;42(3):536–43.

12. Aarts M, Rovers M, van der Veen E, et al. The diagnostic value of diffusion-weighted magnetic resonance imaging in detecting a residual cholesteatoma. Otolaryngol Head Neck Surg 2010;143:12–6.

13. Le Bihan D. Diffusion MRI: what water tells us about the brain. EMBO Mol Med 2014;6:569–73.

14. De Foer B, Vercruysse J, Bernaerts A, et al. Middle ear cholesteatoma: non-echo-planar diffusion-weighted MR imaging versus delayed gadolinium-enhanced T1-weighted MR imaging value in detection. Radiology 2010;255:866–72.

15. Sasaki M, Yamada K, Watanabe Y, et al. Variability in absolute apparent diffusion coefficient values across different platforms may be substantial: a multivendor, multi-institutional comparison study. Radiology 2008;249:624–30.

16. Dornhoffer JL, Friedman AB, Gluth MB. Management of acquired cholesteatoma in the pediatric population. Curr Opin Otolaryngol Head Neck Surg 2013;21(5): 440–5.

17. Stankovic M. Follow-up of cholestatoma surgery; open versus closed tympano-plasty. ORL J Otorhinolaryngol Relat Spec 2007;69(5):299–305.

18. Kazahaya K, Postic WF. Congenital cholesteatoma. Curr Opin Otolaryngol Head Neck Surg 2004;12(5):392–403.

19. Trinidade A, Skingsley A, Yung MW. Pediatric cholesteatoma surgery using a single-staged canal wall down approach: results of a 5 year longitudinal study. Otol Neurotol 2015;36(1):82–5.

20. Vercruysse JP, De Foer B, Somers T, et al. Mastoid and epitympanic bony oblit-eration in pediatric cholesteatoma. Otol Neurotol 2008;29(7):953–60.

21. Godinho RA, Kamil SH, Lubianca JN, et al. Pediatric cholesteatoma: canal wall window alternative to canal wall down mastoidectomy. Otol Neurotol 2005; 26(3):466–71.

22. Ho SY, Kveton JF. Efficacy of the 2-staged procedure in the management of cho-lesteatoma. Arch Otolaryngol Head Neck Surg 2003;129(5):541–5.

23. Ueda H, Nakashima T, Nakata S. Surgical strategy for cholesteatoma in children. Auris Nasus Larynx 2001;28(2):125–9.

24. Dornhoffer JL. Retrograde mastoidectomy with canal wall reconstruction: a single-stage technique for cholestatoma removal. Ann Otol Rhinol Laryngol 2000;109(11):1033–9.

25. Dodson EE, Hashisaki GT, Hobgood TC, et al. Intact canal wall mastoidectomy with tympanoplasty for cholesteatoma in children. Laryngoscope 1998;108(7): 977–83.

26. Parisier SC, Hanson MB, Han JC, et al. Pediatric cholesteatoma: an individual-ized single-stage approach. Otolaryngol Head Neck Surg 1996;115(1):107–14.

27. Shirazi MA, Muzaffar K, Leonetti JP, et al. Surgical treatment of pediatric choles-teatomas. Laryngoscope 2006;116(9):1603–7.

28. Scraff SA, Strasnick B. Pediatric cholesteatoma: a retrospective review. Int J Pe-diatr Otorhinolaryngol 2006;70(3):385–93.

29. Tos M, Lau T. hearing after surgery for cholesteatoma using various techniques. Auris Nasus Larynx 1989;16(2):61–73.

30. Osborn AJ, Papsin BC, James AL. Clinical indications for canal wall-down mas-toidectomy in a pediatric population. Otolaryngol Head Neck Surg 2012;147(2): 316–21.

31. Gantz B, Wilkinson E, Hansen M. Canal wall reconstruction tympanomastoidec-tomy with mastoid obliteration. Laryngoscope 2005;115(10):1734–40.

32. Mercke U. The cholesteatomatous ear one year after surgery with obliteration technique. Am J Otol 1987;8:534–6.

33. Poe DS, Rebeiz EE, Pankratov MM, et al. Trans-tympanic endoscopy of the middle ear. Laryngoscope 1992;102(9):993–6.

34. Tarabichi M. Endoscopic management of acquired cholesteatoma. Am J Otol 1997;18(5):544–9.

35. Isaacson G. Endoscopic anatomy of the pediatric middle ear. Otolaryngol Head Neck Surg 2014;140(1):6–15.

36. Kiringoda R, Kozen ED, Lee DJ. Outcomes in endoscopic ear surgery. Otolaryngol Clin North Am 2016;49(5):1271–90.

37. Tarabichi M, Kapadia M. Principles of endoscopic ear surgery. Curr Opin Otolaryngol Head Neck Surg 2016;24(5):382–7.

38. Sajjadi H. Endoscopic middle ear and mastoid surgery for cholesteatoma. Iran J Otorhinolaryngol 2013;25(71):63–70.

39. Sarcu D, Isaacson G. Long-term results of endoscopically assisted pediatric cholesteatoma surgery. Otolaryngol Head Neck Surg 2015;154(3):535–9.

40. Badr-el-Dine M. Surgery of sinus tympani cholesteatoma: endoscopic necessity. J Int Adv Otol 2009;5:158–65.

41. Presutti L, Marchioni D, Mattioli F, et al. Endoscopic management of acquired cholesteatoma: our experience. J Otolaryngol Head Neck Surg 2008;37(4): 481–7.

42. Bennet M, Wanna G, Francis D, et al. Clinical and cost utility of intraoperative endoscopic second look in cholesteatoma surgery. Laryngoscope 2018; 128(12):2867–71.

43. Han SY, Lee DY, Chung J, et al. Comparison of endoscopic and microscopic ear surgery in pediatric patients: a meta-analysis. Laryngoscope 2019;129(6): 1444–52.

44. Park JH, Ahn J, Moon IJ. Transcanal endoscopic ear surgery for congenital cholesteatoma. Clin Exp Otorhinolaryngol 2018;11(4):233–41.

45. Kim BJ, Kim JH, Park MK, et al. Endoscopic visualization to the anterior surface of the malleus and tensor tympani tendon in congenital cholesteatoma. Eur Arch Otorhinolaryngol 2018;275(5):1069–75.

46. Ghadersoh S, Carter JM, Hoff SR. Endoscopic transcanal approach to the middle ear for management of pediatric cholesteatoma. Laryngoscope 2017;127(11): 2653–8.

47. Kobayashi T, Gyo K, Komori M, et al. Efficacy and safety of transcanal endoscopic ear surgery for congenital cholesteatomas: a preliminary report. Otol Neurotol 2015;36(10):1644–50.

48. Marchioni D, Rubini A, Gazzini L, et al. Complications in endoscopic ear surgery. Otol Neurotol 2018;39(8):1012–7.

49. Ito T, Kubota T, Watanabe T, et al. Transcanal endoscopic ear surgery for pediatric population with a narrow external auditory canal. Int J Pediatr Otorhinolaryngol 2015;79(12):2265–9.

50. James AL. Endoscopic middle ear surgery in children. Otolaryngol Clin North Am 2013;46(2):233–44.

51. Marchioni D, Soloperto D, Rubini A, et al. Endoscopic exclusive transcanal approach to the tympanic cavity cholesteatoma in pediatric patients: our experience. Int J Pediatr Otorhinolaryngol 2015;79(3):316–22.

52. Presutti L, Anschuetz L, Rubini A, et al. The impact of the transcanal endoscopic approach and mastoid preservation on recurrence of primary acquired attic cholesteatoma. Otol Neurotol 2018;39(4):445–50.

53. Cohen MS, Basonbul RA, Kozen ED, et al. Residual cholesteatoma during second-look procedures following primary pediatric endoscopic ear surgery. Otolaryngol Head Neck Surg 2017;157(6):1034–40.
54. Hanna BM, Kivekas I, Wu YH, et al. Minimally invasive functional approach for cholesteatoma surgery. Laryngoscope 2014;124(10):2386–92.
55. Magliulo G, Iannella G. Endoscopic versus microscopic approach in attic cholesteatoma surgery. Am J Otolaryngol 2018;39(1):25–30.
56. Kakehata S, Furukawa T, Ito T, et al. Comparison of postoperative pain in patients following transcanal endoscopic versus microscopic ear surgery. Otol Neurotol 2018;39(7):847–53.
57. Landegger LD, Cohen MS. Use of the flexible fiber CO_2 laser in pediatric transcanal endoscopic middle ear surgery. Int J Pediatr Otorhinolaryngol 2016;85:154–7.
58. Kakehata S, Watanabe T, Ito IT, et al. Extension of indications for transcanal endoscopic ear surgery using an ultrasonic bone curette for cholesteatomas. Otol Neurotol 2014;35(1):101–7.
59. Sheehy JL, Crabtree JA. Tympanoplasty: staging the operation. Laryngoscope 1973;83:1594–621.
60. Shelton C, Sheehy JL. Tympanoplasty: review of 400 staged cases. Laryngoscope 1990;100(7):679–81.
61. Tos M. Late results in tympanoplasty: staging the operation. Acta Otolaryngol 1976;82:282–5.
62. Crowson M, Ramprasad V, Chapurin N, et al. Cost analysis and outcomes of a second-look tympanoplasty-mastoidectomy strategy for cholesteatoma. Laryngoscope 2016;126:2574–9.
63. Kim H, Battista R, Kumar A, et al. Should ossicular reconstruction be staged following tympanomastoidectomy. Laryngoscope 2010;116(1):47–51.
64. Albu S, Babighian G, Trabalzini F. Prognostic factors in tympanoplasty. Am J Otol 1998;19:136–40.
65. Redaelli Z, Tonni D, Barezzani M. Single-stage canal wall-down tympanoplasty: long-term results and prognostic factors. Ann Otol Rhinol Laryngol 2010;119(5):304–12.
66. Bennet ML, Zhang D, Labadie RF, et al. Comparison of middle ear visualization with endoscopy and microscopy. Otol Neurotol 2016;37(4):362–6.
67. Dornhoffer JL, Gardner E. Prognostic factors in ossiculoplasty: a statistical staging system. Otol Neurotol 2001;22:299–304.
68. Brackmann DE, Sheehy JL, Luxford WM. TORPs and PORPs in tympanoplasty: a review of 1042 operations. Otolaryngol Head Neck Surg 1984;92:32–7.
69. O'Reilly R, Cass S, Hirsch B, et al. Ossiculoplasty using incus interposition: hearing results and analysis of the middle ear risk index. Otol Neurotol 2005;26:853–8.

Principles of Pediatric Endoscopic Ear Surgery

Kimberly A. Miller, MD[a], Manuela Fina, MD[b,c], Daniel J. Lee, MD[d,*]

KEYWORDS

- Pediatric • Children • Endoscope • Endoscopic ear surgery • Transcanal
- Tympanoplasty • Congenital • Cholesteatoma

KEY POINTS

- Pediatric ears are ideally suited for endoscopic ear surgery (EES) because small diameter rigid telescopes with wide-angle lenses enable superior transcanal visualization of the tympanic membrane and middle ear compared with the operating microscope.
- In the setting of disease limited to the tympanic membrane and middle ear, the transcanal endoscopic approach can avoid the need for a postauricular incision. This reduces postoperative morbidity and avoids the need for a bulky mastoid dressing.
- Transcanal EES is a safe and effective minimally invasive approach for the management of congenital or attic cholesteatoma and, in most cases, avoids a postauricular incision or significant bony dissection.
- In cases of extensive cholesteatoma involving the tympanic space, improved visualization of the epitympanic, protympanic, retrotympanic, and hypotympanic recesses reduces the need for a canal wall up mastoidectomy.
- When disease extends to the antrum, transmastoid endoscopic ear surgery allows for visualization of the posterior attic and aditus ad antrum to ensure gross total resection of disease and avoids a canal wall down mastoidectomy. The senior authors have not performed a canal wall down mastoidectomy for primary pediatric cholesteatomata since introducing the endoscope to their surgical practice.

Disclosure Statement: Dr M. Fina and Dr K.A. Miller have no relevant conflicts of interest or financial ties to disclose. Dr D.J. Lee has financial relationships with Akouos, Auregen Bio-Therapeutics, Agilis, Frequency Therapeutics, and 3NT Medical, Ltd. None of these entities have commercialized products that are relevant to the topic of pediatric endoscopic ear surgery.
^a Department of Otolaryngology, University of Minnesota, Minneapolis, MN, USA; ^b Department of Otolaryngology, University of Minnesota, 420 Delaware Street Southeast, MMC 396, Minneapolis, MN 55455, USA; ^c HealthPartners Medical Group, 401 Phalen Blvd, St Paul, MN 55130, USA; ^d Pediatric Otology and Neurotology, Department of Otology and Laryngology, Harvard Medical School, Massachusetts Eye and Ear Infirmary, 243 Charles Street, Boston, MA 02114, USA
* Corresponding author.
E-mail address: Daniel_lee@meei.harvard.edu

Otolaryngol Clin N Am 52 (2019) 825–845
https://doi.org/10.1016/j.otc.2019.06.001
0030-6665/19/© 2019 Elsevier Inc. All rights reserved.

INTRODUCTION

The binocular microscope is the workhorse of the otologic surgeon and provides excellent optics, true depth of field, and allows for 2-handed dissection. Where the microscope falters is the ability to visualize complex middle ear disease transcanal and nowhere is this more apparent than in children. An endaural or postauricular incision and bony dissection are often required during cases in which the external auditory canal (EAC) is small or tortuous. Disease that extends superiorly or anteriorly (eg, congenital cholesteatoma) is especially challenging to access using a speculum-assisted microscopic dissection owing to the limitations of line-of-sight surgery.

Over the past three decades, rigid endoscopy has gradually entered the field of middle ear surgery. Initially, endoscopes were used only as adjunct tools to rule out residual disease (otoendoscopy) following cholesteatoma resection performed with the binocular microscope.[1] Endoscopes were first used to perform middle ear surgery (ie, endoscopic ear surgery [EES] or transcanal endoscopic ear surgery) in the 1990s by Tarabichi, Thomassin, and Poe; this work mirrored improvements in both endoscopic and video technology.[2–4] Adoption has been slow since these first steps because few training programs offer exposure to EES in the United States and abroad; however, the availability of training courses continues to increase. Although few would question the advantages of the Hopkins rod-lens telescope over the microscope in transcanal visualization of the middle ear, EES does have limitations, which are often cited by critics of this approach. First, a single-handed technique (no suction in the other hand) and the relative ratio of the diameter of the scope to the ear canal can be challenging, especially in children and in narrow or tortuous canals. Second, modern high-definition video cameras are 2-dimensional and do not offer true depth perception. The surgeon must rely on motion parallax to assess the relative position of landmarks in a 3-dimensional (3D) space (current 3D systems are still unwieldly). Third, there is a limited selection of endoscopes and dissectors designed for pediatric EES. Fourth, learning EES is challenging and only a few surgical residency and fellowship programs offer significant exposure to EES.

This article provides a rationale for EES in children, describes differences in pediatric and adult anatomy and the implications for EES, reviews the basic principles of EES, and summarizes outcomes in pediatric EES for chronic ear disease.

WHY IS ENDOSCOPIC EAR SURGERY AN IDEAL APPROACH IN CHILDREN?

The authors believe that the routine use of endoscopes to perform transcanal surgery greatly enhances the care of children with chronic ear disease. The main advantages of EES over the microscope in the pediatric population are (1) transcanal visual access to the hidden recesses of the middle ear, especially the protympanum (eg, congenital cholesteatoma), epitympanum, and retrotympanum (eg, acquired cholesteatoma) that reduces the need for soft tissue and bony dissection, including canal wall up mastoidectomy; (2) incision avoidance to reduce issues such as dysesthesia or anesthesia of the auricle, hypertrophic scars or keloids, wound infections, and the challenges of dressing changes or suture removal in young children; and (3) avoidance of canal wall down mastoidectomy for extensive disease (using transmastoid endoscopic-assisted dissection, **Fig. 1**).

Overall, EES enables a more conservative surgical approach in children with chronic ear disease compared with the microscope. The authors hypothesize that EES provides similar rates of disease control to traditional microscope dissection while

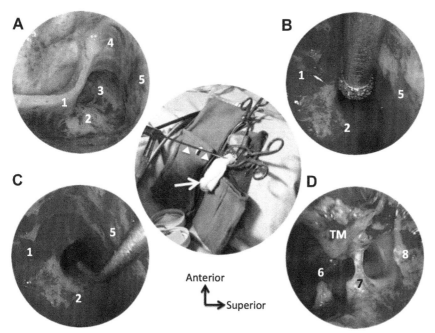

Fig. 1. Endoscopic-assisted transmastoid dissection can reduce the need for canal wall down mastoidectomy in cases of extensive cholesteatoma. Middle: the rigid endoscope (*arrowheads*) should be resting against a moist gauze sponge placed in the mastoid cavity (*arrow*) to stabilize the image and prevent unnecessary movement. (*A*) Left ear canal wall up mastoidectomy can be completed with the surgical microscope to provide access to the aditus ad antrum and epitympanum for a rigid angled endoscope and curved suction or dissecting instrument. (*B*) Powered surgical drill (3-mm coarse diamond burr shown) can be used transmastoid with 30° endoscopic visualization to widen the atticotomy. (*C*) A curved #3 or #5 suction and 30° endoscope can be used to debride residual disease in the epitympanum. (*D*) Transmastoid 30° endoscopic view looking down into the middle ear (and toward the Eustachian tube) enables a surgical perspective not possible through the ear canal to ensure gross total resection of chronic ear disease. 1, EAC; 2, horizontal semicircular canal; 3, aditus ad antrum; 4, zygomatic root; 5, tegmen mastoideum; 6, stapes; 7, cochleariform process and tensor tympani tendon; 8, cog, TM, tympanic membrane.

improving quality of life by reducing postoperative morbidity, the need for frequent debridement postoperatively, and the challenges of water precautions in active children. Prospective studies are ongoing to quantify these benefits.

HOW DOES PEDIATRIC TEMPORAL BONE ANATOMY INFLUENCE THE ENDOSCOPIC APPROACH?

The tympanic membrane (TM), middle ear, and inner ear in pediatric patients are similar in size to adults but the morphology of the pinna and EAC is smaller.[5] This can dictate the diameter of the endoscope needed to successfully visualize the middle ear in younger children (**Fig. 2**). Although a traditional 4-mm rigid Hopkins rod-lens sinus telescope can be used for older children and adults with non-tortuous canals, most younger children require a 3-mm, 2.7-mm, or 1.9-mm diameter endoscope during EES for visualization and dissection of the TM and middle ear.[6,7]

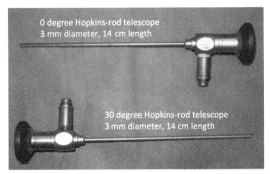

Fig. 2. Hopkins rod-lens telescopes less than 4 mm in diameter are ideal for pediatric endoscopic ear surgery. Pictured are 3 mm × 14 cm rigid endoscopes (smaller than traditional sinus endoscopes that are 4 mm × 18 cm).

External Auditory Canal

The EAC undergoes significant changes during the first 10 years of life. At birth, the cartilaginous canal abuts the tympanic ring. There is substantial lateral growth in the first 5 years, with ossification of the lateral part of the tympanic ring and bony ear canal.[8] Between ages 5 and 18 years, the bony canal doubles in length. During this period of development, the height and width of the EAC also increase from a neonatal (1–6 months) size of approximately 4.4 to 6.3 mm in width and approximately 5.4 mm in height, reaching an adult size of approximately 6.1 mm to 10.4 mm in width, and 6.9 mm in height.[9,10] Based on a computed tomography (CT) study, 84% of a pediatric cohort (40 subjects, 80 ears, ages 0–18 years, median age 8.5 years) would be able to undergo transcanal endoscopic ear surgery with a 3-mm diameter endoscope.[10] However, some children may require smaller endoscopes to navigate the bony EAC, especially in congenital cholesteatoma when patients present at younger ages.[6,7]

Tympanic Membrane Anatomy in Children

The TM is adult size at birth (roughly 9 mm in diameter) but the anatomic plane of the tympanic annulus will not reach maturity until later. The neonatal tympanic annulus is only 34° from horizontal, becoming 63° from horizontal in adulthood[11] (**Fig. 3**). This change in tympanic annulus orientation is due to growth of the temporal lobe and skull base rather than change to middle ear morphology. The more acute angle of the TM relative to the plane of the bony EAC in younger children (see **Fig. 3**) makes endoscopic or microscope visualization of the epitympanum and retrotympanum more challenging. Angled telescopes, ranging from 30° to 45° (see **Fig. 2**), and curved or angled suctions and dissectors (**Fig. 4**) can help to overcome these anatomic challenges but should only be used by experienced surgeons. New designs are available with steerable lenses ranging from 10° to 90° without changing endoscopes; however, these are only available in 4.5-mm diameter and are therefore too large for EES in children or adults.

Ossicles and Middle Ear Cleft

Although the ossicles are adult size at birth, morphologic changes still occur during childhood. The bone density of the neonatal ossicular chain increases over the first decade of life as marrow-containing spaces involute into cancellous bone. The axis of the ossicles also shifts due to growth of the middle cranial fossa, similar to the tympanic annulus.[8]

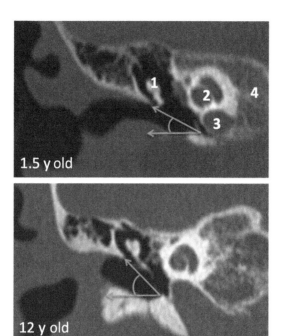

Fig. 3. Coronal CT of the right temporal bone in an infant (upper panel, 1.5 years old) and older child (lower panel, 12 years old) highlighting differences in tympanic membrane (TM) orientation. In otherwise normal temporal bones, infants and younger children have a more acute angle of the TM relative to the bony EAC compared with older children.[12] This makes visualization of the hidden recesses of the middle ear even more challenging with microscope but this can be overcome by using small-diameter right-angled endoscopes. 1, malleus; 2, cochlea; 3, carotid artery; 4, petrous apex.

The middle ear cleft undergoes more subtle changes during development. The neonatal mesotympanum, including sinus tympani and facial recess, are nearly adult size, but the epitympanum and hypotympanum grow apart, increasing the height of the middle ear space. As a result, the adult tympanic cavity has a volume that is 1.5 times larger than in the neonate.[12] Pediatric temporal bone sections commonly demonstrate residual mesenchyme between middle ear mucosa and bone. This additional layer could, in theory, blunt the retrotympanic recess in neonatal patients. Mesenchyme also fills the Prussak space at birth and is resorbed slowly over the first 5 years of life. This presence of mesenchyme in the neonatal Prussak space may be a factor contributing to the low incidence of pars flaccida cholesteatoma in younger children.[13]

INDICATIONS FOR ENDOSCOPIC EAR SURGERY IN CHILDREN

The endoscope can be used in any transcanal (or transmastoid) pediatric middle ear procedure that traditionally requires the microscope. One exception would be a chronic ear with inflammatory changes associated with significant bleeding that would be more efficiently managed with 2-handed dissection under microscope-assisted visualization (or with a new technology called an exoscope-extracorporeal digital microscope). In many routine or complex middle ear cases, such as an anterior TM perforation, deep retraction pocket, or cholesteatoma, the endoscope enables a transcanal approach that would ordinarily require a postauricular incision (**Fig. 5**).

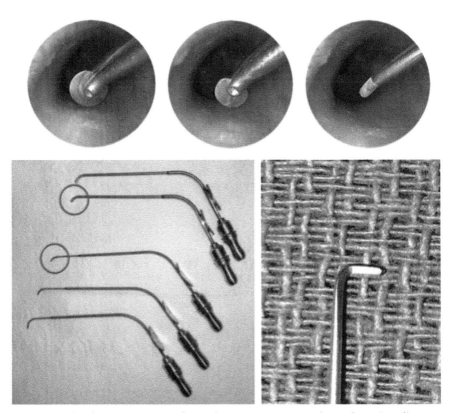

Fig. 4. Specialized instrumentation for endoscopic ear surgery. (*Upper*) Suction dissectors are modified round or joint knives and are useful for (1) novice surgeons when elevating a tympanomeatal flap and (2) during chronic ear cases when vasoconstriction is difficult to achieve. (*Lower left*) Curved suctions (shown are #3 and #5 Fraser tip suctions) with swivel connectors to reduce torque associated with tubing are essential for removal of disease in the retrotympanic or epitympanic recesses when visualized with a 0° or angled endoscope. Please begin with the less graduated curved suctions (*red circles*) because the more severely curved suctions are more difficult to use and, in some cases, cannot be placed through a pediatric EAC. (*Lower right*) The Crabtree dissector is an ideal instrument for removing disease from the hidden recesses of the middle ear and is found in most otologic instrument sets.

Finally, after a microscope-assisted canal wall up mastoidectomy for extensive cholesteatoma, a transmastoid endoscopic approach can also be used to visualize and remove residual disease from the aditus ad antrum and attic to avoid a canal wall down mastoidectomy (see **Fig. 1**).

PEDIATRIC OTOENDOSCOPY IN THE OFFICE

The examination of the ear in a child is particularly challenging because it requires a degree of trust and cooperation with the patient and family. The ear is first examined with an otoscope or microscope and debrided as needed to visualize the medial EAC and TM (debridement of the ear using an endoscope can be challenging and only reserved for the experienced endoscopic ear surgeon). Although the pediatric sinus 0° endoscopes (2.7 mm diameter × 18 cm) that are readily available in a pediatric otolaryngology office can be used, the longer length makes them challenging for

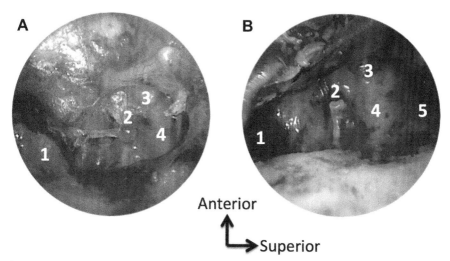

Fig. 5. Intraoperative images taken using a 0° endoscope from a 7-year-old child with a left ear complex par tensa retraction pocket and chronic otitis media. (*A*) Deep posterior drum retraction adherent to a prominent or dehiscent jugular bulb (1), stapes (2), cochleariform process (3), and facial nerve (4). (*B*) Following transcanal endoscopic tympanotomy, a fully dehiscent jugular bulb (1) is seen, with an eroded stapes (2), intact cochleariform process (3), bony covered tympanic facial nerve (4), and horizontal semicircular canal (5). EES enabled successful dissection of this complex pars tensa retraction pocket with preservation of the sac followed by cartilage graft tympanoplasty with stapes columella. A microscopic approach would have required a posterior canalplasty and postauricular incision to visualize these same structures.

otoendoscopy. The authors favor the 0° 2.7 mm by 11 cm rigid telescope for office otoendoscopy, and strongly recommend that the child is placed supine to ensure maximum stability of the head during the procedure, with the light cord and camera cord tucked under the patient's neck. The endoscope provides a panoramic view of the entire eardrum with enhanced depth of field compared with the microscope, with which, at high magnification, only a small portion of distal anatomy can be appreciated. Do not use an angled 30° or 45° endoscope in the clinic setting because this greatly increases the risk of contacting the bony EAC with the instruments and causing pain and bleeding. Office otoendoscopy is feasible in infants as young as 1.5 years old, based on the experience of the authors, but may not be possible in some children.

Specialized Instrumentation for Pediatric Endoscopic Ear Surgery

Because of the shorter EAC in children, a reported advantage with an endoscopic-assisted approach is a greater range of mobility that enhances both visualization and dissection of middle ear disease.[14] Owing to a more narrow canal in younger patients, however, a standard sinus scope (4-mm diameter, 18-cm length) may present significant limitations for transcanal EES. Pediatric sinus telescopes are generally 2.7 mm in diameter but the length (18-cm) makes them both fragile and unwieldy for routine use. Most endoscopic ear surgeons favor a 3 mm by 14 cm telescope (in 0° and 30°, 45° for advanced surgeons) for transcanal dissection in both children and adults (see **Fig. 2**). Importantly, most endoscopic cases can be performed exclusively with a 0° endoscope because the lens offers a wide field of view. In cases of disease that involve the retrotympanic, epitympanic, or protympanic recesses, a 30° telescope is needed to ensure gross total resection.

When beginning endoscopic ear surgery for TM perforation or a small attic cholesteatoma, standard otologic instrumentation is adequate (eg, Crabtree dissector [see **Fig. 4**] and straight Fraser tip suctions can be hand-bent to reach cholesteatoma in the epitympanum). Generous use of cotton balls or cottonoids soaked with concentrated epinephrine can be used topically for chemical vasoconstriction, as well as wicking of secretions during 1-handed surgery. For more experienced surgeons, specialized middle ear dissection instruments are now offered by several manufacturers. These include suction-dissectors to reduce the frustration of 1-handed ear surgery (especially during flap elevation, a great option for beginners), precurved suctions (up and down) of varying degrees with swivel connectors to reduce kinking of suction tubing, and right-angle curettes and dissectors of different lengths to reach disease when working with angled vision endoscopy (see **Fig. 4**).

Special attention is needed to ensure that the intensity of the xenon or light-emitting diode (LED) light source is kept to a minimum because the endoscope lens can rapidly warm the middle ear within 1 minute of use (when not using a suction dissector).[15] If possible, the lowest possible light intensity (50% or less) should be used to maximize image quality while avoiding potential thermal injury to outer, middle, and inner ear structures.[15] Suction rapidly cools the middle ear and the continued development of novel suction-dissectors is essential to ensure safe and prolonged endoscopic-assisted dissection.[15] McCallum and colleagues[16] have demonstrated that keeping the light intensity at 10% does not affect the image quality of the surgical field when using a Hopkins rod-lens telescope. New technologies incorporating distal chip technology offer excellent illumination with minimal radiant energy levels and may offer a safer alternative to EES.

Operating Room Set up, Ergonomics, and Right Versus Left Ear Surgery

The operating room setup for endoscopic ear surgery is important for both efficiency and surgeon's ergonomics (**Fig. 6**). Three common errors in surgeon posture are forward head position, improper shoulder elevation, and pelvic girdle asymmetry.[17] Heads-up surgery with endoscopes (and digital microscopes or exoscopes for mastoidectomy and lateral skull base surgery) overcome the inherent ergonomic limitations of traditional microscope-assisted dissection.[18] Successful transition from the microscope to transcanal endoscopic dissection includes (1) taking 1 or several hands-on dissection courses, (2) positioning the video monitor directly in front of the surgeon and at eye level, and (3) stabilization of both the camera hand and dissection hand (see **Fig. 6**). The operating room layout for EES necessitates clear communication and agreement with the surgical team before the patient is brought into the room. When starting endoscopic ear surgery, selecting a left-ear case for a right-hand dominant surgeon (or right ear case for a left hand dominant surgeon) is recommended. Right-handed surgeons will hold the scope in their nondominant left hand while performing dissection with the right. Rest the endoscope gently against the external auditory meatus posteroinferiorly to stabilize the video image.

Is There a Role for Endoscopic-Assisted Tympanostomy Tube Placement?

The binocular microscope is better-suited for routine and uncomplicated myringotomy and tympanostomy tube placement in children. Using an undraped microscope is more efficient and cost-effective than an endoscope because (1) a new sterile endoscope would be required for each case and (2) for bilateral tube placement, a boom-mounted video screen or 2 screens are needed to address both the left and right ears.

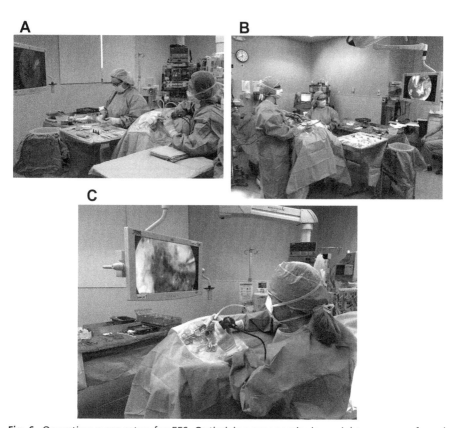

Fig. 6. Operating room setup for EES. Optimizing ergonomics is crucial to ensure safe and successful endoscopic ear dissection. Key elements for proper ergonomics while standing or sitting during EES include (1) stability of both hands and forearms using a Mayo stand or a chair with armrests, (2) video monitor should be as close to eye level as possible, and (3) surgical assistant should be positioned across from the surgeon and as close to the foot of the bed as possible to avoid blocking the video monitor. (A) Right ear, with surgeon sitting. (B) Left ear, with surgeon standing. A few surgeons perform EES while standing and the biggest advantage is greater maneuverability, which is an important factor when changing the vector of the surgical approach to reach complex middle ear disease. (C) Right ear, with surgeon sitting during transmastoid endoscopic portion of the procedure.

The authors reserve the use of the endoscope for myringotomy in specialized cases, such as a deep retraction pocket that has a depth that cannot be easily assessed with the otoscope or microscope or if there is concern for severe atelectasis. Endoscopes are also useful in children with small EACs. In children with trisomy 21, the EAC is narrow, often only accommodating a 2-mm speculum. This size constraint will complicate successful completion of a myringotomy and tube insertion. In these situations, a 3-mm or 2.7-mm rigid telescope positioned in the lateral bony EAC is often sufficient to visualize the posteroinferior TM and to complete tube placement.

Pediatric Endoscopic Tympanoplasty

In most children, a speculum or endaural-assisted transcanal microscopic approach is feasible for the repair of a posterior central perforation owing to the shorter length of the EAC. For anterior perforations with poorly defined margins based on otoscopic or microscopic examination, a postauricular incision is often needed. Because the endoscope provides an improved field of view of the anterior tympanic margin, a posterior skin incision and canalplasty are not necessary for a medial graft tympanoplasty. EES is ideal for uncomplicated cartilage graft myringoplasty in children with anterior perforations following tube extrusion (**Fig. 7**). Although infections and keloid formation of the skin incision are infrequent complications, families and children always welcome a less invasive approach, with minimal wound care issues and avoidance of a bulky mastoid dressing.

Several studies have examined the feasibility of endoscopic-assisted tympanoplasty and compared outcomes between endoscopic and microscopic cohorts in adults.[19,20] Similar studies in children are more limited but have shown similar results for rate of perforation closure.[14,21–24] In addition, endoscopic-assisted tympanoplasty is associated with similar postoperative hearing improvements compared with microscopic cases, but patients tend to be discharged earlier from the hospital following surgery.[6,21,22]

Graft Materials

The most common autologous graft material for tympanoplasty includes temporalis fascia, conchal or tragal cartilage, and perichondrium. From experience, the authors favor the use of cartilage and perichondrium. A cartilaginous graft offers a thicker, more stable graft with the added advantage of reducing the risk of TM retraction. In addition, when performing an exclusive endoscopic transcanal tympanoplasty, harvesting of cartilage and perichondrium from a tragal incision (or posterior conchal incision) offers a small and hidden incision compared with a postauricular incision to harvest temporalis fascia. Two main limitations of tragal cartilage harvest are (1) the tragus is not fully developed in very young children and so a large perforation may be difficult to close if the graft size is small and (2) aggressive harvesting of tragus without preservation of the rim is cosmetically unacceptable. If a sizable cartilage graft

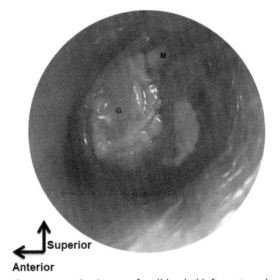

Superior

Anterior

Fig. 7. Otoendoscopic postoperative image of well-healed left ear tragal cartilage butterfly graft myringoplasty. This child had a chronic anterior central perforation not easily seen with the microscope following extrusion of a tympanostomy tube. A transcanal endoscopic approach is well-suited for the primary management of an anterior central perforation using a button or butterfly cartilage graft. G, cartilage graft; M, malleus.

is needed, a small incision along the posterior surface of the auricle overlying the conchal bowl provides access to a large surface area of perichondrium, as well as cartilage with an invisible scar.

Nonautologous grafts materials may be useful in revision surgery when there is insufficient fascia, perichondrium, or cartilage. Human cadaveric acellular dermal grafts, such as Alloderm (Life-Cell Corp, Bridgewater, NJ, USA) have been used for tympanoplasty with some success.[25,26] Newer engineered biological materials provide lower cost options for tympanoplasty with the advantage of avoiding cadaveric tissue. Extracellular collagen matrix derived acellular porcine small intestinal submucosa (SIS) (Biodesign; Cook Medical Inc., Bloomington, IN) has been used to repair tympanic perforations with reasonable outcomes.[27,28] This porcine-based graft retains the natural composition of matrix molecules such as collagen, glycosaminoglycans (hyaluronic acid, chondroitin sulfate A and B, heparin, and heparin sulfate), proteoglycans, and fibronectin. This technology has the advantage of providing a thin graft that, when moistened with water, retains more stiffness than a traditional fascia graft, and yet is soft and pliable when used during a medial graft tympanoplasty. Ideally, a small piece of autologous tissue (eg, split-thickness skin graft, perichondrium, or fascia should be used to cover the exposed collagen graft).

SURGICAL TECHNIQUES
Pediatric Endoscopic Cartilage Button or Butterfly Graft Myringoplasty

Endoscopic repair of small central pars tensa perforations using a myringoplasty technique is a reasonable initial surgical procedure to sharpen transcanal endoscopic dexterity and skills before advancing to more challenging EES cases (see **Fig. 7**). Tiny persistent perforations can be repaired with an earlobe fat graft, whereas larger central perforations can be repaired with a cartilage graft shaped with a circumferential rimming modeled as a spool or bobbin or butterfly.[29]

The technique for cartilage button myringoplasty varies. The cartilage graft must be larger than the perforation (at least 1–2 mm larger than the defect) and should be difficult to place because a graft that easily slips into the defect will fail and fall into the middle ear during the recovery phase. Cartilage can be harvested from the conchal bowl or tragus. A disposal dermal punch of appropriate diameter (usually 4–5 mm) is then used on the back table to create a circular graft and then this new graft is incised circumferentially under magnification with a tympanoplasty blade #6900 (Beaver -Visitec International, Waltham, MA) to create a button or butterfly shape. An overlying layer of perichondrium can be left attached as a tuft to the cartilage graft to provide an island of perichondrium as the cartilage graft is inserted within the edges of the perforation. The edges of the perforation are freshened with a sickle knife or a Rosen needle, and the butterfly graft is placed with an alligator and snapped into place with a pick or Rosen needle. The edges are checked to ensure good placement (see **Fig. 7**). Some surgeons place a small split-thickness skin graft over the exposed cartilage after placement, harvested from the posterior auricular skin.

Pediatric Endoscopic Tympanoplasty: Medial Versus Lateral Graft Techniques

Performing a medial versus a lateral graft (relative to the annular ligament) technique is primarily the surgeon's choice and depends on the location and size of the perforation, as well as the surgeon's preference and level of experience. The authors perform underlay tympanoplasty in most cases of central perforations. Usually, when the TM defect abuts the manubrium, a lateral-to-malleus underlay tympanoplasty with degloving of the malleus is preferred[30] (**Fig. 8**). The malleus supports medial

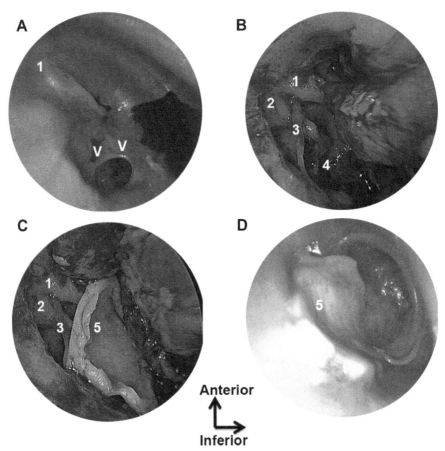

Fig. 8. Intraoperative right ear tragal cartilage graft tympanoplasty. (*A*) Posterior central perforation (*arrowheads*) at the bottom of a pars tensa retraction. 1, malleus. (*B*) Following tympanotomy, minimal erosion of distal incus observed. 1, malleus; 2, incus; 3, chorda tympani; 4, stapes. (*C*) Tragal cartilage graft with skirt of perichondrium (5) is positioned lateral to the malleus, and medial to defect. (*D*) Well healed postoperative result. The cartilage graft (5) is visible and well-integrated.

placement of the graft to reduce the risk of medial displacement or retraction. When repairing an anterior TM perforation, graft suspension over the manubrium facilitates improved contact of the graft to the anterior perforation margin. Dissection of the TM from the manubrium of the malleus can be performed with a sharp Rosen needle or the tip of a sickle knife, with extreme caution not to leave epithelial remnants attached to manubrium that can remain medial to the graft.

In larger perforations that directly involve the annulus (especially in complex revision cases) a lateral graft approach is favored. Because postoperative blunting of the anterior sulcus is a known complication of the overlay technique, a canalplasty is needed to increase the angle between the TM and medial bony EAC. In a transcanal endoscopic approach, this can be completed using a sharp bony curette or small microdrill, and does not have to be as aggressive as a traditional microscopic lateral graft tympanoplasty. Preliminary results suggest excellent closure rates with transcanal overlay repair that are comparable to larger microscopic series and that avoid a large postauricular incision.[31]

Pediatric Endoscopic Ossiculoplasty

The increased depth of field with endoscopic visualization is a distinct advantage over the microscope during ossiculoplasty. The surgeon can place the prosthesis with a clear view of the overlying graft laterally and the ossicular remnant medially for precise placement. One-handed placement of a partial ossicular replacement prosthesis (PORP) or a total ossicular replacement prosthesis (TORP) can be more challenging, however, and should not be performed except after gaining proficiency in basic transcanal dissection skills.

Ossiculoplasty is most often performed during primary or second-look surgery following removal of cholesteatoma or repair of retraction pocket (**Figs. 9** and **10**; see **Fig. 12**). For chronic ear disease involving an extensive infiltrative matrix cholesteatoma, the senior author favors staging the ossiculoplasty at the second-look and placing a cartilage graft stapes columella reconstruction, or performing an incus interposition if there was no matrix adherent to the stapes superstructure.

Currently, most middle ear prostheses are made of titanium, a material that has replaced plastipore for its decreased extrusion rate, lighter size, and thinner profile. Modern titanium PORPs have the ability to grab the stapes superstructure for greater stability (see **Fig. 10**), and TORPs have optional shoes to provide a larger footprint against the footplate, as well as greater degrees of freedom to pivot around a ball joint at the TORP-shoe interface (not shown). A hydroxyapatite incudostapedial joint prosthesis provides a bridge between an eroded incus and stapes, maintains a more physiologic lever mechanism, and restores conductive hearing loss, even in young children.[32] Bone cement can also be used to address erosion of the long process of incus associated with a retraction pocket or limited pars tensa cholesteatoma. All of these techniques can be completed using a transcanal endoscopic approach; the increased depth of field enables more precise placement and assessment of the position of the prosthesis or extent of repair.

Use of autologous incus as an interposition graft is an attractive option with almost no risk of extrusion, although displacement can occur over time. Results of autologous incus interposition grafts compared with nonautologous prostheses show comparable

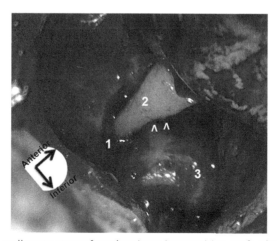

Fig. 9. Right ear, malleus-to-stapes footplate incus interposition graft. The diseased ossicles are removed. The incus has been refashioned with a blunt end to rest on the stapes footplate and a notched end to hold the manubrium of the malleus. 1, footplate; 2, incus; 3, cochlea.

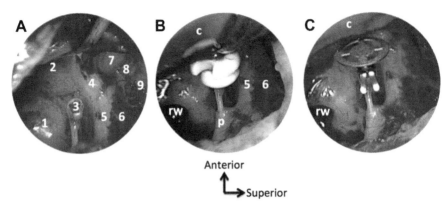

Fig. 10. Primary left ear endoscopic ossiculoplasty following resection of attic cholesteatoma. A 3-mm diameter 0° endoscope offers a superior depth of field (compared with binocular microscopy) for visualization of both the medial ossicular remnant (stapes superstructure), overlying cartilage graft, and the entire length of the prosthesis. (*A*) Following atticotomy, resection of attic cholesteatoma, removal of eroded incus, resection of malleus head, and transection of tensor tympani tendon are performed to facilitate medial graft placement. The 0° endoscope provides a panoramic view of the mesotympanic and epitympanic recesses and confirms gross total resection of disease. (*B*) Endoscopic placement of PORP sizer, confirming 2.0-mm height. (*C*) Appropriate position of titanium PORP with specialized fingers that articulate around the capitulum, crurae, and stapedial tendon. 1, cochlea; 2, Eustachian tube; 3, stapes; 4, cochleariform process; 5, tympanic facial nerve; 6, horizontal semicircular canal; 7, supratubal recess; 8, cog; 9, tegmen tympani; rw, round window; c, cartilage graft; p, pyramidal process.

results for hearing gain.[33,34] The second author favors the utilization of autologous incus for ossicular reconstruction over a titanium prosthesis if (1) the incus remnant is robust and (2) there is a close relationship of the manubrium to stapes capitulum or footplate (to reduce the risk of displacement). In the case of the presence of an intact stapes, the incus is sculpted with a notch to articulate with the stapes capitulum and a shorter notched arm placed under the manubrium (see **Fig. 12**). If the stapes is missing, the incus is sculpted as a club with a small flat end to rest over the footplate and a distal broader notched end to cradle the manubrium (see **Fig. 9**).

One initial perceived disadvantage of using the incus as an interposition graft is the added time required to prepare the graft and the need for high magnification to complete this task. When performing middle ear surgery through an exclusive transcanal endoscopic approach, this may require the draping of an operative microscope that can add cost and time to the surgical procedure. One can use surgical loupes and a battery-powered microdrill to shape the remnant incus with reasonable time and cost containment. Hovering the endoscope to provide magnification and light during incus sculpting is not useful. Being able to place and position a middle ear prosthesis or a sculpted incus interposition graft with a single hand endoscopically may be perceived as challenging initially; however, with experience, this is an acquirable skill.[35,36]

Cholesteatoma Surgery

Cholesteatoma in children is considered an aggressive disease with higher recidivism compared with chronic ear disease in adults, more often involves the pars tensa than the pars flaccida region of the TM, and can spread to the retrotympanic recess. Several studies have demonstrated that the addition of endoscopes during cholesteatoma surgery significantly reduces the rate of recidivism.[37,38] When disease is limited to the tympanic cavity and does not extend past the horizontal canal, a transcanal endoscopic resection is feasible.

For more advanced cholesteatoma that involves the aditus ad antrum and antrum, the endoscope is a powerful tool that enables transmastoid visualization of residual disease in the aditus ad antrum and epitympanum (not reachable transcanal) (see **Fig. 1**). An aggressive canal wall up or canal wall down mastoidectomy can be avoided when using a 30° endoscope and a curved #3 or #5 suction to debride matrix not accessible from the transcanal approach.

Congenital cholesteatoma is ideally suited for transcanal EES. Early disease is often limited to the anterosuperior (stage 1) quadrant of the tympanic cavity (**Fig. 11**). Transcanal endoscopic gross total resection of congenital cholesteatoma is feasible in most cases, with preservation of the ossicular chain and no bone removal needed (see **Fig. 11**). Following resection, a 30° endoscope provides an excellent view of the supratubal recess and protympanum to detect residual matrix. When congenital cholesteatoma involves the ossicular chain (stages 2–4) (**Fig. 12**), the tensor tympani tendon and cochleariform process are often affected. These are areas of great challenge in dissection because matrix is often found wrapped around the tensor tympani tendon and in close proximity to the geniculate ganglion. When cholesteatoma involves the mastoid, a combined approach is necessary and can be significantly assisted with a transmastoid endoscopic survey to avoid the need for a canal wall down procedure (see **Fig. 1**). Outcome studies on congenital cholesteatoma confined to the middle ear and treated surgically with EES report a residual rate of 8.3%.[7] This compares favorably with traditional microscopic techniques, which range from 10.5% to 45.5%.[39]

When removal of noninfiltrative matrix cholesteatoma requires removal of the eroded ossicular chain, an ossiculoplasty using an incus interposition is a reasonable option at the time of primary resection, followed by reconstruction of the pars tensa and the attic defect with cartilage (see **Fig. 12**). For highly infiltrative matrix cholesteatoma, the incus can be banked in the attic or posterior EAC and used as an interposition graft at second-look surgery. Second-look surgery is reserved for more aggressive cases with disease extending to the mastoid or to regions that harbor a high risk of residual disease (eg, cochleariform process and tensor tympani tendon).

Cholesteatoma limited to the tympanic cavity and without infiltrative matrix can be followed closely with serial examinations, CT imaging, and/or diffusion-weighted MRI to assess for residual or recurrent disease.

Pediatric Stapes Fixation

Microscopic or endoscopic-assisted stapes surgery in children should not be performed except by experienced surgeons with a substantial stapedectomy practice. Most specialists will delay discussion of stapedectomy in children until adolescence or older to receive assent from the child, in addition to formal consent from the parents, due to the risk of sensorineural hearing loss with surgery. Increasingly, with the concept of amblyaudia and a greater awareness of the long-term impact of uncorrected, reversible unilateral hearing loss in children, the option of surgical repair is being discussed at younger ages.[40] Pediatric stapes surgery has been shown to be safe and effective and comparable to most adult series.[40-46] A conservative approach, however, is best when reviewing options for elective repair of a condition that could result in profound hearing loss, a small but known risk that may be higher in children than in adults.[43] In addition, congenital ossicular fixation based on hearing testing may be associated with greater abnormalities of the malleus and incus,[44] and so a careful

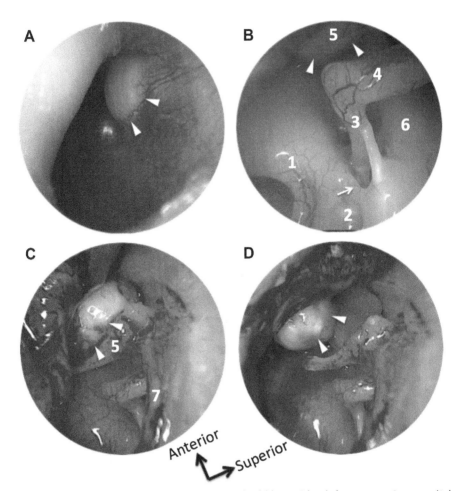

Fig. 11. Intraoperative images from an 18-month-old boy with a left ear stage 1 congenital cholesteatoma (*arrowheads*). Transcanal endoscopic resection is an ideal technique for gross total resection of congenital cholesteatoma (especially stages 1–3) and does not require a postauricular incision except in stage 4 cases in which disease has extended into the mastoid. (*A*) White mass seen in the anterosuperior quadrant of the mesotympanum, and abutting the malleus. (*B*) Following transcanal tympanotomy, the mass is barely visible and is anterior and medial to the malleus. Arrow points to the ponticulus. (*C*) Degloving of the malleus reveals a cholesteatoma abutting the anterior border of the manubrium and undersurface of the TM. (*D*) Fully degloving the manubrium and umbo enables access to the entire cholesteatoma, which is mobilized and removed. 1, cochlea; 2, sinus tympani; 3, stapes; 4, incus; 5, malleus; 6, tympanic facial nerve; 7, chorda tympani.

review of imaging is imperative. A child with Crouzon, Treacher Collins, Pierre Robin, Apert, or other syndrome will be at greater risk for ossicular head fixation rather than isolated stapes fixation,[45] complicating stapes surgery and favoring bone conduction amplification over middle ear surgery.

Endoscopic stapes surgery should not be attempted (aside from flap elevation and completion of tympanotomy) until there is significant experience performing endoscopic chronic ear surgery. The 2 most consistent fallacies mentioned by EES course participants are (1) endoscopic stapedectomy is easier than

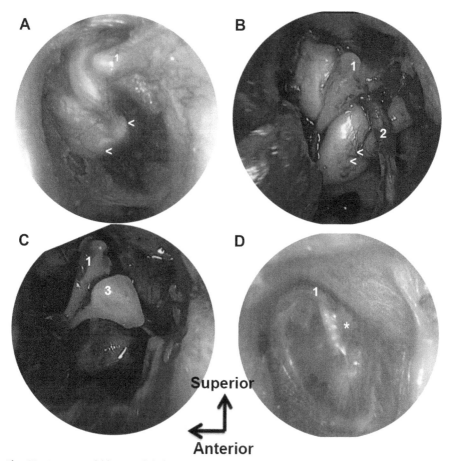

Fig. 12. A 7-year-old boy with left ear congenital cholesteatoma involving the upper meso-tympanum and ossicular chain (stage 2), intraoperatively. (*A*) White mass in anterosuperior mesotympanum (*arrowheads*) with extension posteriorly past the manubrium (1). (*B*) On tympanotomy and degloving of malleus, cholesteatomata (*arrowheads*) are found wedged between the malleus (1) and an eroded incus, engulfing the chorda tympani nerve (2). (*C*) Following resection of cholesteatoma, an incus interposition graft (3) is fashioned and placed between the manubrium (1) and stapes capitulum. (*D*) Postoperative otoendoscopy demonstrates a stable incus interposition graft (*asterisk*) cradling the malleus (1) and well-integrated with the TM.

microscopic stapes surgery and (2) endoscopic stapedectomy does not require scutum removal due to improved visualization of the ossicular chain. Nothing could be further from the truth. First, all surgeons today were trained using microscopic techniques to perform stapes surgery, and all otologic instruments and lasers and prostheses were designed for line-of-sight, microscope-assisted transcanal procedures. Second, 90% of endoscopic stapes surgery necessitates generous curetting of the scutum unless the chorda tympani is sacrificed, resulting in higher rates of dysgeusia. Safe navigation around an intact chorda tympani requires generous bone removal to work below AND above the nerve to access the entire footplate. A straight pick is the best instrument to use to determine whether adequate access to the entire stapes and footplate are possible (**Fig. 13**).

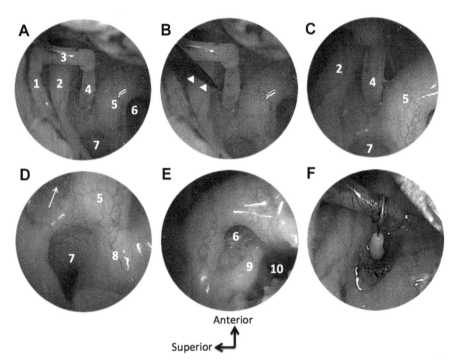

Anterior

Superior

Fig. 13. Intraoperative photos from a 10 year old with right ear conductive hearing loss. This child had normal tympanometry and absent acoustic reflexes, suggesting ossicular fixation and grossly normal CT. (*A*) Right transcanal tympanotomy revealed isolated stapes fixation with a rare congenital absence of the stapedial tendon and pyramidal process, not clearly noted on imaging (0°, 3-mm diameter endoscope, held with right hand). (*B*) Straight pick (*arrowheads*) is essential to assess surgical access to footplate (the endoscope provides a wide-angle view but all otologic instruments are designed for line-of-sight). Unlike this patient, however, most endoscopic stapes cases require curetting of scutum for adequate access to the entire footplate. (*C*) A 30°endoscopic view of the oval window niche showing a prominent but otherwise normal stapes superstructure. (*D*) A 30° endoscopic view rotated posteriorly toward the retrotympanum or sinus tympani. There is no ponticulus because there is congenital absence of the pyramidal eminence. (*E*) A 30° endoscopic view, rotated superiorly, toward the round window niche. (*F*) Following carbon-dioxide (CO_2) laser small fenestra stapedotomy and placement of nitinol alloy piston prosthesis. Due to the complexity and elective nature of these cases, pediatric endoscopic stapes surgery should only be performed by experienced surgeons. 1, chorda tympani; 2, facial nerve; 3, incus; 4, stapes; 5, cochlear promontory; 6, round window niche; 7, sinus tympani; 8, subiculum; 9, fustis; 10, subcochlear canaliculus. Arrow: stapes footplate.

What is the rationale for endoscopic stapes surgery in children? For the experienced surgeon there are several:

1. Superior visualization of the entire ossicular chain to rule out malleus and/or incus fixation; to exclude the presence (and document for patient and family) the more subtle findings in pediatric ossicular fixation, such as a bony bar between the incus and tympanic nerve, or ossification of the stapedial tendon; and to accurately assess the round window reflex to confirm fixation and exclude a third window from superior canal dehiscence or large vestibular aqueduct[46]
2. Endoscopic visualization of the anterior crus, in some cases

3. A more accurate measurement of the height between the footplate and incus due to enhanced depth of field with the endoscope
4. Teaching the steps of stapes surgery to residents and fellows can be done with greater fidelity: visualization of the flap elevation, identification of individual land-marks, and surgical technique is more easily conveyed during heads-up high-defi-nition video-assisted endoscopic ear surgery.

Future Directions in EES

1. Prospective studies of quality of life measures to quantify benefits of endoscopic ear surgery over traditional approaches in children
2. Refinements in suction dissectors, curved suctions, and angled dissectors to lower barriers to adoption, enhance patient safety, and improve outcomes in pe-diatric EES
3. Task-driven 3D-printed temporal bones with conformable left and right ear pinna, and realistic EAC morphology and middle ear anatomy to resemble children younger than 5 years of age will be critical for skills training of pediatric otologists (temporal bone courses have adult specimens)
4. Next-generation distal chip technology with smaller scope diameters and light-weight designs will offer a greater degree of visualization while providing more de-grees of freedom with dissection instruments; this innovation will have its greatest impact in the pediatric population
5. Microrobotic technology with steerable suction, dissector, and distal chip camera or light source for 2-handed pediatric middle ear surgery.

SUMMARY

Endoscopic ear surgery is ideally suited for the management of routine and complex middle ear disease in children. A graduated approach to ensure patient safety is essential when incorporating the endoscope into a pediatric otology practice for tym-panoplasty, cholesteatoma, and ossiculoplasty. The rigid endoscope enables a minimally invasive transcanal approach and can often spare the child a postauricular incision when disease involves the middle ear and not the mastoid. In advanced cases of cholesteatoma, a transmastoid endoscopic-assisted debridement of residual dis-ease with curved suctions can help avoid a canal wall down mastoidectomy. Finally, stapes surgery in children should only be performed by surgeons with an extensive stapes surgery practice. The microscope should be used for safe and efficient completion of a pediatric stapedectomy until the surgeon gains considerable exper-tise with endoscopic management of complex chronic ear disease.

REFERENCES

1. Thomassin JM, Inedjian JM, Rud C, et al. Otoendoscopy: application in the mid-dle ear surgery. Rev Laryngol Otol Rhinol (Bord) 1990;111(5):475–7 [in French].
2. Tarabichi M. Endoscopic middle ear surgery. Ann Otol Rhinol Laryngol 1999; 108(1):39–46.
3. Thomassin JM, Korchia D, Duchon Doris JM. Endoscopic-guided otosurgery in the prevention of residual cholesteatomas. Laryngoscope 1993;103(8):939.
4. Poe DS, Rebeiz EE, Pankratov MM, et al. Transtympanic endoscopy of the middle ear. Laryngoscope 1992;102(9):993–6.
5. Dahm MC, Shepherd RK, Clark GM. The postnatal growth of the temporal bone and its implications for cochlear implantation in children. Acta Otolaryngol Suppl 1993;505:1–39.

6. Ito T, Kubota T, Watanabe T, et al. Transcanal endoscopic ear surgery for pediatric population with a narrow external auditory canal. Int J Pediatr Otorhinolaryngol 2015;79(12):2265–9.

7. Kobayashi T, Gyo K, Komori M, et al. Efficacy and safety of transcanal endoscopic ear surgery for congenital cholesteatomas: a preliminary report. Otol Neurotol 2015;36(10):1644–50.

8. Isaacson G. Endoscopic anatomy of the pediatric middle ear. Otolaryngol Head Neck Surg 2014;150(1):6–15.

9. Keefe DH, Bulen JC, Arehart KH, et al. Ear-canal impedance and reflection coefficient in human infants and adults. J Acoust Soc Am 1993;94(5):2617–38.

10. Sun WH, Kuo CL, Huang TC. The anatomic applicability of transcanal endoscopic ear surgery in children. Int J Pediatr Otorhinolaryngol 2018;105:118–22.

11. Ikui A, Sando I, Sudo M, et al. Postnatal change in angle between the tympanic annulus and surrounding structures. Computer-aided three-dimensional reconstruction study. Ann Otol Rhinol Laryngol 1997;106(1):33–6.

12. Ikui A, Sando I, Haginomori S, et al. Postnatal development of the tympanic cavity: a computer-aided reconstruction and measurement study. Acta Otolaryngol 2000;120(3):375–9.

13. Yoon TH, Schachern PA, Paparella MM, et al. Pathology and pathogenesis of tympanic membrane retraction. Am J Otolaryngol 1990;11(1):10–7.

14. James AL. Endoscopic middle ear surgery in children. Otolaryngol Clin North Am 2013;46(2):233–44.

15. Kozin E, Lee D. Staying safe during endoscopic ear surgery. ENT Audiol News 2016;25(2):1–4.

16. McCallum R, McColl J, Iyer A. The effect of light intensity on image quality in endoscopic ear surgery. Clin Otolaryngol 2018;43(5):1266–72.

17. Rosenblatt P, McKinney J, Adams S. Ergonomics in the operating room: protecting the surgeon. J Minim Invasive Gynecol 2013;20(6).

18. Smith S, Kozin ED, Kanumuri VV, et al. Initial experience with 3-dimensional exoscope-assisted transmastoid and lateral skull base surgery. Otolaryngol Head Neck Surg 2019;160(2):364–7.

19. Choi N, Noh Y, Park W, et al. Comparison of endoscopic tympanoplasty to microscopic tympanoplasty. Clin Exp Otorhinolaryngol 2017;10(1):44–9.

20. Lade H, Choudhary SR, Vashishth A. Endoscopic vs microscopic myringoplasty: a different perspective. Eur Arch Otorhinolaryngol 2014;271(7):1897–902.

21. James AL. Endoscope or microscope-guided pediatric tympanoplasty? Comparison of grafting technique and outcome. Laryngoscope 2017;127(11):2659–64.

22. Nassif N, Berlucchi M, Redaelli de Zinis LO. Tympanic membrane perforation in children: endoscopic type I tympanoplasty, a newly technique, is it worthwhile? Int J Pediatr Otorhinolaryngol 2015;79(11):1860–4.

23. Cohen MS, Landegger LD, Kozin ED, et al. Pediatric endoscopic ear surgery in clinical practice: lessons learned and early outcomes. Laryngoscope 2016; 126(3):732–8.

24. Dündar R, Kulduk E, Soy FK, et al. Endoscopic versus microscopic approach to type 1 tympanoplasty in children. Int J Pediatr Otorhinolaryngol 2014;78(7):1084–9.

25. Lai P, Propst EJ, Papsin BC. Lateral graft type 1 tympanoplasty using AlloDerm for tympanic membrane reconstruction in children. Int J Pediatr Otorhinolaryngol 2006;70(8):1423–9.

26. Vos JD, Latev MD, Labadie RF, et al. Use of AlloDerm in type I tympanoplasty: a comparison with native tissue grafts. Laryngoscope 2005;115(9):1599–602.

27. Basonbul RA, Cohen MS. Use of porcine small intestinal submucosa for pediatric endoscopic tympanic membrane repair. World J Otorhinolaryngol Head Neck Surg 2017;3(3):142–7.
28. D'Eredità R. Porcine small intestinal submucosa (SIS) myringoplasty in children: a randomized controlled study. Int J Pediatr Otorhinolaryngol 2015;79(7):1085–9.
29. Eavey RD. Inlay tympanoplasty: cartilage butterfly technique. Laryngoscope 1998;108(5):657–61.
30. Yawn RJ, Carlson ML, Haynes DS, et al. Lateral-to-malleus underlay tympanoplasty: surgical technique and outcomes. Otol Neurotol 2014;35(10):1809–12.
31. Creighton FX, Kozin E, Rong A, et al. Outcomes following transcanal endoscopic lateral graft tympanoplasty. Otology and Neurotology, in press.
32. Schwetschenau EL, Isaacson G. Ossiculoplasty in young children with the Applebaum incudostapedial joint prosthesis. Laryngoscope 1999;109(10):1621–5.
33. O'Reilly RC, Cass SP, Hirsch BE, et al. Ossiculoplasty using incus interposition: hearing results and analysis of the middle ear risk index. Otol Neurotol 2005;26(5):853–8.
34. Amith N, Rs M. Autologous incus versus titanium partial ossicular replacement prosthesis in reconstruction of Austin type A ossicular defects: a prospective randomised clinical trial. J Laryngol Otol 2017;131(5):391–8.
35. Yawn RJ, Hunter JB, O'Connell BP, et al. Audiometric outcomes following endoscopic ossicular chain reconstruction. Otol Neurotol 2017;38(9):1296–300.
36. Kakehata S, Futai K, Sasaki A, et al. Endoscopic transtympanic tympanoplasty in the treatment of conductive hearing loss: early results. Otol Neurotol 2006;27(1):14–9.
37. Hunter JB, Zuniga MG, Sweeney AD, et al. Pediatric endoscopic cholesteatoma surgery. Otolaryngol Head Neck Surg 2016;154(6):1121–7.
38. Ghadersohi S, Carter JM, Hoff SR. Endoscopic transcanal approach to the middle ear for management of pediatric cholesteatoma. Laryngoscope 2017;127(11):2653–8.
39. Chen JM, Schloss MD, Manoukian JJ, et al. Congenital cholesteatoma of the middle ear in children. J Otolaryngol 1989;18(1):44–8.
40. Kaplan AB, Kozin ED, Remenschneider A, et al. Amblyaudia: review of pathophysiology, clinical presentation, and treatment of a new diagnosis. Otolaryngol Head Neck Surg 2016;154(2):247–55.
41. Vincent R, Wegner I, Vonck BM, et al. Primary stapedotomy in children with otosclerosis: a prospective study of 41 consecutive cases. Laryngoscope 2016;126(2):442–6.
42. Lippy WH, Burkey JM, Schuring AG, et al. Short- and long-term results of stapedectomy in children. Laryngoscope 1998;108(4 Pt 1):569–72.
43. Neilan RE, Zhang RW, Roland PS, et al. Pediatric stapedectomy: does cause of fixation affect outcomes? Int J Pediatr Otorhinolaryngol 2013;77(7):1099–102.
44. De la Cruz A, Angeli S, Slattery WH. Stapedectomy in children. Otolaryngol Head Neck Surg 1999;120(4):487–92.
45. Markou K, Stavrakas M, Karkos P, et al. Juvenile otosclerosis: a case presentation and review of the literature. BMJ Case Rep 2016;2016. https://doi.org/10.1136/bcr-1110.11362015.
46. Merchant SN, Nakajima HH, Halpin C, et al. Clinical investigation and mechanism of air-bone gaps in large vestibular aqueduct syndrome. Ann Otol Rhinol Laryngol 2007;116(7):532–41.

Advances in Management of Pediatric Sensorineural Hearing Loss

C. Carrie Liu, MD, MPH[a], Samantha Anne, MD, MS[b,*],
David L. Horn, MD, MS[a]

KEYWORDS

- Sensorineural hearing loss • Cochlear implant • Bone conduction sound processor
- Auditory brainstem implant

KEY POINTS

- The work-up of children with sensorineural hearing loss has evolved, with genetic and cytomegalovirus testing becoming increasingly available.
- Congenital infections account for half of nongenetic hearing loss, with the most prevalent currently being cytomegalovirus.
- Genetic testing should be considered in children with hearing loss of unknown cause.
- Aural rehabilitation should be offered to children in a timely manner.
- At present, the main surgical options for the management of sensorineural hearing loss are bone conduction sound processors and cochlear implants.

INTRODUCTION

Over the past 30 years, there has been a steady growth in understanding of the causes and optimal management of sensorineural hearing loss (SNHL) in children. With the rapid introduction and refinement of devices for aural rehabilitation and more precise, cost-effective methods to determine causes, it would be beneficial to have an evidence-based investigative algorithm and keep abreast of the evidence for management of these patients. This article reviews the recent advances in medical evaluation and surgical management of children presenting with SNHL, with a focus on the expanded indications for cochlear implants and bone conduction sound processors.

Disclosures: The authors do not have any commercial or financial conflicts of interest to declare.
[a] Pediatric Otolaryngology – Head and Neck Surgery, Seattle Children's Hospital, 4800 Sand Point Way NE, OA9.329, Seattle, WA 98105, USA; [b] Department of Otolaryngology–Head and Neck Surgery, Otolaryngology, Head & Neck Institute, The Cleveland Clinic, 9500 Euclid Avenue A71, Cleveland, OH 44195, USA
* Corresponding author.
E-mail address: annes@ccf.org

Otolaryngol Clin N Am 52 (2019) 847–861
https://doi.org/10.1016/j.otc.2019.05.004
0030-6665/19/© 2019 Elsevier Inc. All rights reserved.

MEDICAL EVALUATION OF CHILDREN PRESENTING WITH SENSORINEURAL HEARING LOSS

SNHL occurs in 0.2% to 0.4% of infants.[1] The goals of medical evaluation are to identify the cause of hearing loss with possible associated syndromes and medical conditions, to estimate speech and language outcomes, and to offer appropriate aural rehabilitation in order to optimize communication and language development.

Advances in Genetic Hearing Loss Work-up

Genetic testing should be considered in children with hearing loss of unknown cause. Among causal testing options, genetic testing has the highest yield, with the identification of a genetic cause in 44% of patients with bilateral SNHL.[2] Children presenting with asymmetric or unilateral SNHL can also have genetic causes, with diagnostic yields of 22% and 1% on genetic testing, respectively.[2] Identifying a genetic cause is important in the prognostication of hearing loss and language development as well as in the choice of management. For example, children with Usher syndrome may benefit from cochlear implantation because loss of vision renders patients reliant on braille and/or verbal communication.[3] Identifying an underlying genetic cause also provides guidance for additional investigations; children with Usher syndrome require ophthalmologic assessments given the association with retinitis pigmentosa, and those with Jervell and Lange-Nielsen syndrome need cardiac assessment and intervention because they may benefit from an implanted cardioverter-defibrillator.

Comprehensive genetic testing has been more accessible and attainable since the advent of new genetic testing platforms based on massively parallel sequencing (MPS) in 2010. MPS allows the sequencing of billions of DNA base pairs simultaneously, which is helpful with diagnosis of SNHL because it allows the sequencing of all known deafness genes simultaneously.[4] Options also exist for more targeted testing in which a particular syndrome or genetic cause is strongly suggested by patient and family history, such as testing for SLC26A4 mutations in Pendred syndrome. In addition, comprehensive genetic testing for deafness has recently been able to be completed on fresh and archived dried blood spots.[5] Dried blood spots are retained for years and this allows further testing at a later time if needed.

Referral for genetic counseling and/or medical genetics should be considered. First, patients and families should be informed of the ethical and social issues related to genetic testing, including the psychological impact of obtaining a genetic diagnosis, the implications for family members, and the potential for discrimination relating to employment and insurance.[6] Second, patients and families should be prepared for the possibility of uncertain findings. Specifically, genetic testing may not identify a causal mutation, or it may identify mutations of unknown significance. Further, the failure of genetic testing to identify an causal mutation does not rule out the presence of a genetic basis for SNHL; certain mutations can also be associated with both syndromic and nonsyndromic phenotypes. In the setting of uncertain results, follow-up is recommended because features related to certain mutations may only be apparent as the child grows, at which point additional testing may be indicated.[7] Follow-up is also recommended because medical advances may make additional genetic tests available for further causal work-up.

Nongenetic Hearing Loss Work-up

Half of nongenetic hearing loss cases occur as a result of fetal exposure to infectious diseases.[8] Specifically, TORCHES (toxoplasmosis, rubella, cytomegalovirus [CMV], herpes, and syphilis) infections are risk factors for congenital SNHL.[9] In addition to hearing loss, these infections are associated with other neurologic and ophthalmologic sequelae; therefore, recognition is important for both treatment and counseling. As congenital toxoplasmosis, rubella, herpes, and syphilis have decreased in incidence, congenital CMV infection has emerged as the most prevalent infectious cause of congenital SNHL.[10]

CMV infection is estimated to occur in 0.7% of newborn infants in the United States.[11] Historical methods of CMV detection predominantly used viral culture techniques,[12] including shell vial urine culture, which was the gold standard for many years. At present, methods for CMV diagnosis include polymerase chain reaction (PCR) on urine, saliva, blood, or cerebrospinal fluid (CSF) samples. Postnatal infections are common given the ubiquity of this virus; therefore, the accepted diagnostic window of a congenital infection is 21 days.[13] The identification of congenital infection is important in hearing prognosis, because postnatal CMV acquisition is not associated with SNHL.[14] Outside the 21-day time window, dried blood spot testing has been investigated as a method of retrospectively diagnosing congenital CMV (cCMV) infection. However, the sensitivity of dried blood spot testing ranges from 28.3% using a single-primer PCR assay to 34.4% using a 2-primer assay, with a specificity of 99.9%.[15] Given the poor sensitivity, dried blood spot real-time PCR is not recommended as a primary test to diagnose or screen for CMV. Instead, it is useful in the work-up of children who present with SNHL. However, because of the poor sensitivity, a negative result does not rule out cCMV as the cause.

Even if detected, the treatment of children with isolated SNHL is unclear. In a valganciclovir trial on children with symptomatic cCMV that included children who had SNHL as the sole presenting symptom, only 1 child was enrolled that met this criteria; therefore, no meaningful conclusion could be made regarding the role of antiviral treatment in this population.[16] The consensus recommendations for prevention, diagnosis, and treatment of cCMV published in 2017 states that "antiviral therapy is not routinely recommended for cCMV infection with isolated SNHL and otherwise asymptomatic."[13] However, the most recent study, published in 2018, was a retrospective review showing that valganciclovir is beneficial in these children.[17] Specifically, in the series reported by Pasternak and colleagues,[17] 76% of children with bilateral SNHL experienced improved hearing after receiving long-term antiviral therapy. Overall, antiviral treatment in children with isolated SNHL, as well as initiating treatment beyond 1 month of life, are areas of ongoing investigation.[13] At present, treatment of these children should be determined on a case-by-case basis and referral to an infectious disease specialist is recommended to review the risks and benefits of antiviral therapy.

Imaging

The goals of imaging are to identify anatomic causes of hearing loss, assess for candidacy for surgical intervention, and assess for surgical planning. Computed tomography (CT) and MRI are the main imaging modalities used in children with hearing loss.

The diagnostic yield of CT and MRI is associated with the symmetry and severity of the hearing loss.[18,19] A recent retrospective cohort study of children who had undergone imaging for SNHL found an overall diagnostic yield of 34% for MRI and 20% for CT.[18] In their cohort, 52% of children with asymmetric SNHL and 30% with symmetric SNHL had a causative abnormality on imaging. Children with more severe SNHL were also more likely to have an abnormality on imaging. In addition, MRI had a significantly higher diagnostic yield, identifying abnormalities in 14% of children who had normal CT findings. In a similar retrospective study of children with unilateral SNHL, abnormalities were found in 43% and 37% of children who underwent MRI and CT, respectively,[19] although the difference was not statistically significant.

Two systematic reviews have been published that evaluate the overall diagnostic yields of CT and MRI in pediatric hearing loss.[20,21] The pooled diagnostic yield of CT scans was 30%; therefore, the number of patients needed to be imaged to yield 1 diagnosis is 4.[20] Compared with MRI, CT scans have a higher yield in identifying enlarged vestibular aqueducts and cochlear anomalies.[21] It seems that MRI is preferable to evaluate the cochlear nerve and brain; however, the results were not significant.[21] There is no clear answer to which test is superior for any specific diagnosis of hearing loss. Choice of imaging should include consideration of suspected cause and discussion with family regarding the exposure to radiation, possible need for sedation, and the diagnostic yield of each study.

Additional Investigations

Additional testing should be based on medical and family history, clinical examination findings, imaging results, and audiometric results. A so-called shotgun approach for all patients has been shown to have extremely low diagnostic yield.[22] Electrocardiogram should be considered to rule out Jervell and Lange-Nielsen syndrome, seen in approximately 4% of children with profound SNHL, particularly for children with bilateral profound hearing loss or family history of childhood arrhythmia or sudden death of unknown cause.[23] Ophthalmology referrals should be made for all children with SNHL.[24] First, ophthalmologic disorder is common in syndromic causes of SNHL.[25,26] Second, children with hearing loss should have early diagnosis and intervention for possible vision impairment, to optimize other means of communication.

Auditory Rehabilitation

The Joint Committee on Infant Hearing recommends hearing screening by 1 month of age, definitive diagnosis of hearing loss by 3 months of age in those who fail their newborn screen, and early intervention by 6 months of age in those who are diagnosed with hearing loss.[9] Early interventions, including hearing aid fitting, is important in children with bilateral hearing loss.[9] Children with unaided bilateral hearing loss, from mild to profound, are known to have significant language and academic delays.[27] If amplification is provided before 6 months of age, children can experience improved language development compared with children who are diagnosed and treated after 6 months of age.[27,28] Similarly, children who receive early cochlear implantation are more likely to undergo speech and language development that are comparable with their normal-hearing peers.[29]

Although the need for intervention in bilateral SNHL is accepted, the need for timely amplification of unilateral hearing loss (UHL) was not emphasized until recent years.[30] It is now established that children with UHL have lower oral language scores, are more likely to show behavioral issues in the classroom, and are more likely to require academic assistance.[30,31] In a recent systematic review, most of the included studies showed worsened speech and language scores and skills in children with UHL, especially in those with profound UHL.[32] Treatment of UHL is designed to either amplify the affected ear when feasible or to maximize the ability to hear in noise. Interventions designed to improve hearing in noise include preferential seating, frequency-modulating (FM) systems, bone conduction sound processors, and contralateral routing of sound (CROS) aids. Appachi and colleagues[33] performed a systematic review that examined the audiologic outcomes of various aural rehabilitation methods for UHL. Conventional hearing aids and FM systems are likely of benefit, especially for hearing in noise. Two studies examined CROS aids and their findings were variable. Studies examining the use of implanted bone conduction hearing devices showed a consistent benefit in audiologic outcomes, including pure tone average (PTA), speech reception threshold, and hearing in noise. More recently, cochlear implants have also been explored as an option for unilateral SNHL; this is discussed later.

BONE CONDUCTION SOUND PROCESSORS
Indications

Since their commercial introduction in 1987, osseointegrated implants have become a common treatment option for patients with conductive hearing loss who cannot be fitted with conventional hearing aids, as well as for single-sided deafness (SSD).[34] They represent an improvement compared with historical bone conduction hearing aids given the direct transduction of sound to the skull via the osseointegrated implant. Specific indications include patients with chronic otitis media or externa, congenital ear anomalies, and allergic reactions to standard hearing aids.[35]

Surgical Considerations

Numerous skin incisions and flaps have been described for osseointegrated implants, each with its own advantages and disadvantages.[36–38] Most of the techniques involve creating skin flaps and subsequently thinning them to allow the abutment to reach the skin surface. Over the past decade, longer abutments have been introduced, thereby decreasing the need to thin the subcutaneous tissue. In 2013, Wilson and Kim[39] introduced a minimally invasive technique whereby a biopsy punch is used to excise the skin and underlying tissues, with placement of the implant through this opening. This technique removes the need for a skin flap and may decrease the rates of soft tissue complications.

A meta-analysis by Kiringoda and Lustig[40] found that the most common complications seen in children are soft tissue reactions (77.8%), implant infection (5.6%–44.4%), soft tissue overgrowth of the abutment (10%–22.2%), failure of osseointegration (0%–14.3%), need for revision surgery (0%–44.4%), and loss of the implant (0%–25%). A complication that has only been reported in the pediatric population is overgrowth of bone at the abutment site, which occurs in 3.6% to 14.8% of children. The most common indications for revision surgery are soft tissue overgrowth, implant loss, and recurrent infections. The complication rates associated with bone conduction hearing aid implantation are comparable between children and adults.[33]

Transcutaneous bone conduction sound processor systems were introduced in 2013.[41] In these systems, an osseointegrated implant vibrates either passively via transcutaneous magnetic connection[41,42] or actively via a vibratory element in the implant itself.[43] The proposed benefit of the active system is that the vibratory energy originates at the implant and directly onto bone, thereby circumventing the soft tissue attenuation that can be seen with the passive systems.[44–46] For the passive systems, a skin flap is raised to facilitate placement of the implant; the flap is then placed back over the magnet and the sound processor is fitted transcutaneously opposite the magnet once healing has occurred. The active system is placed most commonly via a mastoidectomy.[45] In patients with insufficient space in the mastoid, the implant may also be placed via a retrosigmoid or middle cranial fossa approach.[45] In the absence of a percutaneous abutment, the transcutaneous systems have been found to carry a lower risk of postoperative soft tissue complications compared with percutaneous implant systems.[47] At present, passive systems are US Food and Drug Administration (FDA) approved for children aged 5 years and older, whereas the active system is approved for children aged 12 years and older.

There are 2 studies that evaluate the outcomes of the transcutaneous implant system in small series of pediatric patients.[48,49] In the study by Dimitriadis and colleagues,[48] wound complications were seen in 24%; most resolved with conservative measures, but 2 required conversion to the percutaneous system. Of those who completed the Speech, Spatial and Qualities of Hearing Scale, a 22% improvement was noted. Nine children previously had a percutaneous bone conduction hearing aid and were converted to the transcutaneous system because of ongoing soft tissue reactions with the percutaneous abutment. These children expressed their contentment with the new magnet system because of the ease of care. However, a commonly raised concern was that the sound from the transcutaneous system seemed quieter compared with the previous percutaneous system. Baker and colleagues[49] described their experience with two types of passive implant systems. Both implant systems were associated with improvements in the PTA postoperatively compared with preoperative assessments. The complication rate in this cohort was 18%, with 1 patient experiencing headaches that required explantation; the remaining patients had complications that resolved with conservative management.

COCHLEAR IMPLANTATION

Approved for use in adults in 1985 and in children in 1990, cochlear implants represent one of the most important developments in the management of severe to profound pediatric SNHL.

Indications

FDA criteria for cochlear implantation differ depending on the age of the patient and the device manufacture. Specifically, cochlear implantation is indicated in children 12 to 24 months of age with bilateral profound SNHL and in children older than 24 months with bilateral severe to profound SNHL. At present, there is no FDA approval for implantation in children less than 12 months of age. Beyond FDA criteria, implant candidacy is determined through a comprehensive audiologic and developmental evaluation. These children must experience minimal benefit from a trial of appropriately fitted hearing aids. In young children, this requires a 3-month to 6-month trial with close monitoring of auditory skills and language development. In older children who can undergo speech audiometry, hearing aid benefit is determined by aided speech perception scores using age-appropriate materials.

Recently, implant candidacy has broadened to include patients with lower audiometric thresholds than the current FDA criteria.[50] Specifically, children with pure tone thresholds less than 70 dBHL are increasingly being considered for cochlear implantation, particularly when aided speech understanding is disproportionately poor. These children may not experience as much benefit from conventional hearing aids compared with children with similar PTAs, but may experience better speech discrimination. In one retrospective review, 51 children received cochlear implants and had pure tone thresholds greater than 70 dBHL and aided speech recognition scores greater than 30%.[50] Postoperatively, significant improvements in speech recognition and language outcomes were seen, suggesting that there is a group of children with less severe pure tone thresholds but poor aided speech discrimination that may benefit from cochlear implants.

Another area of investigation is whether children can benefit from electric acoustic stimulation (EAS) in the setting of residual hearing. Studies of adolescents and adults suggest that electrical stimulation from the cochlear implant combined with residual hearing may lead to improved speech perception.[51,52] However, EAS and hearing preservation techniques are less studied in children. In general, surgeons advocate an atraumatic insertion technique, including care to not manipulate the ossicles, avoidance of perilymph suctioning, slow electrode insertion, and minimizing cochlear bony drilling.[53] In addition to surgical technique, hearing preservation may also be associated with younger age at implantation, electrode length and insertion depth, and the use of perioperative steroids.[54–56] Even in the absence of residual hearing, hearing preservation techniques may be beneficial because the preservation of cochlear microanatomy may allow the patients to participate in treatment and technological advances in the future.

SSD is defined as severe to profound hearing loss in 1 ear, with little benefit from ipsilateral amplification, whereas the contralateral ear has normal hearing.[57] Current treatments of SSD are meant to minimize the impact on hearing in noise for these patients, which include, as discussed earlier for UHL, preferential seating, FM system, contralateral routing hearing aids, and bone conduction sound processors. However, the only currently available method to reestablish binaural auditory input for these patients is cochlear implantation. Data from postlingually deaf adults suggests that many patients obtain improved speech understanding in noise and sound localization; however, the degree of benefit is highly variable. Perhaps most importantly, most of these patients actively use the device despite the impoverished signal relative to their unaffected ears. At present, SSD is not an FDA-approved indication for cochlear implantation in children.

Generalization of these findings to children with prelingual SSD is limited by a paucity of data to small case series with short-term follow-up. A recent systematic review concluded that, although some evidence exists for improved speech perception in noise and sound localization following cochlear implantation in children with SSD, no definitive conclusion could be made because of study heterogeneity and small samples.[57] Nevertheless, more recent studies continue to suggest a modest benefit from cochlear implantation in these children.[58–61] Perhaps most importantly, as with adults with postlingual SSD, children with SSD have a high rate of device use, especially in noisy environments.[59] Further investigations are required before cochlear implantation is routinely recommended in children with SSD.

Surgical Considerations

The site of insertion, specifically round window versus cochleostomy, is an area of discussion. Insertion via a cochleostomy is proposed to have a more favorable angle and therefore be less traumatic[62] In contrast, advocates of round window insertion cite a decreased risk of violating the basilar membrane, as well as avoiding acoustic and mechanical trauma to the cochlea from drilling a fenestra.[63–65] Studies examining these two techniques have not found any significant difference in audiologic outcomes.[66–68] A systematic review examining the outcomes of cochleostomy versus the round window approach found that low-frequency hearing loss can be seen with both techniques and that the rates of hearing preservation are similar.[69] At present, conclusions cannot be drawn regarding the superiority of either the round window or cochleostomy approach.

As discussed briefly earlier, surgeons advocate a soft technique when placing cochlear implants. The goal of the soft technique is to minimize cochlear reaction to the implant, such as fibrosis, osteoneogenesis, fluid pressure changes, and the inflammatory response, all of which may lead to loss of residual hearing.[70] Components of the soft technique include preventing blood and bone dust from entering the scala tympani as well as avoidance of suctioning perilymph; however, the effectiveness of these measures in hearing preservation is not well established.[70] Applying topical steroids to the cochleostomy or round window at the time of implant placement likely minimizes cochlear inflammation, thereby improving hearing preservation.[70] The concern of topical application is that there will be a concentration gradient, thereby decreasing the amount of steroid being delivered to the apex.[71] The administration of systemic steroids may circumvent this issue and be more effective in delivering steroids to all parts of the cochlea. Using lubricant such as hyaluronic acid at the site of implantation and on the electrode array has also been an area of investigation. In small amounts, hyaluronic acid does not seem to be ototoxic,[70] has been found to decrease electrode insertion force, and may also act as a barrier to keep blood from entering the cochlea.[70,72] Studies suggest that using Healon during implant insertion may be beneficial for hearing preservation.[53,73,74]

Special Populations

Inner ear malformation
Approximately 20% of pediatric SNHL is associated with inner ear malformations on temporal bone imaging.[75,76] The most common inner ear anomalies seen clinically are enlarged vestibular aqueduct, incomplete partition, cochlear hypoplasia, and common cavity.[77,78] Inner ear malformations were historically considered a contraindication to cochlear implantation, because of the risk of CSF leak, facial nerve injury, and poor audiologic outcomes.[77,79] However, there has been an emergence of literature discussing the placement of implants in these children with satisfactory outcomes.[77] In a systematic review that examined both cochlear malformations and enlarged vestibular aqueducts, the rate of intraoperative perilymphatic gusher ranged from 9.5% to 40.3%; there was no significant association between the rate of perilymphatic gusher and the severity of the malformation.[77] The same review found an anomalous facial nerve rate of 25%, with more severe malformations associated with an increased rate of an anomalous facial nerve.[77]

Following cochlear implantation, children with inner ear anomalies show significant improvements in speech perception compared with baseline[80]; however, children with cochlear or vestibular hypoplasia seem to experience less improvement compared with those with isolated enlarged vestibular aqueducts.[81] On average, children with mild cochlear anomalies or isolated enlarged vestibular aqueduct experience benefits from cochlear implantation that are comparable with children with normal anatomy. However, outcomes for those with more severe cochlear anomalies are highly variable and difficult to predict. In addition, absence of a cochlear nerve on MRI, regardless of cochlear development, is generally considered a poor predictor for auditory outcome, particularly in the absence of measurable auditory brainstem response or behavioral responses to sound. However, auditory benefit from a cochlear implantation in cases of cochlear nerve hypoplasia or absence have been reported.[82,83]

Auditory neuropathy spectrum disorder
Auditory neuropathy spectrum disorder (ANSD) is estimated to occur in 8% of pediatric SNHL.[84] ANSD is differentiated from SNHL by the presence of evoked otoacoustic emissions, absence of auditory brainstem response, and fluctuating behavioral audiometric thresholds and speech discrimination. Often, speech perception is poorer than pure tone thresholds would predict. This pattern of findings is thought to suggest disorder at the level of the inner hair cell synapse with the spiral ganglion cells or more

centrally at the level of the auditory nerve.[85] The result is dyssynchrony in the stimulus evoked auditory nerve action potentials. Risk factors for ANSD include neonatal hypoxia and hyperbilirubinemia.[86,87] Syndromic and nonsyndromic genetic associations with ANSD have been described.[88]

Children with ANSD are less likely to benefit from conventional amplification, possibly because amplification of the acoustic signal does not address the dyssynchrony.[85] Cochlear implants have been proposed as a treatment of ANSD in patients who do not benefit from amplification. The available data from observational studies show that cochlear implant outcomes are more variable in children with ANSD than in children with SNHL.[89] Roush and colleagues[90] performed a systematic review on aural rehabilitation methods in children with ANSD. In the studies reporting cochlear implant outcomes, most cases were of children who failed a trial of conventional hearing aids, with most children showing severe to profound hearing loss. All children experienced improved pure tone thresholds postimplantation. There was also general agreement among studies that cochlear implantation leads to improved speech perception outcomes; however, the methods of assessing speech varied across studies and not all studies include preimplantation assessments. As such, no firm conclusions could be made regarding the benefit of cochlear implants in ANSD.

A group of children that have been shown to have improved outcomes with early cochlear implantation are those with ANSD caused by mutations in the *OTOF* gene (DNFB9).[91] The *OTOF* gene encodes otoferlin, a transmembrane protein at the synapse of inner hair cells. Mutations lead to impaired neurotransmitter release and auditory nerve dyssynchrony.[92] In a recent study, all included patients with *OTOF* mutations who underwent cochlear implantation experienced improvements in Categories of Auditory Performance (CAP), speech intelligibility, and speech perception.[91] Improved speech perception and auditory skills have also been reported in other studies examining cochlear implant recipients with *OTOF*-related ANSD.[92–94] For the remainder of patients with ANSD from other causes, it is difficult to predict who will benefit from a cochlear implant; therefore, a trial of amplification is necessary before determining candidacy.

AUDITORY BRAINSTEM IMPLANTATION

Auditory brainstem implants (ABIs) provide direct electric stimulation to the cochlear nucleus in the brainstem. Because it bypasses the inner ear and cochlear nerve, auditory brainstem implantation is an option for auditory rehabilitation when the patient is not a candidate for a cochlear implant. Although initially conceived for patients with neurofibromatosis type 2 (NF2), indications for ABI have expanded and are divided into congenital and acquired indications.[95] Congenital indications include cochlear nerve aplasia, complete labyrinthine aplasia, cochlear aplasia, and cochlear aperture aplasia. Acquired indications include severe cochlear ossification, bilateral temporal bone fractures with cochlear nerve avulsion, advanced cochlear otosclerosis, and intractable facial nerve stimulation with cochlear implantation.[95] Both labyrinthine and retrosigmoid approaches have been described for ABI placement.[96,97] Complications are those seen in cerebellopontine angle surgery, such as facial nerve palsy, cerebellar edema, bleeding, CSF leak, and meningitis.[98] Auditory brainstem implants were initially approved by the FDA in 2000 for use in patients 12 years of age or older. In 2013, the FDA gave approval for ABI clinical trials in children younger than 12 years of age.[99]

The outcome data for ABIs in children are limited to small case series. A 2015 systematic review of these studies showed that, after 5 years, 47.9% of children without

NF2 with ABI achieved a CAP score of greater than 4, reflecting the ability to comprehend common phrases without lip reading.[100] In more recent studies, sound detection was obtained in most or all children after ABI placement.[101,102] Speech perception was found to progress slowly, taking up to 5 years.[102] Open-set word recognition was obtained in either none or only a small percentage of children.[101,102] Children without a history of NF2 tend to have better audiologic outcomes compared with children with NF2-related SNHL.[103]

ABI placement can be considered in certain patients who are not candidates for cochlear implantation. Investigations are ongoing in terms of technological advancement of the implants as well as identifying patients who may benefit the most from this technology.

SUMMARY

The approach to children with SNHL is evolving. The diagnostic process is becoming refined with the availability of genetic and CMV testing. At present, the main surgical modalities for SNHL are cochlear implantation and bone conduction sound processors placement. With advancing technology, the indications for surgical intervention and the surgical techniques will likely continue to change.

ACKNOWLEDGMENTS

The authors would like to thank Dr Dylan Chan for his review and comments on the article.

REFERENCES

1. White KR. Early hearing detection and intervention programs: opportunities for genetic services. Am J Med Genet A 2004;130A(1):29–36.

2. Sloan-Heggen CM, Bierer AO, Shearer AE, et al. Comprehensive genetic testing in the clinical evaluation of 1119 patients with hearing loss. Hum Genet 2016; 135(4):441–50.

3. Liu X. Cochlear implants in genetic deafness. J Otol 2014;9(4):156–62.

4. Shearer AE, Black-Ziegelbein EA, Hildebrand MS, et al. Advancing genetic testing for deafness with genomic technology. J Med Genet 2013;50(9): 627–34.

5. Shearer AE, Frees K, Kolbe DL, et al. Comprehensive genetic testing for deafness from fresh and archived dried blood spots. Otolaryngol Head Neck Surg 2018. https://doi.org/10.1177/0194599818797291. 194599818797291.

6. Arnos KS. The implications of genetic testing for deafness. Ear Hear 2003;24(4): 324–31.

7. Alford RL, Arnos KS, Fox M, et al. American College of Medical Genetics and Genomics guideline for the clinical evaluation and etiologic diagnosis of hearing loss. Genet Med 2014;16(4):347–55.

8. Mehta D, Noon SE, Schwartz E, et al. Outcomes of evaluation and testing of 660 individuals with hearing loss in a pediatric genetics of hearing loss clinic. Am J Med Genet A 2016;170(10):2523–30.

9. American Academy of Pediatrics JCoIH. Year 2007 position statement: principles and guidelines for early hearing detection and intervention programs. Pediatrics 2007;120(4):898–921.

10. Kimberlin DW, Lin CY, Sanchez PJ, et al. Effect of ganciclovir therapy on hearing in symptomatic congenital cytomegalovirus disease involving the central nervous system: a randomized, controlled trial. J Pediatr 2003;143(1):16–25.

11. Dollard SC, Grosse SD, Ross DS. New estimates of the prevalence of neurological and sensory sequelae and mortality associated with congenital cytomegalovirus infection. Rev Med Virol 2007;17(5):355–63.

12. Ross SA, Novak Z, Pati S, et al. Overview of the diagnosis of cytomegalovirus infection. Infect Disord Drug Targets 2011;11(5):466–74.

13. Rawlinson WD, Boppana SB, Fowler KB, et al. Congenital cytomegalovirus infection in pregnancy and the neonate: consensus recommendations for prevention, diagnosis, and therapy. Lancet Infect Dis 2017;17(6):e177–88.

14. Schleiss MR. Role of breast milk in acquisition of cytomegalovirus infection: recent advances. Curr Opin Pediatr 2006;18(1):48–52.

15. Boppana SB, Ross SA, Novak Z, et al. Dried blood spot real-time polymerase chain reaction assays to screen newborns for congenital cytomegalovirus infection. JAMA 2010;303(14):1375–82.

16. Kimberlin DW, Jester PM, Sanchez PJ, et al. Valganciclovir for symptomatic congenital cytomegalovirus disease. N Engl J Med 2015;372(10):933–43.

17. Pasternak Y, Ziv L, Attias J, et al. Valganciclovir is beneficial in children with congenital cytomegalovirus and isolated hearing loss. J Pediatr 2018;199:166–70.

18. van Beeck Calkoen EA, Merkus P, Goverts ST, et al. Evaluation of the outcome of CT and MR imaging in pediatric patients with bilateral sensorineural hearing loss. Int J Pediatr Otorhinolaryngol 2018;108:180–5.

19. Shah J, Pham GN, Zhang J, et al. Evaluating diagnostic yield of computed tomography (CT) and magnetic resonance imaging (MRI) in pediatric unilateral sensorineural hearing loss. Int J Pediatr Otorhinolaryngol 2018;115:41–4.

20. Chen JX, Kachniarz B, Shin JJ. Diagnostic yield of computed tomography scan for pediatric hearing loss: a systematic review. Otolaryngol Head Neck Surg 2014;151(5):718–39.

21. Kachniarz B, Chen JX, Gilani S, et al. Diagnostic yield of MRI for pediatric hearing loss: a systematic review. Otolaryngol Head Neck Surg 2015;152(1):5–22.

22. Preciado DA, Lim LH, Cohen AP, et al. A diagnostic paradigm for childhood idiopathic sensorineural hearing loss. Otolaryngol Head Neck Surg 2004;131(6):804–9.

23. Chang RK, Lan YT, Silka MJ, et al. Genetic variants for long QT syndrome among infants and children from a statewide newborn hearing screening program cohort. J Pediatr 2014;164(3):590–5.e1-3.

24. De Leenheer EM, Janssens S, Padalko E, et al. Etiological diagnosis in the hearing impaired newborn: proposal of a flow chart. Int J Pediatr Otorhinolaryngol 2011;75(1):27–32.

25. Johnston DR, Curry JM, Newborough B, et al. Ophthalmologic disorders in children with syndromic and nonsyndromic hearing loss. Arch Otolaryngol Head Neck Surg 2010;136(3):277–80.

26. Nikolopoulos TP, Lioumi D, Stamataki S, et al. Evidence-based overview of ophthalmic disorders in deaf children: a literature update. Otol Neurotol 2006;27(2 Suppl 1):S1–24 [discussion: S20].

27. Yoshinaga-Itano C, Sedey AL, Coulter DK, et al. Language of early- and later-identified children with hearing loss. Pediatrics 1998;102(5):1161–71.

28. Robinshaw HM. Early intervention for hearing impairment: differences in the timing of communicative and linguistic development. Br J Audiol 1995;29(6): 315–34.

29. Leigh J, Dettman S, Dowell R, et al. Communication development in children who receive a cochlear implant by 12 months of age. Otol Neurotol 2013; 34(3):443–50.

30. Lieu JE. Speech-language and educational consequences of unilateral hearing loss in children. Arch Otolaryngol Head Neck Surg 2004;130(5):524–30.

31. Lieu JE, Tye-Murray N, Karzon RK, et al. Unilateral hearing loss is associated with worse speech-language scores in children. Pediatrics 2010;125(6): e1348–55.

32. Anne S, Lieu JEC, Cohen MS. Speech and language consequences of unilateral hearing loss: a systematic review. Otolaryngol Head Neck Surg 2017;157(4): 572–9.

33. Appachi S, Specht JL, Raol N, et al. Auditory outcomes with hearing rehabilitation in children with unilateral hearing loss: a systematic review. Otolaryngol Head Neck Surg 2017;157(4):565–71.

34. Tjellstrom A, Hakansson B, Granstrom G. Bone-anchored hearing aids: current status in adults and children. Otolaryngol Clin North Am 2001;34(2):337–64.

35. Liu CC, Chadha NK, Bance M, et al. The current practice trends in pediatric bone-anchored hearing aids in Canada: a national clinical and surgical practice survey. J Otolaryngol Head Neck Surg 2013;42:43.

36. Stalfors J, Tjellstrom A. Skin reactions after BAHA surgery: a comparison between the U-graft technique and the BAHA dermatome. Otol Neurotol 2008; 29(8):1109–14.

37. Mylanus EA, Cremers CW. A one-stage surgical procedure for placement of percutaneous implants for the bone-anchored hearing aid. J Laryngol Otol 1994;108(12):1031–5.

38. de Wolf MJ, Hol MK, Huygen PL, et al. Clinical outcome of the simplified surgical technique for BAHA implantation. Otol Neurotol 2008;29(8):1100–8.

39. Wilson DF, Kim HH. A minimally invasive technique for the implantation of bone-anchored hearing devices. Otolaryngol Head Neck Surg 2013;149(3):473–7.

40. Kiringoda R, Lustig LR. A meta-analysis of the complications associated with osseointegrated hearing aids. Otol Neurotol 2013;34(5):790–4.

41. Siegert R, Kanderske J. A new semi-implantable transcutaneous bone conduction device: clinical, surgical, and audiologic outcomes in patients with congenital ear canal atresia. Otol Neurotol 2013;34(5):927–34.

42. Clamp PJ, Briggs RJ. The Cochlear Baha 4 Attract System - design concepts, surgical technique and early clinical results. Expert Rev Med Devices 2015; 12(3):223–30.

43. Manrique M, Sanhueza I, Manrique R, et al. A new bone conduction implant: surgical technique and results. Otol Neurotol 2014;35(2):216–20.

44. Briggs R, Van Hasselt A, Luntz M, et al. Clinical performance of a new magnetic bone conduction hearing implant system: results from a prospective, multicenter, clinical investigation. Otol Neurotol 2015;36(5):834–41.

45. Zernotti ME, Chiaraviglio MM, Mauricio SB, et al. Audiological outcomes in patients with congenital aural atresia implanted with transcutaneous active bone conduction hearing implant. Int J Pediatr Otorhinolaryngol 2019;119:54–8.

46. Zernotti ME, Di Gregorio MF, Galeazzi P, et al. Comparative outcomes of active and passive hearing devices by transcutaneous bone conduction. Acta Otolaryngol 2016;136(6):556–8.

47. Steehler MW, Larner SP, Mintz JS, et al. A comparison of the operative techniques and the postoperative complications for bone-anchored hearing aid implantation. Int Arch Otorhinolaryngol 2018;22(4):368–73.

48. Dimitriadis PA, Carrick S, Ray J. Intermediate outcomes of a transcutaneous bone conduction hearing device in a paediatric population. Int J Pediatr Otorhinolaryngol 2017;94:59–63.

49. Baker S, Centric A, Chennupati SK. Innovation in abutment-free bone-anchored hearing devices in children: updated results and experience. Int J Pediatr Otorhinolaryngol 2015;79(10):1667–72.

50. Carlson ML, Sladen DP, Haynes DS, et al. Evidence for the expansion of pediatric cochlear implant candidacy. Otol Neurotol 2015;36(1):43–50.

51. Gantz BJ, Turner CW. Combining acoustic and electrical hearing. Laryngoscope 2003;113(10):1726–30.

52. Gantz BJ, Dunn C, Walker E, et al. Outcomes of adolescents with a short electrode cochlear implant with preserved residual hearing. Otol Neurotol 2016; 37(2):e118–25.

53. Kiefer J, Gstoettner W, Baumgartner W, et al. Conservation of low-frequency hearing in cochlear implantation. Acta Otolaryngol 2004;124(3):272–80.

54. Huarte RM, Roland JT Jr. Toward hearing preservation in cochlear implant surgery. Curr Opin Otolaryngol Head Neck Surg 2014;22(5):349–52.

55. Nguyen Y, Mosnier I, Borel S, et al. Evolution of electrode array diameter for hearing preservation in cochlear implantation. Acta Otolaryngol 2013;133(2): 116–22.

56. Santa Maria PL, Gluth MB, Yuan Y, et al. Hearing preservation surgery for cochlear implantation: a meta-analysis. Otol Neurotol 2014;35(10):e256–69.

57. Peters JP, Ramakers GG, Smit AL, et al. Cochlear implantation in children with unilateral hearing loss: a systematic review. Laryngoscope 2016;126(3): 713–21.

58. Tavora-Vieira D, Rajan GP. Cochlear implantation in children with congenital and noncongenital unilateral deafness. Otol Neurotol 2015;36(8):1457–8.

59. Polonenko MJ, Papsin BC, Gordon KA. Children with single-sided deafness use their cochlear implant. Ear Hear 2017;38(6):681–9.

60. Arndt S, Prosse S, Laszig R, et al. Cochlear implantation in children with single-sided deafness: does aetiology and duration of deafness matter? Audiol Neurootol 2015;20(Suppl 1):21–30.

61. Rahne T, Plontke SK. Functional result after cochlear implantation in children and adults with single-sided deafness. Otol Neurotol 2016;37(9):e332–40.

62. Hamamoto M, Murakami G, Kataura A. Topographical relationships among the facial nerve, chorda tympani nerve and round window with special reference to the approach route for cochlear implant surgery. Clin Anat 2000;13(4):251–6.

63. Meshik X, Holden TA, Chole RA, et al. Optimal cochlear implant insertion vectors. Otol Neurotol 2010;31(1):58–63.

64. Pau HW, Just T, Bornitz M, et al. Noise exposure of the inner ear during drilling a cochleostomy for cochlear implantation. Laryngoscope 2007;117(3):535–40.

65. Nadol JB Jr, Eddington DK. Histologic evaluation of the tissue seal and biologic response around cochlear implant electrodes in the human. Otol Neurotol 2004; 25(3):257–62.

66. Kang BJ, Kim AH. Comparison of cochlear implant performance after round window electrode insertion compared with traditional cochleostomy. Otolaryngol Head Neck Surg 2013;148(5):822–6.

67. Gudis DA, Montes M, Bigelow DC, et al. The round window: is it the "cochleostomy" of choice? Experience in 130 consecutive cochlear implants. Otol Neurotol 2012;33(9):1497–501.

68. Adunka OF, Dillon MT, Adunka MC, et al. Cochleostomy versus round window insertions: influence on functional outcomes in electric-acoustic stimulation of the auditory system. Otol Neurotol 2014;35(4):613–8.

69. Havenith S, Lammers MJ, Tange RA, et al. Hearing preservation surgery: cochleostomy or round window approach? A systematic review. Otol Neurotol 2013; 34(4):667–74.

70. Friedland DR, Runge-Samuelson C. Soft cochlear implantation: rationale for the surgical approach. Trends Amplif 2009;13(2):124–38.

71. Plontke SK, Biegner T, Kammerer B, et al. Dexamethasone concentration gradients along scala tympani after application to the round window membrane. Otol Neurotol 2008;29(3):401–6.

72. Kontorinis G, Paasche G, Lenarz T, et al. The effect of different lubricants on cochlear implant electrode insertion forces. Otol Neurotol 2011;32(7): 1050–6.

73. Skarzynski H, Lorens A, D'Haese P, et al. Preservation of residual hearing in children and post-lingually deafened adults after cochlear implantation: an initial study. ORL J Otorhinolaryngol Relat Spec 2002;64(4):247–53.

74. Garcia-Ibanez L, Macias AR, Morera C, et al. An evaluation of the preservation of residual hearing with the Nucleus Contour Advance electrode. Acta Otolaryngol 2009;129(6):651–64.

75. Jackler RK, Luxford WM, House WF. Congenital malformations of the inner ear: a classification based on embryogenesis. Laryngoscope 1987;97(3 Pt 2 Suppl 40):2–14.

76. Park AH, Kou B, Hotaling A, et al. Clinical course of pediatric congenital inner ear malformations. Laryngoscope 2000;110(10 Pt 1):1715–9.

77. Pakdaman MN, Herrmann BS, Curtin HD, et al. Cochlear implantation in children with anomalous cochleovestibular anatomy: a systematic review. Otolaryngol Head Neck Surg 2012;146(2):180–90.

78. Madden C, Halsted M, Benton C, et al. Enlarged vestibular aqueduct syndrome in the pediatric population. Otol Neurotol 2003;24(4):625–32.

79. Luntz M, Balkany T, Hodges AV, et al. Cochlear implants in children with congenital inner ear malformations. Arch Otolaryngol Head Neck Surg 1997;123(9): 974–7.

80. Pritchett C, Zwolan T, Huq F, et al. Variations in the cochlear implant experience in children with enlarged vestibular aqueduct. Laryngoscope 2015;125(9): 2169–74.

81. Isaiah A, Lee D, Lenes-Voit F, et al. Clinical outcomes following cochlear implantation in children with inner ear anomalies. Int J Pediatr Otorhinolaryngol 2017; 93:1–6.

82. Young NM, Kim FM, Ryan ME, et al. Pediatric cochlear implantation of children with eighth nerve deficiency. Int J Pediatr Otorhinolaryngol 2012;76(10):1442–8.

83. Zanetti D, Guida M, Barezzani MG, et al. Favorable outcome of cochlear implant in VIIIth nerve deficiency. Otol Neurotol 2006;27(6):815–23.

84. Vlastarakos PV, Nikolopoulos TP, Tavoulari E, et al. Auditory neuropathy: endocochlear lesion or temporal processing impairment? Implications for diagnosis and management. Int J Pediatr Otorhinolaryngol 2008;72(8):1135–50.

85. Rance G. Auditory neuropathy/dys-synchrony and its perceptual consequences. Trends Amplif 2005;9(1):1–43.

86. Amin SB, Wang H, Laroia N, et al. Unbound bilirubin and auditory neuropathy spectrum disorder in late preterm and term infants with severe jaundice. J Pediatr 2016;173:84–9.

87. Sawada S, Mori N, Mount RJ, et al. Differential vulnerability of inner and outer hair cell systems to chronic mild hypoxia and glutamate ototoxicity: insights into the cause of auditory neuropathy. J Otolaryngol 2001;30(2):106–14.

88. Manchaiah VK, Zhao F, Danesh AA, et al. The genetic basis of auditory neuropathy spectrum disorder (ANSD). Int J Pediatr Otorhinolaryngol 2011;75(2): 151–8.

89. Humphriss R, Hall A, Maddocks J, et al. Does cochlear implantation improve speech recognition in children with auditory neuropathy spectrum disorder? A systematic review. Int J Audiol 2013;52(7):442–54.

90. Roush P, Frymark T, Venediktov R, et al. Audiologic management of auditory neuropathy spectrum disorder in children: a systematic review of the literature. Am J Audiol 2011;20(2):159–70.

91. Wu CC, Hsu CJ, Huang FL, et al. Timing of cochlear implantation in auditory neuropathy patients with OTOF mutations: our experience with 10 patients. Clin Otolaryngol 2018;43(1):352–7.

92. Santarelli R, del Castillo I, Cama E, et al. Audibility, speech perception and processing of temporal cues in ribbon synaptic disorders due to OTOF mutations. Hear Res 2015;330(Pt B):200–12.

93. Rouillon I, Marcolla A, Roux I, et al. Results of cochlear implantation in two children with mutations in the OTOF gene. Int J Pediatr Otorhinolaryngol 2006;70(4): 689–96.

94. Runge CL, Erbe CB, McNally MT, et al. A novel otoferlin splice-site mutation in siblings with auditory neuropathy spectrum disorder. Audiol Neurootol 2013; 18(6):374–82.

95. Sennaroglu L, Colletti V, Manrique M, et al. Auditory brainstem implantation in children and non-neurofibromatosis type 2 patients: a consensus statement. Otol Neurotol 2011;32(2):187–91.

96. Colletti V, Sacchetto L, Giarbini N, et al. Retrosigmoid approach for auditory brainstem implant. J Laryngol Otol Suppl 2000;(27):37–40.

97. Brackmann DE, Hitselberger WE, Nelson RA, et al. Auditory brainstem implant: I. Issues in surgical implantation. Otolaryngol Head Neck Surg 1993;108(6): 624–33.

98. Colletti V, Carner M, Miorelli V, et al. Auditory brainstem implant (ABI): new frontiers in adults and children. Otolaryngol Head Neck Surg 2005;133(1):126–38.

99. da Costa Monsanto R, Bittencourt AG, Neto NJB, et al. Auditory brainstem implants in children: results based on a review of the literature. J Int Adv Otol 2014; 10(2):284–90.

100. Noij KS, Kozin ED, Sethi R, et al. Systematic review of nontumor pediatric auditory brainstem implant outcomes. Otolaryngol Head Neck Surg 2015;153(5): 739–50.

101. Teagle HFB, Henderson L, He S, et al. Pediatric auditory brainstem implantation: surgical, electrophysiologic, and behavioral outcomes. Ear Hear 2018;39(2): 326–36.

102. Sung JKK, Luk BPK, Wong TKC, et al. Pediatric auditory brainstem implantation: impact on audiological rehabilitation and tonal language development. Audiol Neurootol 2018;23(2):126–34.

103. Colletti V. Auditory outcomes in tumor vs. nontumor patients fitted with auditory brainstem implants. Adv Otorhinolaryngol 2006;64:167–85.

Allergy and the Pediatric Otolaryngologist

Victoria S. Lee, MD, Sandra Y. Lin, MD*

KEYWORDS

- Food allergy • Oral food challenge • Skin prick testing • Specific IgE • Avoidance
- Allergic rhinitis • Sublingual immunotherapy • Subcutaneous immunotherapy

KEY POINTS

- Food allergy is a specific, reproducible immune-mediated response to a food that results in an adverse health outcome.
- The history is key in determining the diagnosis of a food allergy, and strict avoidance is the mainstay of treatment.
- There is a growing amount of evidence that suggests nondelayed and even early introduction of high-risk foods may reduce the risk of developing an allergy.
- Intranasal corticosteroids are the most effective treatment of allergic rhinitis.
- Allergen immunotherapy is generally indicated for the treatment of allergic rhinitis if conventional pharmacotherapy fails or is not an option.

INTRODUCTION

The atopic march refers to the tendency of the typical progression of allergic disease first manifesting in infants as atopic dermatitis and advancing to other allergic diseases as they grow older. The most common allergic diseases with relevance to the pediatric otolaryngologist are food allergy and allergic rhinitis (AR). In particular, food allergy is increasing in prevalence and, therefore, is likely to be more frequently encountered in clinical practice. It is also a main cause of anaphylaxis presenting to the emergency department. For the pediatric otolaryngologist, a solid understanding of these diseases is critical to effectively identifying and managing these children. This article summarizes the epidemiology, pathophysiology, diagnosis, and management of both food allergy and AR. It also highlights exciting new areas of research in diagnostic testing, treatment, and prevention of these diseases, including early

Disclosures: Dr V.S. Lee has no disclosures. Dr S.Y. Lin is a consultant for Aerin Medical and Redesign Health.
Department of Otolaryngology–Head and Neck Surgery, Johns Hopkins University School of Medicine, Johns Hopkins Outpatient Center, 6th Floor, 601 North Caroline Street, Baltimore, MD 21287-0910, USA
* Corresponding author.
E-mail address: slin30@jhmi.edu

introduction of allergen-containing foods as a prevention strategy and sublingual immunotherapy (SLIT) for the treatment of AR.

FOOD ALLERGY
Definition

Food allergy is a specific, reproducible immune-mediated response to a food that results in an adverse health outcome. In contrast, food intolerance is in response to mechanisms that are not immune-mediated, such as metabolic, toxic, and pharmacologic mechanisms.[1]

Epidemiology

The prevalence of food allergy has been estimated to be as high as 10% and is believed to be increasing in the past couple decades. It is more common in children. Of the hundreds of food allergens that have been reported, milk, wheat, egg, soy, peanuts, tree nuts, shellfish, and fish are the most common. Peanuts, tree nuts, shellfish, and fish allergies are often lifelong. Peanuts and tree nuts are responsible for the most severe allergic reactions. There is a higher prevalence of food allergy in children with atopic dermatitis, AR, and asthma.[2,3]

Genetics are believed to play a significant role in the development of a food allergy. Studies have demonstrated that children with parents or siblings who have an allergic condition are more likely to have a food allergy. There are also a growing number of genomic studies identifying corresponding common allergy-specific loci among family members.[2,4,5] Studies also suggest additional risk factors of living in an industrialized area, African and Asian descent, and male sex.[2,6]

Pathophysiology

Food allergy reactions can generally be divided into IgE-mediated, non–IgE-mediated, and mixed processes. In a correctly functioning immune response, induction of food antigen–specific regulatory T cells maintains tolerance. In IgE-mediated food allergy reactions, induction of food antigen–specific type 2 T helper (T_H2) cells drive IgE antibody production, which in turn bind to basophils and mast cells that release inflammatory mediators. Active investigations are underway to elucidate the specific cytokines and other factors involved in this deviated response. Both interleukin (IL)-33 and IL-9 have been identified as potential key cytokines associated with allergic responses to foods, acting through a variety of mechanisms.[2,6]

Non–IgE-mediated processes, such as food protein–induced enterocolitis syndrome, food protein–induced proctocolitis, celiac disease, and dermatitis herpetiformis, as well as mixed processes, such as eosinophilic esophagitis and atopic dermatitis, are poorly understood. T_H2 cells, eosinophils, and components of the innate immune system are some of the factors believed to play a role. The specific immuno mochanioms for thoco proococcos aro ourrontly a oubjoot of aotivo rocoarch.[7]

Diagnosis

Clinical presentation
In IgE-mediated processes, the clinical sequelae tend to occur within minutes to a couple of hours after ingestion. Oral allergy syndrome, the mildest reaction, is related to the cross-reaction of pollen-specific IgE antibodies and proteins found in fresh vegetables and fruit, manifesting as oral cavity and oropharyngeal itchiness and tingling. IgE-mediated reactions can have cutaneous, respiratory, gastrointestinal, and cardiovascular symptoms, with cutaneous being the most common. In contrast, non–IgE-mediated processes tend to be more delayed or chronic in nature. These

reactions tend to have primarily cutaneous and gastrointestinal symptoms. **Table 1** summarizes the key clinical manifestations of Ig-mediated and non–IgE-mediated processes.

Diagnostic algorithm and tests

Fig. 1 outlines a general algorithm for diagnosing food allergies. The algorithm begins with a careful history; identifying suspected foods and their manner of preparation, as well as route of exposure; symptoms and their reproducibility, as well as exacerbating factors; onset and duration of the reaction; and response to treatment. This history is key in determining whether it truly represents a food allergy and, if so, whether it is an IgE-mediated, non–IgE-mediated, or mixed process.[2,6] A thorough physical examination should also be performed, assessing for signs and symptoms if an allergic reaction is actively occurring, and evidence of atopic and allergic disease, such as atopic dermatitis. In children especially, overall health, growth, and nutrition status should be evaluated.

Table 1		
Key clinical manifestations of Ig-mediated and non–IgE-mediated processes		
	IgE-Mediated (Immediate Reactions)	**Non–IgE-mediated (Delayed or Chronic Reactions)**
Skin		
Urticaria	√	—
Angioedema	√	—
Erythema	√	√
Pruritus	√	√
Eczematous rash or lesions	√	√
Respiratory		
Laryngeal edema	√	—
Rhinorrhea	√	—
Bronchospasm	√	—
Nasal congestion	√	—
Cough	√	—
Chest tightness	√	—
Wheezing	√	—
Dyspnea	√	—
Gastrointestinal		
Angioedema of the lips, tongue, palate	√	—
Oral pruritus	√	—
Tongue swelling	√	—
Vomiting	√	√
Diarrhea	√	√
Pain	√	√
Cardiovascular		
Presyncope or syncope	√	—
Hypotension	√	—
Tachycardia	√	—

From Waserman S, Watson W. Food allergy. Allergy Asthma Clin Immunol 2011;7 Suppl 1:S7; with permission.

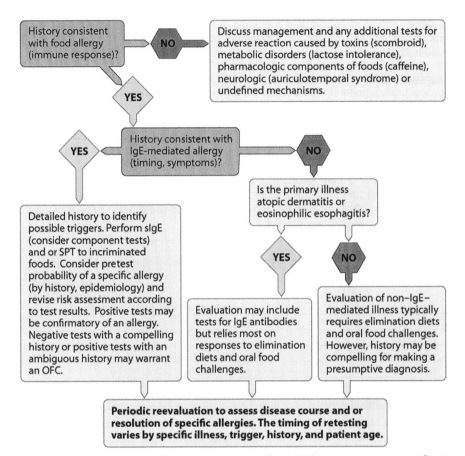

Fig. 1. Diagnostic approach to food allergy. OFC, oral food challenge; sIgE, serum-specific IgE; SPT, skin prick testing. (*From* Sicherer SH, Sampson HA. Food allergy: a review and update on epidemiology, pathogenesis, diagnosis, prevention, and management. J Allergy Clin Immunol 2018;141(1):41–58; with permission.)

At this point, diagnostic tests can be used to further hone the diagnosis of specific food allergies. There are numerous diagnostic modalities that are currently available, with ongoing research focused on developing newer ones. In suspected IgE-mediated processes, skin prick testing (SPT) and serum-specific IgE testing are reasonable initial modalities to pursue. SPT is performed by applying food extract to the skin, followed by a prick, with a positive result exhibiting a wheal and flare response. It is rapid and safe and has a high sensitivity of around 90% but a specificity of only around 50%.[3] Interestingly, SPT is often negative in oral allergy syndrome. Serum-specific IgE testing involves quantifying specific IgE antibodies to foods via in vitro methods. Compared with SPT, it is more expensive and less sensitive.[3] It is especially useful when SPT is not available or cannot be performed. Given the lower specificity of both types of testing and the lack of a simple dichotomous result but, instead, a positive result reported on a spectrum open to interpretation, it is important to avoid indiscriminate testing and focus on suspected foods based on the history.[2]

Oral food challenge (OFC) involves consuming gradually increasing portions of the suspected food and is considered the gold standard for diagnosis of food allergy.

Because it is time-consuming and requires close physician supervision, it is typically reserved for situations in which the diagnosis is still uncertain.[6] There is a growing amount of research looking at improved surrogate testing to avoid performing OFCs, including molecular or component-resolved diagnostics tests and basophil activation tests.[2] It is important to regularly reassess food allergies because some may resolve over time.

Management

Strict avoidance is the mainstay food allergy treatment. Food labeling is not standardized and, therefore, can often be interpreted incorrectly. Also, staff at food service establishments may not have had food allergy training, making careful education of children and their families critical. Avoidance may result in nutritional deficiencies and, therefore, nutritional counseling and growth monitoring are important for all children with food allergies.[2] A potential exception to the strict avoidance policy is milk and egg allergy. Approximately 70% of individuals can tolerate these foods when extensively heated as in baking. Therefore, it is important to perform OFCs to see if these foods can be tolerated in baked form. If so, there are data supporting faster resolution of the allergy with ingestion.[8]

It is important that severe allergic reactions are promptly treated with epinephrine. Individuals with a food allergy should always wear a medic alert bracelet and have an epinephrine autoinjector, dosed according to weight for children, stored in the proper conditions, and regularly checked to ensure it has not exceeded its expiration date. Children, their families, and schools should be trained on how to manage an allergic event and use the device properly.[6]

Prevention and Future Research

There is a growing amount of evidence that suggests nondelayed and even early introduction of high-risk foods may reduce the risk of developing an allergy. Based on the results of the Learning Early About Peanut Allergy (LEAP) trial, the National Institutes of Health recommended that infants at high risk of developing a peanut allergy should have these foods introduced as early as 4 to 6 months, infants with mild to moderate eczema should have these foods introduced around 6 months, and that infants who do not have any food allergies or eczema should have these foods freely introduced.[9,10]

The LEAP trial was focused on high-risk infants rather than the general population and peanut allergies specifically. The Enquiring About Tolerance (EAT) trial sought to address these gaps. In exclusively breast-fed infants in the general population, the early introduction of common dietary allergens (cooked egg, peanut, cow's milk, sesame, whitefish, and wheat) from 3 months of age was compared with only receiving breast milk up to 6 months of age. A per-protocol analysis suggested that the early introduction group had a lower prevalence of food allergy for peanut and egg; however, this was not shown in the intention-to-treat analysis.[11] New research is focused on better evaluating the impact of early introduction of these other common dietary allergens. There is currently no recommendation for early introduction of egg-containing foods but there is also no recommendation to avoid it in the early infant diet.[2]

Allergen immunotherapy is being intensely investigated as a potential treatment of food allergy, specifically the oral, epicutaneous, sublingual, and modified subcutaneous routes. Immunotherapy can increase the threshold of reactivity to specific food allergens, referred to as desensitization; however, the level of that threshold varies. It may allow a higher threshold so that an individual can consume normal amounts of an allergen or a lower threshold so that adverse sequelae are minimized in the event of an accidental ingestion. Perhaps among the biggest drawbacks is that desensitization is not permanent, unlike immune tolerance, and requires repeated exposure to the allergen to be maintained. Other disadvantages include typically months to years of treatment, frequent clinic visits, risk of adverse reactions during treatment, and the limitation of current protocols to only address a single allergen at a time, making use in individuals with multiple food allergies impractical.[12]

Current research is focused on addressing these drawbacks, in particular the risk of adverse reactions through the use of adjunctive therapies. Biologics are an area of active investigation. Thus far, most research has focused on omalizumab, an anti-IgE antibody that reduces circulating IgE concentrations. It has the added advantage of not binding to IgE on mast cells and basophils and, therefore, cannot precipitate an allergic response. Recent studies have looked at the use of omalizumab adjunctively with oral immunotherapy and found that it allows beginning at a higher initial dose of the allergy, thereby reducing time to desensitization, and decreases the number of doses required to reach maintenance. Desensitization is also maintained even after discontinuation of omalizumab. Besides omalizumab, there are multiple other biologics that are being considered for the treatment of food allergy, including those directed against IL-33, IL-5 (mepolizumab and reslizumab), IL-5R (benralizumab), IL-4 and IL-13 (dupilumab), and thymic stromal lymphopoietin (tezepelumab).[12]

DNA-based vaccines are also being evaluated. There are ongoing studies looking at other strategies, including vitamin D sufficiency and probiotics. Probiotics have shown promise in trials looking at its adjunctive use with oral immunotherapy. It is an exciting time with many promising new therapies on the horizon that may alter the way food allergies are treated.[2,12,13]

ALLERGIC RHINITIS
Definition

AR is defined as inflammation of the nasal mucosa due to an inappropriate IgE-mediated response to an inhalational allergen.[14]

Epidemiology

AR is uncommon in children younger than 2 years of age because it requires repeated exposure to the allergen to develop. The prevalence in children aged 6 to 7 years and 13 to 14 years is approximately 9% and 15%, respectively, with most having symptoms before 20 years of age.[15] The prevalence is believed to be increasing, having approximately doubled since 1970.[16] Risk factors include family history, male sex, firstborn status, early systemic antibiotics, maternal smoking, exposure to indoor inhalational allergens, serum IgE greater than 100 IU/mL before 6 years of age, and the presence of allergen-specific IgE.[15]

AR is associated with many other conditions. Up to 50% of individuals with AR have asthma. Conjunctivitis is present in up to 60% of individuals with AR, and symptoms consistent with oral allergy syndrome have been reported in 25% of children with AR. AR is also believed to be a contributing factor in the development of sinusitis, eustachian tube dysfunction and subsequent otitis media, hearing loss, and speech delay and sleep-disordered breathing due to nasal obstruction. Therefore, health care practitioners should closely evaluate for these associated conditions in children with AR.[17]

Pathophysiology

During sensitization, exposure to the allergen results in the production of allergen-specific IgE, which binds to receptors on mast cells. On reexposure, the allergen binds to its specific IgE, resulting in the release of inflammatory mediators. This comprises the early response, which occurs within 5 to 10 minutes of exposure and peaks 15 to 30 minutes after exposure. The late response, which occurs 2 to 8 hours after exposure and peaks 6 to 12 hours after exposure, occurs as a result of infiltration of eosinophils and other inflammatory cells.[14,17]

Diagnosis

Clinical presentation

The most common symptom of AR is nasal congestion. Rhinorrhea, sneezing, postnasal drainage, cough, fatigue, irritability, watery eyes, facial pain, and itching are also common. Symptom patterns can be categorized based on temporal characteristics (seasonal or perennial). Allergens with a seasonal pattern include tree, grass, and ragweed pollens, with symptoms typically in the spring, summer, and fall, respectively. Allergens with a perennial pattern include indoor ones, such as dust mites, pet dander, cockroaches, and respiratory irritants. Mold is both an indoor and outdoor allergen but typically exhibits a perennial pattern. Symptoms can also be categorized by severity. These categorizations are used for classification and guidelines.[17] Physical examination should include a thorough examination of the eyes, nose, ears, and throat.[14,17]

Diagnostic tests

Testing is not required to diagnose AR and to start empiric therapy. Like food allergy, the diagnostic tests available include SPT and serum-specific IgE testing as initial modalities. Again, it is important to avoid indiscriminate testing and focus on suspected allergens based on the history and physical examination.

Management

Environmental control measures

Avoidance is an initial step in the management of AR, although the data are lacking.[17–19] With outdoor allergens, which are primarily pollen-related, counts are typically highest in the morning and on hot, windy, and dry days; therefore, avoidance strategies involve counseling individuals to avoid these high pollen count periods and conditions.[14]

Pharmacotherapy

The next step, if environmental control measures are not particularly effective, is to initiate pharmacotherapies. **Table 2** summarizes the main classes used in the treatment of AR.

Intranasal corticosteroids (INCSs) are the most effective pharmacotherapy, treating all symptoms of AR, as well as associated conditions. Maximal benefit may not be achieved for weeks after starting the therapy. Second-generation INCSs have less than 2% systemic bioavailability compared with 10% to 50% for first-generation INCSs; however, studies have not shown any impact on the hypothalamic-pituitary-adrenal axis or growth with topical administration.[17] It is still recommended, however, that in children prescribed INCSs, the lowest effective dose be used, growth be closely monitored, and the need for it be periodically assessed. Oral corticosteroids are rarely used in children for the treatment of AR.[17]

Oral and intranasal antihistamines are also commonly used for the treatment of AR. These are effective for all symptoms except nasal congestion and are typically well tolerated. Second-generation antihistamines are recommended in children because they have minimal anticholinergic side effects and do not cross the blood-brain barrier, having, therefore, less risk of sedation.[14] Montelukast is the only leukotriene modifier approved in the United States for the treatment of pediatric AR and is also commonly

Table 2
Common classes and names of pharmacotherapies for allergic rhinitis

Class		Generic Name (Brand Name)
Corticosteroids	Topical 1st generation	Beclomethasone (Beconase AQ, Qnasl) Budesonide (Rhinocort Aqua[c]) Triamcinolone (Nasacort AQ[a,c])
	Topical 2nd-generation	Ciclesonide (Omnaris, Zetonna) Fluticasone (Veramyst[a], Flonase[c]) Mometasone (Nasonex[a])
Antihistamines	Topical	Azelastine (Astelin, Astepro) Olopatadine (Patanase)
	Oral 2nd-generation	Cetirizine (Zyrtec[b,c]) Desloratadine (Clarinex[b]) Fexofenadine (Allegra[a,c]) Levocetirizine (Xyzal[b]) Loratadine (Claritin[a,c])
Topical corticosteroid or antihistamine		Azelastine or Fluticasone (Dymista)
Leukotriene modifiers		Montelukast (Singulair[b])
Mast cell stabilizers		Cromolyn (NasalCrom[a,c])
Anticholinergics		Ipratropium (Atrovent)
Topical decongestants		Oxymetazoline (Afrin[c])

[a] Approved for age 2 years and older.
[b] Approved for age 6 months and older.
[c] Available over-the-counter.

Data from Liang J, Smith D, Lin S. Chapter 28: Allergic rhinitis. In: Parikh S, ed. Pediatric otolaryngology - head and neck surgery: clinical reference guide, 1st edition. San Diego, CA: Plural Publishing, Inc.; 2014:247–263; and Tharpe CA, Kemp SF. Pediatric allergic rhinitis. Immunol Allergy Clin North Am 2015;35(1):185–198.

used. There have been some reports of mood disturbance; however, the data have not shown a significant difference from placebo.[20] Other less commonly used intranasal therapies include cromolyn, a mast cell stabilizer that may be used as a preventative measure; ipratropium, an anticholinergic that can sometimes be helpful for rhinorrhea; and oxymetazoline, a decongestant used judiciously to avoid rebound effects.[17]

Allergen immunotherapy

Allergen immunotherapy is generally indicated if conventional pharmacotherapy fails or is not an option. The general principle is that the administration of small but increasing amounts of an allergen leads to a downregulation of the immune response. On a pathophysiologic level, this correlates with a shift from a T_H2 to type 1 T helper (T_H1) immune response, a decline in allergen-specific responsiveness, a decrease in allergen-specific IgE, and an increase in allergen-specific IgG blocking antibodies. The result is better symptom control on exposure. The types of allergen immunotherapy currently used clinically are subcutaneous immunotherapy (SCIT), which has a long history of clinical use in the United States, and SLIT, an option more recently introduced to clinical practice.[14]

In SLIT, the allergen extract is placed under the tongue and allowed to locally absorb over a few minutes and then is spit out or swallowed. The theoretic advantage of SLIT is that oral mucosa has a relatively high proportion of tolerogenic myeloid dendritic cells relative to inflammatory cells, suggesting that administration here would optimize efficacy and minimize adverse effects. Other advantages, particularly in the pediatric population, are that administration does not require an office visit and may be better tolerated because it avoids a painful injection. Disadvantages in the pediatric population, however, include volume constraints in the sublingual space and extract potency limitations.

SLIT is available in both aqueous and tablet forms. Currently, the US Food and Drug Administration has not approved the use of the aqueous form for the treatment of AR in either adults or children. It has approved the use of 4 tablet types, ragweed (Ragwitek), timothy grass (Oralair), grass mix (Grastek), and dust mite (Odactra). Only Oralair and Grastek are approved for the pediatric population, those older than the ages of 5 and 10 years, respectively. Therapy is initiated at least 12 and 16 weeks before the start of pollen season for Oralair and Grastek, respectively, and then continued throughout the season for best results. It is recommended that the initial dose be done in the clinic and that individuals should be monitored for 30 minutes after administration. Subsequent therapy relies on compliance at home. It is currently recommended that if more than 7 days of treatment are missed, reinitiation in the clinic should be performed. An epinephrine autoinjector should also be given. SLIT is contraindicated in children with severe asthma, eosinophilic esophagitis, and if taking a beta blocker that cannot be discontinued.[16]

The effectiveness of SLIT is an area of active investigation. The strongest data currently in support of SLIT are for grass and dust mite allergens. Multiple randomized double-blinded placebo-controlled trials have looked at the efficacy of grass pollen SLIT in the pediatric population, and nearly all of them have shown improved symptom burden and medication use.[21–23] Because SLIT is expensive, a recent literature review emphasizes the importance of patient selection and consideration of factors such as the severity of AR, intensity of allergen exposure, and the relationship of symptoms to allergen exposure confirming a true allergy.[24] Compared with grass pollen SLIT, there are much fewer data evaluating the efficacy of dust mite SLIT in the pediatric population, with most studies focused on the adult population and with primary endpoints related to asthma rather than AR. More recently, randomized double-blinded placebo-controlled trials have been published for younger children, with a large trial demonstrating improved symptom burden and medication use with dust mite SLIT.[25,26]

A 2013 systematic review found a moderate strength of evidence that SLIT improves rhinitis and conjunctivitis symptoms.[27] Studies have also demonstrated sustained benefit after SLIT has been discontinued.[6] Regarding its safety profile, local side effects have been commonly reported but there have been no reported severe systemic reactions such as anaphylaxis.[16] There are limited data comparing SLIT and SCIT, and a 2013 meta-analysis combining systematic reviews could not conclude superiority of either in effectiveness or safety.[28] The biggest challenge to drawing conclusions from the current data is its heterogeneity. There are differences in the type of allergens tested, study methodology, and outcome measures, among others. Future research will need to be more standardized to draw meaningful conclusions.

SUMMARY

Food allergy and AR are childhood diseases of special relevance to the pediatric otolaryngologist. Food allergy has been increasing in prevalence over the past couple decades. Much of the diagnosis of food allergy can be made on history alone, and strict avoidance is the mainstay of treatment. Promising investigations are underway on prevention strategies, including whether early introduction of allergen-containing foods is effective, which could dramatically impact the current practice guidelines.

AR is commonly encountered in pediatric otolaryngology. There are a variety of pharmacotherapies currently available, with multiple formulations available within each class, and it is important for the pediatric otolaryngologist to be up-to-date on which are approved for younger children and their over-the-counter availability. If pharmacotherapy fails or is not an option, allergen immunotherapy is a proven treatment option. The effectiveness and safety of the sublingual route is currently an intense area of investigation, given its obvious advantages of home administration and less painful delivery method.

REFERENCES

1. Boyce JA, Assa'ad A, Burks AW, et al. Guidelines for the diagnosis and management of food allergy in the United States: Summary of the NIAID-sponsored expert panel report. J Allergy Clin Immunol 2010;126(6):1105–18.
2. Sicherer SH, Sampson HA. Food allergy: a review and update on epidemiology, pathogenesis, diagnosis, prevention, and management. J Allergy Clin Immunol 2018;141(1):41–58.
3. Waserman S, Watson W. Food allergy. Allergy Asthma Clin Immunol 2011;7(Suppl 1):S7.
4. Gupta RS, Walkner MM, Greenhawt M, et al. Food allergy sensitization and presentation in siblings of food allergic children. J Allergy Clin Immunol Pract 2016; 4(5):956–62.
5. Muraro A, Dreborg S, Halken S, et al. Dietary prevention of allergic diseases in infants and small children. Part II. Evaluation of methods in allergy prevention studies and sensitization markers. Definitions and diagnostic criteria of allergic diseases. Pediatr Allergy Immunol 2004;15(3):196–205.
6. Ciccolini A, French S, Tenn M, et al. Update in pediatric allergy. In: Piteau S, editor. Update in pediatrics. 1st edition. Basel (Switzerland): Springer; 2018. p. 39–59.
7. Sampson HA, O'Mahony L, Burks AW, et al. Mechanisms of food allergy. J Allergy Clin Immunol 2018;141(1):11–9.
8. Lambert R, Grimshaw KEC, Ellis B, et al. Evidence that eating baked egg or milk influences egg or milk allergy resolution: a systematic review. Clin Exp Allergy 2017;47(6):829–37.
9. Du Toit G, Roberts G, Sayre PH, et al. Randomized trial of peanut consumption in infants at risk for peanut allergy. N Engl J Med 2015;372(9):803–13.
10. Togias A, Cooper SF, Acebal ML, et al. Addendum guidelines for the prevention of peanut allergy in the united states: Summary of the national institute of allergy and infectious diseases-sponsored expert panel. J Acad Nutr Diet 2017;117(5):788–93.
11. Perkin MR, Logan K, Tseng A, et al. Randomized trial of introduction of allergenic foods in breast-fed infants. N Engl J Med 2016;374(18):1733–43.
12. Sampath V, Sindher SB, Zhang W, et al. New treatment directions in food allergy. Ann Allergy Asthma Immunol 2018;120(3):254–62.
13. Dantzer JA, Wood RA. Next-generation approaches for the treatment of food allergy. Curr Allergy Asthma Rep 2019;19(1):5.
14. Liang J, Smith D, Lin S. Chapter 28: allergic rhinitis. In: Parikh S, editor. Pediatric otolaryngology - head and neck surgery: clinical reference guide. 1st edition. San Diego (CA): Plural Publishing, Inc.; 2014. p. 247–63.
15. Wallace DV, Dykewicz MS, Bernstein DI, et al. The diagnosis and management of rhinitis: an updated practice parameter. J Allergy Clin Immunol 2008;122(2 Suppl):1.

16. Mener DJ, Lin SY. Sublingual immunotherapy in children. Curr Otorhinolaryngol Rep 2015;3(3):155–61.
17. Tharpe CA, Kemp SF. Pediatric allergic rhinitis. Immunol Allergy Clin North Am 2015;35(1):185–98.
18. Arroyave WD, Rabito FA, Carlson JC, et al. Impermeable dust mite covers in the primary and tertiary prevention of allergic disease: a meta-analysis. Ann Allergy Asthma Immunol 2014;112(3):237–48.
19. Nurmatov U, van Schayck CP, Hurwitz B, et al. House dust mite avoidance measures for perennial allergic rhinitis: An updated cochrane systematic review. Allergy 2012;67(2):158–65.
20. Philip G, Hustad CM, Malice MP, et al. Analysis of behavior-related adverse experiences in clinical trials of montelukast. J Allergy Clin Immunol 2009;124(4):706.e8.
21. Halken S, Agertoft L, Seidenberg J, et al. Five-grass pollen 300IR SLIT tablets: efficacy and safety in children and adolescents. Pediatr Allergy Immunol 2010;21(6):970–6.
22. Wahn U, Tabar A, Kuna P, et al. Efficacy and safety of 5-grass-pollen sublingual immunotherapy tablets in pediatric allergic rhinoconjunctivitis. J Allergy Clin Immunol 2009;123(1):166.e3.
23. Blaiss M, Maloney J, Nolte H, et al. Efficacy and safety of timothy grass allergy immunotherapy tablets in North American children and adolescents. J Allergy Clin Immunol 2011;127(1):4.
24. Poddighe D, Licari A, Caimmi S, et al. Sublingual immunotherapy for pediatric allergic rhinitis: the clinical evidence. World J Clin Pediatr 2016;5(1):47–56.
25. Shao J, Cui YX, Zheng YF, et al. Efficacy and safety of sublingual immunotherapy in children aged 3-13 years with allergic rhinitis. Am J Rhinol Allergy 2014;28(2):131–9.
26. Aydogan M, Eifan AO, Keles S, et al. Sublingual immunotherapy in children with allergic rhinoconjunctivitis mono-sensitized to house-dust-mites: a double-blind-placebo-controlled randomised trial. Respir Med 2013;107(9):1322–9.
27. Kim JM, Lin SY, Suarez-Cuervo C, et al. Allergen-specific immunotherapy for pediatric asthma and rhinoconjunctivitis: a systematic review. Pediatrics 2013;131(6):1155–67.
28. Dretzke J, Meadows A, Novielli N, et al. Subcutaneous and sublingual immunotherapy for seasonal allergic rhinitis: a systematic review and indirect comparison. J Allergy Clin Immunol 2013;131(5):1361–6.

Innovations in Endonasal Sinus Surgery in Children

Sophie G. Shay, MD[a], Taher Valika, MD[b], Robert Chun, MD[a,*],
Jeffrey Rastatter, MD[b,*]

KEYWORDS

- Balloon sinuplasty • Skull base • Anesthesia • Sinus computed tomography
- Rhinosinusitis • Subperiosteal abscess

KEY POINTS

- In young children with chronic rhinosinusitis, the first-line surgical treatment is still adenoidectomy.
- Functional endoscopic sinus surgery (FESS) is still the first-line surgical treatment for refractory pediatric rhinosinusitis following adenoidectomy.
- Balloon sinus dilation may have a role in chronic rhinosinusitis management in children; however, the advantages and accuracy of dilation in children remain to be determined.
- Although FESS is largely safe in children, FESS performed on inpatients and in urgent/emergent settings may be associated with increased morbidity and mortality.
- When indicated, FESS has gained increasing acceptance as a first-line approach for management of orbital and intracranial complications of acute bacterial rhinosinusitis.

INTRODUCTION

Advances in endoscopic sinus surgery have allowed for successful management of many conditions with improved patient outcomes. Pediatric endonasal sinus surgery includes management of choanal atresia, acute and/or chronic rhinosinusitis, skull base surgery, and tumor removal. Although the management and care for pediatric chronic rhinosinusitis have remained relatively unchanged, there have been many advances in new tools and procedures for endonasal sinus surgery in children. This article discusses choanal atresia surgery, management of acute and chronic pediatric rhinosinusitis, and new understanding about the perioperative concerns in children. Additionally, the article discusses recent advances in skull base surgery and tumor removal.

Disclosure Statement: The authors have nothing to disclose.
[a] Medical College of Wisconsin, 9000 West Wisconsin Avenue, ENT Offices Suite 540, Milwaukee, WI 53226, USA; [b] Northwestern University, Ann & Robert H. Lurie Children's Hospital of Chicago, 225 East Chicago Avenue, Box 40, Chicago, IL 60611, USA
* Corresponding authors.
E-mail addresses: Rchun@mcw.edu (R.C.); jrastatter@luriechildrens.org (J.R.)

Otolaryngol Clin N Am 52 (2019) 875–890
https://doi.org/10.1016/j.otc.2019.06.003
0030-6665/19/© 2019 Elsevier Inc. All rights reserved.

CHOANAL ATRESIA

Choanal atresia (CA) is a congenital anomaly in which at least posterior nasal cavities fails to canalize, resulting in nasal obstruction. This occurs in 1 case out of 5000 to 8000 live births, with a female-to-male preponderance of 2:1.[1,2] The underlying pathophysiology is still not clearly understood. The persistence of the buccopharyngeal membrane, failure of the bucconasal membrane to involute, and misdirection of neural crest cell migration are all potential causes resulting in choanal atresia.[3] Other proposed theories include errors in vitamin A metabolism and prenatal use of thionamides. The resulting atresia can be either bony (30%) or mixed membranous-bony (70%).[4]

Unilateral CA accounts for 75% of patients, whereas bilateral CA is seen in 25% of patients.[3] The right choana is more readily affected. Fifty percent of patients with CA may have an associated syndrome (CHARGE, Treacher-Collins).[1,2] Surgical intervention to correct bilateral atresia requires early intervention, as newborns are obligatory nasal breathers. Prompt intervention can also resolve any feeding disruption resultant from CA-associated incoordination of the newborn "suck, swallow, breathe" pattern.[5]

Surgical Evaluation and Management

The goal of any CA repair is to restore the function of the nasal passage. The ideal procedure allows for a safe and effective procedure with minimal risk to adjacent critical structures. Minimizing length of stay is also important, although this can be significantly affected by comorbidities, which are not uncommon in patients with CA. For example, patients with CHARGE syndrome may have associated cardiac disease that requires prolonged hospitalization. Traditionally, the standard technique for CA repair was the transpalatal approach. This approach is associated with increased injury to the palatal mucosa and resulting wound healing complications.[6,7] More recently, an endoscopic, transnasal approach has become the preferred procedure for many CA surgeons.[8] The endoscopic approach allows use of the normal nasal passageway and allows better visualization of the surgical bed. Continuing advancements with endoscopic instrumentation have allowed for refinements in technique, further establishing the endoscopic endonasal technique as the gold standard for CA repair.

Several factors are critical in defining a successful outcome in CA surgery. Individuals have defined success rates based on nasal patency and the need for revision surgery.[1] The factors that influence the outcomes of surgical success in CA are numerous.

Age/Sex/Weight

Bilateral CA repair is often undertaken in the neonatal period, sometimes as early as the first few days after birth. Studies have shown that patients undergoing surgery at less than 6 months of age have an increased probability of requiring revision surgery. Surgeries in these young patients are also associated with a longer hospital stay.[1] These young patients often have low weights, and being under 5 kg at the time of surgery has been shown to be associated with requiring more revision procedures, longer hospital stays, and an overall higher risk of recurrent stenosis and failure to maintain nasal patency.[1,5,9,10] There are no differences in outcomes between boys and girls.[1]

Unilateral/Bilateral

Bilateral CA versus unilateral CA results in significantly different outcomes. Patients with bilateral atresia require more surgical procedures and have longer hospital stays.

Additionally, patients with bilateral atresia have less odds of successful repair compared to patients with unilateral atresia.[1,7] The surgical techniques vary for bony or membranous atresia, with the latter requiring less complex intervention at times. Despite this, the odds for successful nasal patency show no difference in final outcome.

Syndromes

The presence of bilateral CA demands a work-up for a possible underlying abnormality or syndrome. In nearly 50% of patients with bilateral CA, there is either an underlying syndrome or other abnormality.[1,2,8,9] Syndromes commonly with bilateral CA include CHARGE, Crouzon, or Treacher-Collins. Other congenital associations include heart disease, laryngomalacia, cleft palate, laryngeal cleft, and tracheoesophageal fistula. Renal ultrasounds and cardiac echo should be considered in patients with CA prior to surgical intervention. Despite syndromic children requiring further operations to obtain nasal patency, the potential for ultimately achieving stable and prolonged choanal patency remains the same as for nonsyndromic children.[2,7,9]

Surgical Approach and Therapies

Endoscopic repair is currently the gold standard in management of CA. There is a variety of powered instrumentation available to assist with this approach, including the microdebrider, drill, CO_2 laser, and balloons for dilation.[11–13] Much debate exists on the various techniques of the initial surgery including mucosal flaps, stenting, and use of mitomycin. No single endoscopic technique or instrument has demonstrated superior outcomes, and choices among the many instruments and subtleties in endoscopic surgical technique often come down to surgeon preference.[5] Postoperative care often employs the use of steroid or saline drops to allow for clearance of secretions and reduce the inflammatory burden.

The challenge of a successful endoscopic repair is preventing granulation tissue formation and resulting nasal stenosis. Adequate identification of critical landmarks is vital and thus arguably safer with use of endoscopes and image guidance. The goal is to identify the atretic plate and subsequently the posterior nasopharynx. The surrounding bone or mucosa is removed, and functional neochoanae created. Employing tools to permit patency of this area has shown variable success.

After the neochoanae is created, ensuring prevention of granulation tissue can lead to better patency and overall outcome. Use of mucosal flaps overlying the exposed bone has been shown to have reduced granulation tissue formation and better nasal patency.[1,6,7,10] These flaps are based most commonly off the nasoseptal flap and can be split in 2 or 3 flaps (**Fig. 1**) to ensure bony coverage. Multiple flaps can help prevent lateral and medial stenosis and ensure patency.

Stenting of the choana postoperatively was traditionally done to allow for a functional nasal passage and prevent restenosis. The stent was classically created from an endotracheal tube and secured to the septum. Despite the popular use of stents among many surgeons, no difference has been shown in the final outcome or number of revision procedures with the use of stenting.[1,13–15] In recent years, the focus of research has shifted to the use of steroid-eluting stents (**Fig. 2**). Currently, these stents are not approved by the US Food and Drug Administration (FDA) for use in the pediatric population. The stents contain 370 µg of mometasone furoate and allow for delivery of the steroid locally over 30 days and then dissolve. The literature is sparse, but the stents have been shown to result in less granulation tissue formation.[10,14,15]

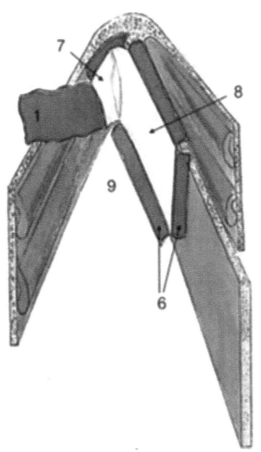

Fig. 1. Representation of various surgical flaps utilized in correcting the atretic plate. (1) Main septal flap. (6) Secondary flaps. (7) Medial pterygoid. (8) vomer. (9) Floor of right nostril. (*From* Brihaye P, Delpierre I, De Villé A, Johansson A-B, Biarent D, Mansbach A-L. Comprehensive management of congenital choanal atresia. *International journal of pediatric otorhinolaryngology.* 2017;98:9–18; with permission.)

Mitomycin functions by altering the function of fibroblasts and thus results in decreased scar tissue formation. Classically, it is used in revision CA repair to potentially prevent further surgical interventions.[1,16] Unfortunately, the data are unclear, and whether a significant benefit exists is difficult to ascertain. No long-term prospective study exists in demonstrating its efficacy and final outcomes.

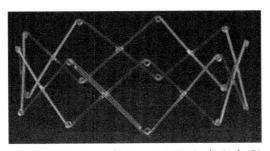

Fig. 2. Steroid-eluting stent. (*Courtesy of* Intersect ENT, Menlo Park, CA; with permission.)

ACUTE AND CHRONIC RHINOSINUSITIS
Management of Pediatric Chronic Rhinosinusitis

The most recent clinical consensus statement on pediatric chronic rhinosinusitis (PCRS) defined it is at least 90 continuous days of 2 or more symptoms of purulent rhinorrhea, nasal obstruction, facial pressure/pain, or cough and either endoscopic signs of mucosal edema, purulent drainage, or nasal polyposis and/or computed tomography (CT) scan changes showing mucosal changes within the osteomeatal complex and/or sinuses in a pediatric patient.[17] It is important to emphasize that management of pediatric nasal polyposis with or without cystic fibrosis is different than PCRS and outside the scope of this article. Prior to consideration for surgical management of PCRS, initiation of medical management including nasal irrigation, topical nasal steroid, and 10 to 20 days of culture-directed antibiotics, is recommended.

For children younger than 12 years of age who fail medical management, adenoidectomy without tonsillectomy is an effective first-line surgical procedure for PCRS, with a beneficial effect independent from FESS. It is the authors' opinion that CT of the sinuses should only be considered in the routine pediatric patient in consideration for FESS after failure of medical management and adenoidectomy. In a meta-analysis of 1301 pediatric patients, FESS was found to be an effective treatment for PCRS with a low complication rate of 1.4% and improved quality of life.[18,19] Postsurgical operative debridement is not essential for successful treatment of PCRS. Although there were previous concerns regarding the effects of FESS on midface growth in children, there is an overall lack of evidence that FESS causes a clinically significant change in facial growth in children, and it is generally viewed as safe to perform in children.[20]

Role of Balloon Sinuplasty

Balloon sinuplasty (BCS) as a tool has been shown to be effective in children who have failed adenoidectomy in 81% of a cohort of 26 children.[21] In another study of 50 children with BCS, with and without concomitant other procedures like turbinate coblation or adenoidectomy, 92% were shown to have significant improvement of the Sinus and Nasal Quality of Life Survey up to 1 year following the procedure.[22] In a prospective, randomized study looking at adenoidectomy with BCS or maxillary sinus irrigation via inferior metal puncture, both groups had significant improvement of quality of life, but BCS did not provide additional improvement in quality of life versus inferior metal puncture. There have been cases demonstrating the benefit of frontal balloon dilation in children with complicated frontal sinusitis with intracranial abscess to avoid the need for frontal trephination.[23] Nonetheless, there has been no study to directly compare FESS versus BCS alone for PCRS without adenoidectomy. Thus, although BCS appears to be effective, at this time it is difficult to draw conclusions on its usefulness compared with more established surgical approaches to PCRS, particularly in regard to management of maxillary PCRS.

The safety of BCS is much more well-studied in the adult population. However, even among adults, there are concerns regarding the accuracy of maxillary ostia dilation in patients, with only 62% dilating the correct maxillary ostia.[24] The accuracy of BCS in children has not been studied. Furthermore, complications can occur with adult BCS in 5.6% of cases, such as bleeding, cerebrospinal fluid CSF leak, and orbital hematoma.[25] In adults, BCS can be performed in the clinic, but in the pediatric population, this is not an option. Therefore, the clinician and family must weigh the benefit of BCS versus FESS as the treatment after the failure of adenoidectomy in PCRS.

Complications of Acute Rhinosinusitis in Children

Orbital complications

Orbital complications represent up to 91% of all complications of acute bacterial rhinosinusitis (ABRS) and are more prevalent among the pediatric population.[26] Without prompt diagnosis and treatment, orbital complications can lead to blindness, intracranial extension, cavernous sinus thrombosis, and even death. The spread of infection is often from ipsilateral acute ethmoiditis through the lamina papyracea or via hematogenous spread.[26,27]

In 1970, Chandler and colleagues classically described the severity of orbital infections (**Table 1**).[28] Chander and colleagues recognized the orbital septum as a distinct fascial plane separating the preseptal and postseptal orbital compartments, preventing lymphatic or venous spread between the two. Diagnosis and classification of an orbital complication of ABRS are usually made with the Chandler classification in conjunction with CT findings. Contrast-enhanced CT is the imaging modality of choice to evaluate acute sinusitis and suspected complications.[29] In light of concerns regarding radiation exposure, recent studies have suggested the utility of MRI to further investigate the presence of an orbital abscess in the setting of a negative CT.[30,31]

In a review of 136 patients with orbital cellulitis, Smith and colleagues reported that children older than 9 years of age, extraocular motility restriction, proptosis, and elevated intraocular pressure were more likely to require surgery.[32] For subperiosteal abscesses (SPAs), the last several decades have seen a shift in management for orbital complications of ARS, moving toward increased medical management. Traditionally, SPAs have involved *Streptococcus* species, but recently there has been a reported rise of *Streptococcus anginosus,* anaerobic bacteria, and *Staphylococcus aureus*, with potentially an 11% incidence of methicillin-resistant *Staphylococcus aureus*.[27,33,34] Garcia and Harris published a landmark, prospective study delineating criteria for selecting patients for medical management; they reported a 93.1% success rate in children under 9 years of age with small, medially based SPAs.[35] In a critical review of the literature, Coenraad and Buwalda reported that surgical drainage was warranted for nonmedial abscesses, signs of systemic infection, impaired visual acuity, or lack of improvement or worsening of symptoms after 48 to 72 hours of intravenous antibiotics.[36] In a 7-year review of 450 patients, Ryan and colleagues found that nonmedial abscesses and large medial abscesses defined as wider than 10 mm on CT were significantly more likely to require surgical drainage.[37]

Multiple recent studies have attempted to demonstrate specific CT measurements of SPA size, although there remains a clear consensus guiding size criteria for surgical management. Todman and Enzer reported that abscesses measuring less than 1250 mm³ were less likely to require surgical management, while Le and colleagues

Table 1	
Chandler classification of orbital complications	
I	Preseptal cellulitis
II	Orbital (postseptal) cellulitis
III	Subperiosteal abscess
IV	Orbital abscess
V	Cavernous sinus thrombosis

Adapted from Chandler JR, Langenbrunner DJ, Stevens ER. The pathogenesis of orbital complications in acute sinusitis. The Laryngoscope. 1970;80(9):1414–1428; with permission.

found that the cutoff of 3800 mm^3 in abscess size predicted likelihood of surgical drainage.[38,39] Finally, in a retrospective case series of SPA in 48 patients by Nation and colleagues, children with SPA volume greater than 500 mm^3 had longer inpatient admissions, increased duration of antibiotics, and higher likelihood of peripherally inserted central catheter placement.[40] Using the American College of Surgeons National Surgical Quality Improvement Program (NSQIP) database from 2012 to 2015 to evaluate the 30-day outcomes of FESS for orbital complications of pediatric ARS, Cheng and colleagues reported that although adverse events were common (61.4%), serious adverse events were rare, and overall FESS for orbital complications in children was safe.[41] Prolonged hospitalization longer than 5 days was the most common adverse event, and predicted by delayed surgical intervention (odds ratio 25.65).

Intracranial complications

Intracranial involvement is estimated to have a prevalence of approximately 3% of pediatric patients admitted for ARS.[42,43] Intracranial complications include abscess, empyema, meningitis, encephalitis, and dural sinus thrombophlebitis. The presence of acute frontal sinusitis significantly increases the risk of intracranial involvement by twentyfold, with the infection spreading directly via the frontal sinus posterior table, valveless diploic veins, or septic emboli.[23,44,45] Given the high association with frontal sinusitis, intracranial complications often occur in older children and adolescents. In a systematic review of 180 patients, Patel and colleagues reported the following frequencies of intracranial complications: subdural empyema (49%), epidural abscess (36%), cerebral abscess (21%), and meningitis (10%).[46] The most common presenting symptoms were headache, fever, nausea, and vomiting.

A high index of suspicion and prompt management are critical to preventing long-term complications. Preoperative imaging often includes both CT and MRI, although MRI tends to allow for increased visualization of the intracranial infection. Management often requires involvement of both otolaryngology and neurosurgery and a duration of intravenous antibiotics.[46] Although classically the management of acute frontal sinusitis involved trephination, these infections are increasingly successfully managed endoscopically. Kou and colleagues reported that 27% of patients underwent concurrent neurosurgical intervention with FESS, and that FESS was associated with a lower likelihood of requiring subsequent neurosurgical intervention.[47] With aggressive medical and surgical therapy, Germiller and colleagues suggested that most children and adolescents have a favorable prognosis; among 25 consecutive patients, they reported 1 mortality secondary to meningitis, and a 40% incidence of neurologic deficits, which mostly resolved within 2 months.[48] However, Gitomer and colleagues found a 46% rate of revision surgery, most commonly among patients with subdural abscesses.[49] These authors also reported a 33% rate of long-term complications, with a mean follow-up duration of 92 months. Of note, compared to pediatric patients with orbital complications of ARS, those with intracranial complications are more likely to require pediatric intensive care unit stays and have longer hospital admissions.[50] Additionally, there have been increasing reports of S anginosus-related intracranial infections, which were more likely to require neurosurgical intervention, longer duration of antibiotics, and long-term neurologic sequelae.[51]

POTT PUFFY TUMOR

Pott puffy tumor often arises from acute frontal sinusitis or trauma as an osteomyelitis of the frontal sinus anterior table with a collection of purulent fluid or granulation tissue on the forehead.[52] It often presents with headache, fever, and vomiting. In a recent review of the literature, Koltsidopoulos and colleagues described a high concurrent intracranial complication rate of 72%, and a 50% success rate of using an endoscopic surgical approach.[53] In particular, there is increasing support in the literature for using an endoscopic frontal sinusotomy over traditional external incision and drainage to manage Pott puffy tumor.[54]

PERIOPERATIVE RISK OF PEDIATRIC FUNCTIONAL ENDOSCOPIC SINUS SURGERY

Functional endoscopic sinus surgery in children has been largely established as a safe and effective procedure, with a low complication rate and successful symptomatic improvement.[55] Although there is a 2.9% incidence of minor complications following pediatric FESS, major complications have been reported at occurring between 0.08% and 0.55%.[56,57] Using the American College of Surgeons NSQIP pediatric database, Roxbury and colleagues reported that readmission and reoperation were significantly associated with urgent/emergent procedures and history of a bleeding disorder.[58] Additionally, they reported that age younger than 3 years and history of bleeding disorder were overall associated with a higher incidence of postoperative adverse events. Specifically among pediatric patients with cystic fibrosis, Tumin and colleagues concluded that aside from being more likely to have a prolonged hospital course, FESS was largely safe in this population.[59] Regarding inpatient pediatric FESS, Burton and colleagues reported a higher incidence of morbidity and mortality, at 6% and 1% respectively, with a 2.5% occurrence of respiratory complications.[60] Using the Kids' Inpatient Database (KID), these authors found that inpatient postoperative adverse events were associated with inpatient comorbidities of meningitis, leukemia, benign neoplasm, pneumonia, turbinectomy, and age.

SKULL BASE TUMORS

Skull base lesions in the pediatric population encompass a variety of pathologies. Diagnosis of these lesions requires through understanding of skull base anatomy, presenting symptoms, and disease-specific characteristics. Management of these lesions is often best accomplished with a multidisciplinary approach. Advances in instrumentation have allowed for the improved ability for endoscopic endonasal management. The following sections aim to highlight some of the more commonly encountered skull base lesions in the pediatric population, keeping in mind that pediatric skull base lesions in general are rare. Selected lesions are briefly discussed here, and focus is dedicated to the varied surgical techniques for management. Management of these lesions is particularly illustrative of advanced pediatric sinus surgery techniques and instrumentation.

Congenital Midline Nasal Mass

Midline nasal lesions can occur anywhere from the tip of the nose to the glabella. The most common lesion is a dermoid cyst, followed by a glioma or oncephalocele.[61] The underlying etiology of these lesions is thought to be a developmental failure of separation of the dural diverticulum through the foramen cecum from the overlying skin.[62] As such, these lesions can include an intracranial component in up to 50% of cases.[63,64] CT and MRI can be complementary and help define the diagnosis and plan management (**Fig. 3**).

The surgical approach is decided based on the location and extent of the lesion. Approaches for management include an external approach with pit resection, open rhinoplasty, endoscopy, or craniotomy. Traditionally, an open technique is favored over an endoscopic approach because of the lack of necessary endoscopic instrumentation. The goal of surgery is to recreate the separation between the cranial and

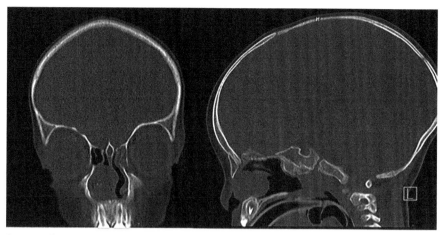

Fig. 3. Right intranasal mass with associated calcification. A thin stalk of tissue extending to the region of the foramen cecum (anterior cranial fossa) is visualized in the sagittal view. This is consistent with a nasal glioma.

sinonasal cavities and remove the underlying lesion. This can be accomplished more easily with an open approach. The ability to successfully dissect a tract can be difficult using endoscopic instrumentation. Newer advances in open excision have led to shorter hospital stays and negligible recurrence rates.[61]

Juvenile Nasopharyngeal Angiofibroma

Juvenile nasopharyngeal angiofibromas (JNAs) are benign, vascular tumors that arise in the region of the sphenopalatine foramen (**Fig. 4**). These lesions have classic growth patterns in the sinonasal cavity.[65] Biopsy should be avoided because of the highly vascular nature of these lesions.

Management is primarily surgical, with utilization of preoperative embolization to limit intraoperative blood loss. An endoscopic approach is practical for a majority of these lesions.[66] Utilization of a coblator provides desiccation and hemostasis,

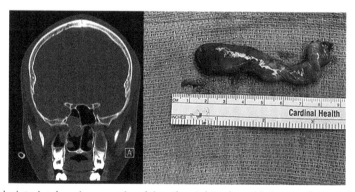

Fig. 4. Lobulated enhancing mass involving the right sphenoid sinus and extending inferiorly to the level of the superior nasopharynx, consistent with juvenile nasopharyngeal angiofibroma. The lesion was resected en bloc with its primary attachment in the pterygopalatine fossa.

although microdebrider may be just as useful. For lesions with extension intracranially or for cases in which complete resection may not be possible, radiation therapy is an option. Consideration for the long-term effects of radiation exposure should be thoughtfully considered in these patients. When experienced surgical teams are utilized, radiation exposure can be avoided in the majority of patients with JNAs.

Sellar/Parasellar Lesions

A craniopharyngioma is the most common pediatric benign tumor in the sellar region (**Fig. 5**). These tumors arise from the epithelial remnants of Rathke pouch, and as such, growth of these lesions can result in significant morbidity causing endocrinopathies and vision changes.

Complete resection is often challenging, and recurrence is a viable risk, even years after treatment.[67] Imaging with MRI is mainstay in defining the lesion and for surgical planning. CT scan can be complementary, particularly if an endoscopic endonasal approach is being planned. Endoscopic resection is possible for most smaller lesions and even many larger lesions (**Fig. 6**). The limits of endoscopic resection are based on the field of view and feasibility of instrumentation. As such, lesions with superior or lateral extension are less likely amenable to complete resection via an endoscopic approach. An open approach, classically via a pterional craniotomy, can be used to access these areas with more ease. Endoscopic and open approaches can also be complementary, and not infrequently both techniques are used in a single patient. Debulking and subtotal resection followed by radiation therapy are options for larger lesions involving cranial nerves or the hypothalamus that are not amenable to complete resection.

The Rathke cleft cyst is a benign cystic lesion that also arises in the region of the anterior pituitary.[68] These lesions are classically slow growing and thus can be followed conservatively. Surgical intervention is undertaken if symptomatic (eg, central nervous system [CNS] changes, vision loss, or endocrinopathy). An endoscopic approach is usually feasible for cyst drainage and resolution of symptoms.

Chordoma

Chordomas are locally aggressive tumors and arise from the embryologic notochord (**Fig. 7**). They most commonly present in the clival region with surrounding osseous destruction. Metastatic disease is present in up to 20% of cases.[69]

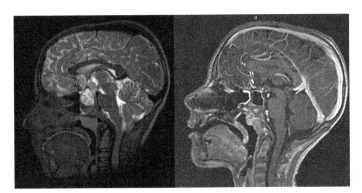

Fig. 5. Heterogeneous enhancing mass centered within the suprasellar cistern, consistent with craniopharyngioma. Postsurgical MRI completed reveals complete resection of lesion, with nasoseptal flap in place over the resulting skull base defect.

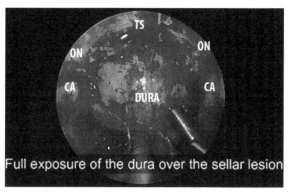

Full exposure of the dura over the sellar lesion

Fig. 6. Exposure of the skull base and sella. The critical landmarks must be well delineated to ensure safety of the patient. CA, internal carotid artery; ON, optic nerve; TS, tuberculum sellae.

An endoscopic approach is a feasible option for complete resection of smaller lesions or partial resection of larger lesions. Complete resection in even smaller lesions can be challenging because of the proximity of lesions to critical CNS structures (eg, the brainstem or basilar artery). Recurrence is frustratingly common with chordomas, even after an apparent complete resection. Multiple procedures, both endoscopic endonasal and open via various craniotomy approaches, may be necessary to eradicate disease. The need for secondary tissue (eg, free vascularized tissue flap, fascia lata, or fat) may be necessary during repair because of the extent of tissue debrided and CSF leak. Radiation and chemotherapy can also help manage residual, recurrent, or metastatic disease.

Fibrous Dysplasia

Fibrous dysplasia is characterized by abnormal growth of fibrous tissue in the place of normal bone (**Fig. 8**). These areas of abnormal growth can occur in multiple locations at the skull base.[70] The expansile nature of this lesion can result in neurovascular compromise, notably optic nerve compression with vision loss or functional neuropathies.[71]

Management is undertaken in situations with functional compromise; otherwise, observation is recommended. Depending on location of lesion, either open or endoscopic approaches are viable options.[72] With either approach, the goals of surgery

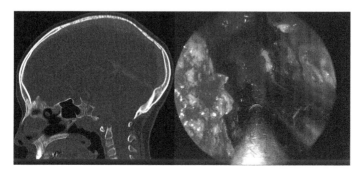

Fig. 7. Large destructive, lytic lesion centered in the inferior aspect of the clivus extending into the posterior fossa, skull base, upper cervical spinal canal, and prevertebral space with focal erosion, consistent with a chordoma. Endoscopic view of the clival lesion.

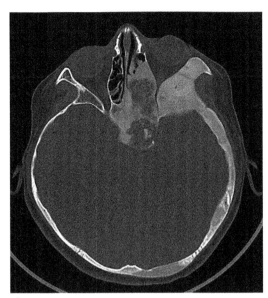

Fig. 8. Axial CT scan revealing multifocal expansile lesions of the anterior skull base, sinonasal cavity, temporal, and parietal bones, consistent with fibrous dysplasia.

should be carefully defined preoperatively. Often the goal is to decompress nerves that are compressed and functionally impaired, particularly when optic nerve compression is leading to visual changes.

Optic nerve decompression is often amenable to an endonasal approach in the hands of experienced surgical teams. Use of image-guidance navigation software is vital because of the aberrant anatomy faced. A combination of drills, microdebrider, and osteotomes can allow for successful debulking via the endonasal approach.

Particularly bulky disease can lead to cosmetic deformities. Surgical indications to address cosmetic deformities with fibrous dysplasia are controversial. Many prefer to address the cosmetic deformities via an open approach, typically in later teenage years when the disease is characteristically less active. This can include use of drills and osteotomes to reshape the normal contour of the facial skeleton. The goal of surgery for fibrous dysplasia is almost never complete excision.

SUMMARY

Advances in endoscopic skull base surgery have opened the door to treat conditions once not manageable through an endoscopic approach. These advances have improved disease management and patient outcomes. Choanal atresia repair, management of pediatric acute and chronic rhinosinusitis, and endonasal skull base procedures have all benefited greatly from advances in endoscopic techniques. Data obtained from multiple centers of excellence have provided invaluable information in advancing the field. Thoughtful consideration of these improvements during the surgical planning process can provide patients the means necessary to ensure a successful outcome.

REFERENCES

1. Moreddu E, Rossi M-E, Nicollas R, et al. Prognostic factors and management of patients with choanal atresia. J Pediatr 2019;204:234–9.e1.

2. Harris J, Robert E, Källén B. Epidemiology of choanal atresia with special reference to the CHARGE association. Pediatrics 1997;99(3):363–7.

3. Patel VA, Carr MM. Transnasal repair of congenital choanal atresia. Oper Tech Otolaryngol Head Neck Surg 2018;29(2):77–82.

4. Brown OE, Pownell P, Manning SC. Choanal atresia. Laryngoscope 1996;106(1): 97–101.

5. Brihaye P, Delpierre I, De Villé A, et al. Comprehensive management of congenital choanal atresia. Int J Pediatr Otorhinolaryngol 2017;98:9–18.

6. Gulşen S, Baysal E, Celenk F, et al. Treatment of congenital choanal atresia via transnasal endoscopic method. J Craniofac Surg 2017;28(2):338–42.

7. Uzomefuna V, Glynn F, Al-Omari B, et al. Transnasal endoscopic repair of choanal atresia in a tertiary care centre: a review of outcomes. Int J Pediatr Otorhinolaryngol 2012;76(5):613–7.

8. Khafagy YW. Endoscopic repair of bilateral congenital choanal atresia. Laryngoscope 2002;112(2):316–9.

9. Eladl HM, Khafagy YW. Endoscopic bilateral congenital choanal atresia repair of 112 cases, evolving concept and technical experience. Int J Pediatr Otorhinolaryngol 2016;85:40–5.

10. Rodríguez H, Cuestas G, Passali D. A 20-year experience in microsurgical treatment of choanal atresia. Acta Otorrinolaringol Esp 2014;65(2):85–92.

11. Bedwell J, Shah RK, Bauman N, et al. Balloon dilation for management of choanal atresia and stenosis. Int J Pediatr Otorhinolaryngol 2011;75(12):1515–8.

12. Riepl R, Scheithauer M, Hoffmann TK, et al. Transnasal endoscopic treatment of bilateral choanal atresia in newborns using balloon dilatation: own results and review of literature. Int J Pediatr Otorhinolaryngol 2014;78(3):459–64.

13. Tzifa KT, Skinner DW. Endoscopic repair of unilateral choanal atresia with the KTP laser: a one stage procedure. J Laryngol Otol 2001;115(4):286–8.

14. Abbeele TVD, François M, Narcy P. Transnasal endoscopic treatment of choanal atresia without prolonged stenting. Arch Otolaryngol Head Neck Surg 2002; 128(8):936–40.

15. Schoem SR. Transnasal endoscopic repair of choanal atresia: why stent? Otolaryngol Head Neck Surg 2004;131(4):362–6.

16. Prasad M, Ward RF, April MM, et al. Topical mitomycin as an adjunct to choanal atresia repair. Arch Otolaryngol Head Neck Surg 2002;128(4):398–400.

17. Brietzke SE, Shin JJ, Choi S, et al. Clinical consensus statement: pediatric chronic rhinosinusitis. Otolaryngol Head Neck Surg 2014;151(4):542–53.

18. Vlastarakos PV, Fetta M, Segas JV, et al. Functional endoscopic sinus surgery improves sinus-related symptoms and quality of life in children with chronic rhinosinusitis: a systematic analysis and meta-analysis of published interventional studies. Clin Pediatr 2013;52(12):1091–7.

19. Makary CA, Ramadan HH. The role of sinus surgery in children. Laryngoscope 2013;123(6):1348–52.

20. Bothwell MR, Piccirillo JF, Lusk RP, et al. Long-term outcome of facial growth after functional endoscopic sinus surgery. Otolaryngol Head Neck Surg 2002;126(6): 628–34.

21. Ramadan HH, Bueller H, Hester ST, et al. Sinus balloon catheter dilation after adenoidectomy failure for children with chronic rhinosinusitis. Arch Otolaryngol Head Neck Surg 2012;138(7):635–7.

22. Soler ZM, Rosenbloom JS, Skarada D, et al. Prospective, multicenter evaluation of balloon sinus dilation for treatment of pediatric chronic rhinosinusitis. Int Forum Allergy Rhinol 2017;7(3):221–9.

23. Roland LT, Wineland AM, Leonard DS. Balloon frontal sinuplasty for intracranial abscess in a pediatric acute sinusitis patient. Int J Pediatr Otorhinolaryngol 2015;79(3):432–4.

24. Jensen BT, Holbrook EH, Chen PG, et al. The intraoperative accuracy of maxillary balloon dilation: a blinded trial. Int Forum Allergy Rhinol 2019;9(5):452–7.

25. Chaaban MR, Rana N, Baillargeon J, et al. Outcomes and complications of balloon and conventional functional endoscopic sinus surgery. Am J Rhinol Allergy 2018;32(5):388–96.

26. Oxford LE, McClay J. Complications of acute sinusitis in children. Otolaryngol Head Neck Surg 2005;133(1):32–7.

27. Coudert A, Ayari-Khalfallah S, Suy P, et al. Microbiology and antibiotic therapy of subperiosteal orbital abscess in children with acute ethmoiditis. Int J Pediatr Otorhinolaryngol 2018;106:91–5.

28. Chandler JR, Langenbrunner DJ, Stevens ER. The pathogenesis of orbital complications in acute sinusitis. Laryngoscope 1970;80(9):1414–28.

29. Bedwell J, Bauman NM. Management of pediatric orbital cellulitis and abscess. Curr Opin Otolaryngol Head Neck Surg 2011;19(6):467–73.

30. McIntosh D, Mahadevan M. Failure of contrast enhanced computed tomography scans to identify an orbital abscess. The benefit of magnetic resonance imaging. J Laryngol Otol 2008;122(6):639–40.

31. Sepahdari AR, Aakalu VK, Kapur R, et al. MRI of orbital cellulitis and orbital abscess: the role of diffusion-weighted imaging. AJR Am J Roentgenol 2009;193(3): W244–50.

32. Smith JM, Bratton EM, DeWitt P, et al. Predicting the need for surgical intervention in pediatric orbital cellulitis. Am J Ophthalmol 2014;158(2):387–94.e1.

33. Hamill CS, Sykes KJ, Harrison CJ, et al. Infection rates of MRSA in complicated pediatric rhinosinusitis: An up to date review. Int J Pediatr Otorhinolaryngol 2018; 104:79–83.

34. Mulvey CL, Kiell EP, Rizzi MD, et al. The microbiology of complicated acute sinusitis among pediatric patients: a case series. Otolaryngol Head Neck Surg 2018; 160(4):712–9.

35. Garcia GH, Harris GJ. Criteria for nonsurgical management of subperiosteal abscess of the orbit: analysis of outcomes 1988-1998. Ophthalmology 2000;107(8): 1454–6 [discussion: 1457–8].

36. Coenraad S, Buwalda J. Surgical or medical management of subperiosteal orbital abscess in children: a critical appraisal of the literature. Rhinology 2009; 47(1):18–23.

37. Ryan JT, Preciado DA, Bauman N, et al. Management of pediatric orbital cellulitis in patients with radiographic findings of subperiosteal abscess. Otolaryngol Head Neck Surg 2009;140(6):907–11.

38. Todman MS, Enzer YR. Medical management versus surgical intervention of pediatric orbital cellulitis: the importance of subperiosteal abscess volume as a new criterion. Ophthalmic Plast Reconstr Surg 2011;27(4):255–9.

39. Le TD, Liu ES, Adatia FA, et al. The effect of adding orbital computed tomography findings to the Chandler criteria for classifying pediatric orbital cellulitis in predicting which patients will require surgical intervention. J AAPOS 2014;18(3):271–7.

40. Nation J, Lopez A, Grover N, et al. Management of large-volume subperiosteal abscesses of the orbit: medical vs surgical outcomes. Otolaryngol Head Neck Surg 2017;157(5):891–7.

41. Cheng J, Liu B, Farjat AE, et al. Adverse events in endoscopic sinus surgery for infectious orbital complications of sinusitis: 30-day NSQIP pediatric outcomes. Otolaryngol Head Neck Surg 2017;157(4):716–21.

42. Clayman GL, Adams GL, Paugh DR, et al. Intracranial complications of paranasal sinusitis: a combined institutional review. Laryngoscope 1991;101(3):234–9.

43. Lerner DN, Choi SS, Zalzal GH, et al. Intracranial complications of sinusitis in childhood. Ann Otol Rhinol Laryngol 1995;104(4 Pt 1):288–93.

44. Hakim HE, Malik AC, Aronyk K, et al. The prevalence of intracranial complications in pediatric frontal sinusitis. Int J Pediatr Otorhinolaryngol 2006;70(8):1383–7.

45. Altman KW, Austin MB, Tom LW, et al. Complications of frontal sinusitis in adolescents: case presentations and treatment options. Int J Pediatr Otorhinolaryngol 1997;41(1):9–20.

46. Patel NA, Garber D, Hu S, et al. Systematic review and case report: intracranial complications of pediatric sinusitis. Int J Pediatr Otorhinolaryngol 2016;86: 200–12.

47. Kou YF, Killeen D, Whittemore B, et al. Intracranial complications of acute sinusitis in children: the role of endoscopic sinus surgery. Int J Pediatr Otorhinolaryngol 2018;110:147–51.

48. Germiller JA, Monin DL, Sparano AM, et al. Intracranial complications of sinusitis in children and adolescents and their outcomes. Arch Otolaryngol Head Neck Surg 2006;132(9):969–76.

49. Gitomer SA, Zhang W, Marquez L, et al. Reducing surgical revisions in intracranial complications of pediatric acute sinusitis. Otolaryngol Head Neck Surg 2018; 159(2):359–64.

50. Padia R, Thomas A, Alt J, et al. Hospital cost of pediatric patients with complicated acute sinusitis. Int J Pediatr Otorhinolaryngol 2016;80:17–20.

51. Deutschmann MW, Livingstone D, Cho JJ, et al. The significance of Streptococcus anginosus group in intracranial complications of pediatric rhinosinusitis. JAMA Otolaryngol Head Neck Surg 2013;139(2):157–60.

52. Palabiyik FB, Yazici Z, Cetin B, et al. Pott puffy tumor in children: a rare emergency clinical entity. J Craniofac Surg 2016;27(3):e313–6.

53. Koltsidopoulos P, Papageorgiou E, Skoulakis C. Pott's puffy tumor in children: a review of the literature. Laryngoscope 2018. [Epub ahead of print].

54. Deutsch E, Hevron I, Eilon A. Pott's puffy tumor treated by endoscopic frontal sinusotomy. Rhinology 2000;38(4):177–80.

55. Hebert RL 2nd, Bent JP 3rd. Meta-analysis of outcomes of pediatric functional endoscopic sinus surgery. Laryngoscope 1998;108(6):796–9.

56. Ramakrishnan VR, Kingdom TT, Nayak JV, et al. Nationwide incidence of major complications in endoscopic sinus surgery. Int Forum Allergy Rhinol 2012; 2(1):34–9.

57. Ramadan HH. Surgical management of chronic sinusitis in children. Laryngoscope 2004;114(12):2103–9.

58. Roxbury CR, Li L, Rhee D, et al. Safety and perioperative adverse events in pediatric endoscopic sinus surgery: an ACS-NSQIP-P analysis. Int Forum Allergy Rhinol 2017;7(8):827–36.

59. Tumin D, Hayes D Jr, Kirkby SE, et al. Safety of endoscopic sinus surgery in children with cystic fibrosis. Int J Pediatr Otorhinolaryngol 2017;98:25–8.

60. Burton BN, Gilani S, Desai M, et al. Perioperative risk factors associated with morbidity and mortality following pediatric inpatient sinus surgery. Ann Otology Rhinology Laryngol 2019;128(1):13–21.

61. Rastatter JC, Snyderman CH, Gardner PA, et al. Endoscopic endonasal surgery for sinonasal and skull base lesions in the pediatric population. Otolaryngol Clin North Am 2015;48(1):79–99.

62. Zapata S, Kearns DB. Nasal dermoids. Curr Opin Otolaryngol Head Neck Surg 2006;14(6):406–11.

63. Pinheiro-Neto CD, Snyderman CH, Fernandez-Miranda J, et al. Endoscopic endonasal surgery for nasal dermoids. Otolaryngol Clin North Am 2011;44(4): 981–7.

64. Rahbar R, Shah P, Mulliken JB, et al. The presentation and management of nasal dermoid: a 30-year experience. Arch Otolaryngol Head Neck Surg 2003;129(4): 464–71.

65. Liu Z-f, Wang D-h, Sun X-c, et al. The site of origin and expansive routes of juvenile nasopharyngeal angiofibroma (JNA). Int J Pediatr Otorhinolaryngol 2011; 75(9):1088–92.

66. Zanation AM, Mitchell CA, Rose AS. Endoscopic skull base techniques for juvenile nasopharyngeal angiofibroma. Otolaryngol Clin North Am 2012;45(3): 711–30.

67. Stamm AC, Vellutini E, Balsalobre L. Craniopharyngioma. Otolaryngol Clin North Am 2011;44(4):937–52.

68. Jagannathan J, Dumont AS, Jane Jr, et al. Pediatric sellar tumors: diagnostic procedures and management. Neurosurg Focus 2005;18(6A):E6.

69. Wold LE, Laws ER. Cranial chordomas in children and young adults. J Neurosurg 1983;59(6):1043–7.

70. Amit M, Fliss DM, Gil Z. Fibrous dysplasia of the sphenoid and skull base. Otolaryngol Clin North Am 2011;44(4):891–902.

71. Tan Y-c, Yu C-c, Chang C-n, et al. Optic nerve compression in craniofacial fibrous dysplasia: the role and indications for decompression. Plast Reconstr Surg 2007; 120(7):1957–62.

72. Pletcher SD, Metson R. Endoscopic optic nerve decompression for nontraumatic optic neuropathy. Arch Otolaryngol Head Neck Surg 2007;133(8):780–3.

Managing the Child with Persistent Sleep Apnea

Andrew E. Bluher, MD[a], Stacey L. Ishman, MD, MPH[b,c], Cristina M. Baldassari, MD[d,e,*]

KEYWORDS

- Pediatric obstructive sleep apnea • Persistent OSA • DISE
- Tongue base obstruction

KEY POINTS

- Pediatric obstructive sleep apnea may persist after adenotonsillectomy and can be challenging to manage.
- Evaluation of persistent disease should focus on identifying the causes of upper airway obstruction—this is often accomplished with drug-induced sleep endoscopy and/or cine MRI.
- Surgical interventions targeted to the site of obstruction may improve polysomnographic parameters.
- Further research is needed to identify which management protocols lead to the best outcomes for children with persistent obstructive sleep apnea.

 Video content accompanies this article at http://www.oto.theclinics.com.

INTRODUCTION

Pediatric obstructive sleep apnea (OSA) affects 2% to 4% of American children, and is associated with metabolic, cardiovascular, and neurocognitive sequelae.[1-5] Children

Disclosure Statement: The authors have no relevant disclosures.
[a] Department of Otolaryngology–Head and Neck Surgery, Eastern Virginia Medical School, 600 Gresham Drive, Suite 1100, Norfolk, VA 23507, USA; [b] Division of Pediatric Otolaryngology–Head and Neck Surgery, Department of Otolaryngology–Head and Neck Surgery, Cincinnati Children's Hospital Medical Center, University of Cincinnati College of Medicine, 3333 Burnet Avenue, MLC# 2018, Cincinnati, OH 45229-2018, USA; [c] Division of Pulmonary Medicine, Cincinnati Children's Hospital Medical Center, University of Cincinnati College of Medicine, 3333 Burnet Avenue, MLC# 2018, Cincinnati, OH 45229-2018, USA; [d] Department of Otolaryngology–Head and Neck Surgery, Eastern Virginia Medical School, 600 Gresham Drive, Suite 1100, Norfolk, VA 23507, USA; [e] Departments of Pediatric Otolaryngology and Pediatric Sleep Medicine, Children's Hospital of the King's Daughters, 601 Children's Lane, 2nd Floor, Norfolk, VA 23507, USA
* Corresponding author. Children's Hospital of the King's Daughters, 601 Children's Lane, ENT Department 2nd Floor, Norfolk, VA 23507.
E-mail address: baldassc@gmail.com

Otolaryngol Clin N Am 52 (2019) 891–901
https://doi.org/10.1016/j.otc.2019.06.004
0030-6665/19/© 2019 Elsevier Inc. All rights reserved.

oto.theclinics.com

with OSA have been shown to have poor quality of life (QOL) and behavioral problems.[6] The gold standard for the diagnosis of OSA in children is overnight polysomnography (PSG) performed in a sleep laboratory. The severity of OSA is typically classified according to the apnea hypopnea index (AHI) obtained from the PSG. The most commonly used pediatric OSA classification system classifies an AHI between 1 and 5 events/h to be mild disease, and an AHI greater than 10 events/h is consistent with severe disease.[7]

Although the pathophysiology of pediatric OSA is multifactorial, adenotonsillar hypertrophy is a common cause of obstruction. Thus, adenotonsillectomy is the primary treatment for children with OSA. The landmark multi-institutional randomized Childhood Adenotonsillectomy Trial found that children with OSA undergoing adenotonsillectomy experienced significant improvements in PSG parameters, QOL, and behavior when compared with children in a watchful waiting group. However, reported PSG-based cure rates are variable, with persistent disease after adenotonsillectomy reported in 15% to 75% of children depending on the presence of comorbidities.[8–10] Risk factors for persistent disease include obesity, black race, higher baseline AHI, craniofacial disorders such as Down syndrome, and neuromuscular diseases. Patients with persistent OSA following adenotonsillectomy can be challenging to manage and thus treatment protocols for these children are still evolving.[11]

ASSESSMENT OF PERSISTENT OBSTRUCTIVE SLEEP APNEA

According to the American Academy of Otolaryngology-Head and Neck Surgery Tonsillectomy in Children guidelines, caregivers of patients undergoing adenotonsillectomy should be counseled about the risk of persistent disease and instructed to present for evaluation if obstructive symptoms return following surgery.[12] In patients returning for evaluation of persistent obstruction following adenotonsillectomy a detailed history and physical examination should be performed. The provider should inquire about signs and symptoms of OSA, including frequency of snoring, presence of gasping or pausing in breathing, daytime sleepiness, and hyperactivity. The provider should also perform a careful assessment of the head and neck anatomy to look for potential causes of airway obstruction. Examples of such findings include turbinate hypertrophy, redundant palatal tissue, large tongue base, and retrognathia (**Fig. 1**). Awake flexible fiberoptic laryngoscopy may also be useful to assess for additional causes of obstruction such as adenoid regrowth, laryngomalacia, or lingual tonsil hypertrophy.

In children presenting with concern for recurrent or persistent obstruction following an adenotonsillectomy, a PSG should be obtained. Additionally, QOL assessments such as the OSA-18, which are completed by caregivers (with input from the child when appropriate) are useful to determine the impact of obstructive symptoms on the child's well-being.[13] Additional caregiver-completed assessments that provide valuable information in children with suspected OSA include a modified version of the Epworth Sleepiness Scale and the Pediatric Sleep Questionnaire.[14,15] To identify sites of obstruction not observed on physical examination, drug-induced sleep endoscopy (DISE) or cine MRI should be considered[16] as these assessments can be very useful in developing treatment plans.

Drug-Induced Sleep Endoscopy

DISE was first described by Croft and Pringle in the early 1990s[17] for the evaluation of adult patients with OSA. In recent years, DISE has been increasingly performed in children, with the most common indication being persistent OSA following adenotonsillectomy. Pediatric DISE involves performing flexible fiberoptic examination of the upper airway while a child is spontaneously breathing and sedated. The ideal

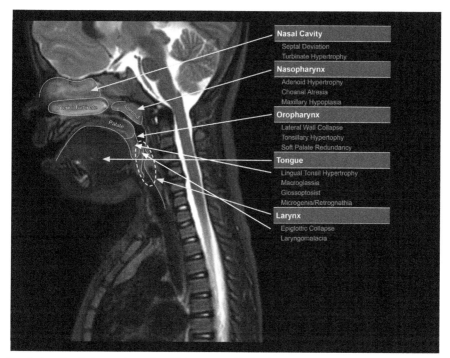

Fig. 1. Levels of obstruction. Cine MRI can provide high-resolution identification of sites of airway collapse during pharmacologically induced sleep.

medication protocol for DISE is debated; however, commonly used agents for this procedure include propofol or dexmedetomidine with or without ketamine.

A recent review article on the evaluation and management of persistent OSA in children found that DISE identified at least 1 site of obstruction in 162 patients.[18] The most common sites of obstruction identified were tongue base, adenoid, inferior turbinates, velum, and lateral oropharyngeal walls; children with severe OSA were more likely to have multi-level obstruction. Recent data have shown that DISE in children impacts surgical decision-making in 35% to 61% of cases.[19,20] However, data demonstrating improved surgical outcomes in children undergoing DISE are lacking, and future prospective trials are needed to confirm that DISE leads to better cure rates in children undergoing sleep surgery.

For adults, there is a widely used, validated DISE scoring system known as the VOTE system.[21] The VOTE scoring system involves identifying both the pattern (anterior-posterior, lateral, or concentric) of collapse and the level of obstruction (velum, oropharynx/lateral walls, tongue base, and epiglottis). In addition it allows for quantification of the severity of the obstruction. However, for children, DISE classification systems are still being developed. For example, Lam and colleagues,[22] developed the Sleep Endoscopy Rating Scale (SERS) to score pediatric DISE. They found the SERS to be reliable and to correlate with pediatric OSA severity.

Cine MRI

Cine MRI is another technique used to identify sites of upper airway obstruction. It allows for dynamic assessment of airway obstruction in children using fast gradient echo sequences that feature axial and sagittal images. Cine MRI can provide high-resolution identification of sites of airway collapse during pharmacologically induced sleep (Video 1). In a recent review article, although 11 studies identified sites of obstruction with DISE, only 3 studies were identified that utilized cine MRI in the evaluation of children with persistent OSA following adenotonsillectomy.[18] In 131 children (many of whom had Down syndrome), cine MRI was able to identify a potential site of obstruction in 93%, and lingual tonsillar hypertrophy was identified in 33% of those with Down syndrome. Proponents of this technique assert that cine MRI has several advantages including recognition of the impact of tongue base obstruction on the palate, quantification of lingual tonsil hypertrophy, and simultaneous assessment of multiple levels of obstruction.[18,23] Cine MRI, however, is not routinely performed at most institutions; this is likely due in part to concern about risks associated with administering sedation to children with severe OSA during an MRI with an unsecured airway. However, these concerns can often be mitigated with the use of continuous positive airway pressure (CPAP) as a backup if the child obstructs and desaturates. Children with metal implants may also be ineligible for cine MRI.

TREATMENT OF PERSISTENT OBSTRUCTIVE SLEEP APNEA

There are numerous treatment options for children with persistent OSA following adenotonsillectomy. Because data comparing different interventions for persistent disease in children are limited, it can be difficult for providers and caregivers to determine the best option for any given child. Because of this, shared decision-making tools may be useful when discussing management options, as it is essential to obtain input from caregivers (and patients when appropriate).[24] Other factors to consider when determining the most appropriate therapy include disease severity, QOL impact, and caregiver/patient preference.

Medical Therapy

Anti-inflammatory medications, including nasal steroids and leukotriene modifiers, can be used to treat children with non-severe persistent OSA following adenotonsillectomy.[25] Gozal and his group reported improvement in the AHI in children with mild persistent OSA (AHI between 1 and 5 events/h) treated with montelukast and/or intranasal budesonide. More recently, Wang and Liang[26] showed that children with mild residual OSA treated with 3 months of montelukast had significantly better PSG and pediatric sleep questionnaire outcomes compared with those treated with a placebo. Further research is needed to determine the appropriate duration of anti-inflammatory therapy in these children.

Positive Airway Pressure

CPAP is also an effective treatment for these children.[27] Marcus and colleagues[28] demonstrated significant improvements in both PSG parameters and daytime sleepiness in children treated with CPAP therapy. Unfortunately many children have significant difficulty tolerating CPAP with adherence reported in only 30% to 50% of children and adolescents.[27,29] Improved compliance among children has been associated with factors such as a family member with a history of CPAP use, maternal education, and young patient age.[30,31]

Surgical Therapy

Physical examination, DISE, and/or cine MRI are typically used to determine sites of obstruction that may direct surgical intervention and it is often useful to frame the discussion of surgical options according to identified anatomic sites of obstruction.

Tongue

The tongue base is identified as a source of obstruction in 35% to 85% of children with persistent OSA.[16,32,33] Anatomic factors that can cause tongue base obstruction include macroglossia, glossoptosis, and enlarged lingual tonsils. Children with trisomy 21 are particularly susceptible to tongue base obstruction and have been found to have a significantly higher incidence of lingual tonsil hypertrophy than non-syndromic children.[34] Surgical options to address tongue base obstruction include lingual tonsillectomy, posterior midline glossectomy, tongue-lip adhesion, hyoid suspension, radiofrequency ablation, tongue suspension, and hypoglossal nerve stimulation.

Of these, lingual tonsillectomy is the most common tongue procedure performed in children with refractory OSA.[18] A variety of techniques including microdebrider, coblation, and laser may be utilized to remove lingual tonsils in children. Complications for lingual tonsillectomy are similar to those for tonsillectomy, with slightly higher need to return to the operating room for control of hemorrhage as bedside control can be more difficult than for tonsillectomy. Oropharyngeal stenosis has also been reported when lingual tonsillectomy is performed as part of multi-level surgery.[35] Lingual tonsillectomy results in significant improvements in PSG parameters such as AHI. A recent review article, however, found that surgical success rates (defined as an AHI < 5) for this surgery were approximately 60%, thus caregivers should be counseled about the possibility of persistent obstruction.[18]

There are very few data regarding outcomes for these children after other tongue base procedures. Wootten and colleagues[36] reported on 16 children who underwent posterior midline glossectomy as part of multi-level sleep surgery. Following surgical intervention, they had significant improvements in the AHI. Coblation is typically utilized to perform midline glossectomy in children, with care being taken to remain in the midline to avoid injury to the lingual artery. There was also a study that reported approximately 60% resolution of OSA in children with recurrent OSA who underwent tongue suspension sutures in combination with radiofrequency ablation.[37] Tongue suspension entails placing a non-absorbable suture anchored to a titanium screw in the genial tubercle to keep the base of the tongue from collapsing. Tongue-lip adhesion has primarily been utilized in children with Pierre Robin sequence, in which the goals include avoidance of mandibular advancement or tracheotomy, and has shown some benefit in reducing AHI in these cases.[38] Hyoid suspension currently lacks evidence in the pediatric literature, but has been shown to improve tongue-base level obstruction in adults.[39]

Hypoglossal nerve stimulation is an emerging therapy that addresses tongue base collapse. The implant stimulates tongue protrusion muscles during inspiration, alleviating tongue base collapse during sleep. Hypoglossal nerve stimulators sense pleural pressure via sensing leads placed between the intercostal muscle layers, and rely on a pulse generator placed inferior to the clavicle to deliver impulses to a stimulation cuff placed around the medial branches of the hypoglossal nerve. The implant has been shown to improve PSG parameters and reduce daytime sleepiness in adults with OSA.[40] The device is now being studied in children with Down syndrome who have persistent OSA following adenotonsillectomy. Initial results are promising, with significant improvement in the AHI with few peri-operative complications.[16,41,42]

Palate

The palate is another common site of obstruction in patients with persistent OSA.[16] Traditionally, uvulopalatopharyngoplasty (UPPP) was the primary procedure performed to address palatal collapse. Indeed, studies have demonstrated improvements in the AHI and other PSG parameters on PSG in children undergoing this procedure.[43,44] However, persistent disease has been identified in many children and adults following UPPP, which has driven the use of DISE to identify all areas of collapse. DISE allows for the determination of pattern of palatal collapse, that is, anterior-posterior or circumferential. In adult sleep surgery, the traditional UPPP has largely been replaced by palatal procedures developed to address specific patterns of palate collapse. For example, expansion pharyngoplasty involves palatal muscle rearrangement including rotation and suspension of the palatopharyngeus muscle from the soft palate.[45] This procedure addresses posterior palatal collapse as well as lateral pharyngeal wall collapse. A recent study showed improvement in AHI in children with severe disease undergoing expansion sphincter pharyngoplasty at the time of initial tonsillectomy.[46] However, data regarding the utilization of this procedure in children with persistent OSA subsequent to adenotonsillectomy are lacking. Risks of palatal surgery are similar to those of tonsillectomy and include velopharyngeal insufficiency and nasopharyngeal stenosis.

Supraglottis
With the increasing utilization of DISE, the supraglottis has increasingly been identified as a site of obstruction in these children. The terms occult laryngomalacia and sleep-dependent laryngomalacia have been used to describe the finding of supraglottic collapse during DISE that is not seen while awake. Unlike children with congenital laryngomalacia, these children are typically older (>2 years) and do not have a history of stridor while awake. Supraglottoplasty, which includes a release of the aryepiglottic folds, has been shown to significantly decrease the AHI and improve the nadir oxygen saturation in children with sleep-dependent laryngomalacia identified on DISE.[47] For patients noted to have an epiglottis that is independently collapsing and obstructive, epiglottopexy can be considered. This procedure involves de-mucosalizing the lingual surface of the epiglottis, vallecula, and adjacent base of the tongue, and then anchoring the epiglottis to the tongue base with a suture.[16]

Nose
The nose has also been identified as a potential cause of obstruction in these children. Nasal findings that may be associated with obstruction, including turbinate hypertrophy and septal deviation, which has resulted in the inclusion of nasal anatomy/patency in a recently proposed pediatric DISE scoring system.[22] Although nasal surgery has been shown to minimally improve PSG parameters in adults with OSA, it has been shown to improve CPAP tolerance and sleep quality.[48–50] In children with OSA, a 2012 retrospective study demonstrated that performing turbinate reduction at the time of adenotonsillectomy conferred additional benefit in terms of AHI and QOL.[51] In addition, 3 studies have demonstrated long-term improvement in nasal obstruction after turbinate surgery.[52–54] In light of these findings, clinicians are increasingly performing turbinate surgery (including either radiofrequency volumetric reduction or microdebrider-assisted turbinoplasty) in children with persistent OSA and nasal obstruction at the time of DISE or with other procedures to treat persistent OSA. Nasal septoplasty may also be useful in select patients, and may improve CPAP tolerance in older children.[55]

Tracheostomy
In some cases of severe persistent OSA, tracheotomy may be considered. Although this surgery does definitively address OSA by bypassing the upper airway entirely, it comes with a host of QOL concerns[56] and potential complications. Because of these concerns, it is most often reserved for patients with substantial cardiopulmonary comorbidities, craniofacial abnormalities, and/or neurologic or neuromuscular disorders.

Dental Therapy

Myofunctional exercises are an alternative non-surgical therapy that has shown benefit in adult sleep apnea, reducing AHI, raising oxygen nadir, decreasing snoring, and improving the Epworth Sleepiness Scale.[57] The therapy has been less frequently studied in children, but there is some evidence to suggest an adjunctive role in patients with persistent OSA post-adenotonsillectomy. A prospective randomized controlled trial reported that performance of thrice-daily myofunctional exercises was associated with a 62% reduction in the AHI of 14 children with mild to moderate residual OSA. This reduction was statistically significant relative to controls.[58] A second study reviewed 24 children who were cured of OSA by a combination of adenotonsillectomy and palatal expansion. Of the 24, 11 received myofunctional exercise therapy, and were found to have a sustained cure over 4 years, compared with a 100% recurrence rate for those who did not perform the exercises.[59] The utility of exercise in children with trisomy 21 is uncertain, as there is only one published study of its use in this population and it was limited to 1 week's duration.[60]

Dental and/or orthodontic treatment can also be considered for children with persistent disease. Oral appliances include mandibular advancement devices, tongue retaining devices, and palatal lift appliances, and may be used most effectively in children with permanent teeth.[61] Additional dental treatment options include rapid maxillary/palatal expansion, or a modified monobloc appliance.[62–64] There are reports of improvement in non-severe AHI with use of dental appliances in children as young as 3 year old.[62,65] There may be some adverse effects on developing dentition. The American Academy of Pediatric Dentistry acknowledges that functional intra-oral appliances alter the position and/or growth of the maxilla or mandible, and recommends that non-surgical intra-oral appliances be considered only after "a complete orthodontic/craniofacial assessment of the patient's growth and development as part of a multidisciplinary approach." The academy recommendations also counsel reassessment throughout treatment to determine whether the appliance is effective in resolving the patient's OSA.[66] Older patients with evident facial skeletal deficiencies and/or malocclusion may, in addition, consider maxillomandibular advancement surgery.

SUMMARY

Persistent OSA in children following adenotonsillectomy can be challenging for providers to manage. Evaluation of persistent disease should focus on identifying the causes of upper airway obstruction using physical examination, DISE, and/or cine MRI. Interventions should be tailored to address the patient's symptoms, sites of obstruction, and preference for surgical versus medical management. Surgical interventions targeted to the site of obstruction may improve PSG and QOL outcomes. Further research, however, is needed to identify which management protocols lead to the best outcomes for children with persistent OSA.

SUPPLEMENTARY DATA

Supplementary data related to this article can be found online at https://doi.org/10.1016/j.otc.2019.06.004.

REFERENCES

1. Lumeng JC, Chervin RD. Epidemiology of pediatric obstructive sleep apnea. Proc Am Thorac Soc 2008;5(2):242–52.

2. Li AM, Au CT, Sung RY, et al. Ambulatory blood pressure in children with obstructive sleep apnoea: a community based study. Thorax 2008;63(9):803–9.
3. Capdevila OS, Kheirandish-Gozal L, Dayyat E, et al. Pediatric obstructive sleep apnea: complications, management, and long-term outcomes. Proc Am Thorac Soc 2008;5(2):274–82.
4. Mitchell RB, Kelly J. Behavior, neurocognition and quality-of-life in children with sleep-disordered breathing. Int J Pediatr Otorhinolaryngol 2006;70(3):395–406.
5. Tan HL, Gozal D, Kheirandish-Gozal L. Obstructive sleep apnea in children: a critical update. Nat Sci Sleep 2013;5:109–23.
6. Baldassari CM, Mitchell RB, Schubert C, et al. Pediatric obstructive sleep apnea and quality of life: a meta-analysis. Otolaryngol Head Neck Surg 2008;138(3): 265–73.
7. Wagner MH, Torrez DM. Interpretation of the polysomnogram in children. Otolaryngol Clin North Am 2007;40(4):745–59.
8. Bhattacharjee R, Kheirandish-Gozal L, Spruyt K, et al. Adenotonsillectomy outcomes in treatment of obstructive sleep apnea in children: a multicenter retrospective study. Am J Respir Crit Care Med 2010;182(5):676–83.
9. Friedman M, Wilson M, Lin HC, et al. Updated systematic review of tonsillectomy and adenoidectomy for treatment of pediatric obstructive sleep apnea/hypopnea syndrome. Otolaryngol Head Neck Surg 2009;140(6):800–8.
10. Tauman R, Gulliver TE, Krishna J, et al. Persistence of obstructive sleep apnea syndrome in children after adenotonsillectomy. J Pediatr 2006;149(6):803–8.
11. Marcus CL, Moore RH, Rosen CL, et al. A randomized trial of adenotonsillectomy for childhood sleep apnea. N Engl J Med 2013;368(25):2366–76.
12. Baugh RF, Archer SM, Mitchell RB, et al. Clinical practice guideline: tonsillectomy in children. Otolaryngol Head Neck Surg 2011;144(1 Suppl):S1–30.
13. Franco RA, Rosenfeld RM, Rao M. First place–resident clinical science award 1999. Quality of life for children with obstructive sleep apnea. Otolaryngol Head Neck Surg 2000;123(1 Pt 1):9–16.
14. Janssen KC, Phillipson S, O'Connor J, et al. Validation of the epworth sleepiness scale for children and adolescents using rasch analysis. Sleep Med 2017; 33:30–5.
15. Chervin RD, Hedger K, Dillon JE, et al. Pediatric sleep questionnaire (PSQ): validity and reliability of scales for sleep-disordered breathing, snoring, sleepiness, and behavioral problems. Sleep Med 2000;1(1):21–32.
16. Ishman SL, Chang KW, Kennedy AA. Techniques for evaluation and management of tongue-base obstruction in pediatric obstructive sleep apnea. Curr Opin Otolaryngol Head Neck Surg 2018;26(6):409–16.
17. Croft CB, Pringle M. Sleep nasendoscopy: a technique of assessment in snoring and obstructive sleep apnoea. Clin Otolaryngol Allied Sci 1991;16(5):504–9.
18. Manickam PV, Shott SR, Boss EF, et al. Systematic review of site of obstruction identification and non-CPAP treatment options for children with persistent pediatric obstructive sleep apnea. Laryngoscope 2016;126(2):491–500.
19. Gazzaz MJ, Isaac A, Anderson S, et al. Does drug-induced sleep endoscopy change the surgical decision in surgically naïve non-syndromic children with snoring/sleep disordered breathing from the standard adenotonsillectomy? A retrospective cohort study. J Otolaryngol Head Neck Surg 2017;46(1):12.
20. Hybášková J, Jor O, Novák V, et al. Drug-induced sleep endoscopy changes the treatment concept in patients with obstructive sleep apnoea. Biomed Res Int 2016;2016:6583216.

21. Kezirian EJ, Hohenhorst W, de Vries N. Drug-induced sleep endoscopy: the VOTE classification. Eur Arch Otorhinolaryngol 2011;268(8):1233–6.

22. Lam DJ, Weaver EM, Macarthur CJ, et al. Assessment of pediatric obstructive sleep apnea using a drug-induced sleep endoscopy rating scale. Laryngoscope 2016;126(6):1492–8.

23. Shott SR, Donnelly LF. Cine magnetic resonance imaging: evaluation of persistent airway obstruction after tonsil and adenoidectomy in children with Down syndrome. Laryngoscope 2004;114(10):1724–9.

24. Bergeron M, Duggins A, Chini B, et al. Clinical outcomes after shared decision-making tools with families of children with obstructive sleep apnea without tonsillar hypertrophy. Laryngoscope 2019. https://doi.org/10.1002/lary.27653.

25. Kheirandish L, Goldbart AD, Gozal D. Intranasal steroids and oral leukotriene modifier therapy in residual sleep-disordered breathing after tonsillectomy and adenoidectomy in children. Pediatrics 2006;117(1):e61–6.

26. Wang B, Liang J. The effect of montelukast on mild persistent OSA after adenotonsillectomy in children: a preliminary study. Otolaryngol Head Neck Surg 2017; 156(5):952–4.

27. Uong EC, Epperson M, Bathon SA, et al. Adherence to nasal positive airway pressure therapy among school-aged children and adolescents with obstructive sleep apnea syndrome. Pediatrics 2007;120(5):e1203–11.

28. Marcus CL, Rosen G, Ward SL, et al. Adherence to and effectiveness of positive airway pressure therapy in children with obstructive sleep apnea. Pediatrics 2006;117(3):e442–51.

29. Beebe DW, Byars KC. Adolescents with obstructive sleep apnea adhere poorly to positive airway pressure (PAP), but PAP users show improved attention and school performance. PLoS One 2011;6(3):e16924.

30. Puri P, Ross KR, Mehra R, et al. Pediatric positive airway pressure adherence in obstructive sleep apnea enhanced by family member positive airway pressure usage. J Clin Sleep Med 2016;12(7):959–63.

31. DiFeo N, Meltzer LJ, Beck SE, et al. Predictors of positive airway pressure therapy adherence in children: a prospective study. J Clin Sleep Med 2012;8(3):279–86.

32. Wilcox LJ, Bergeron M, Reghunathan S, et al. An updated review of pediatric drug-induced sleep endoscopy. Laryngoscope Investig Otolaryngol 2017;2(6): 423–31.

33. Durr ML, Meyer AK, Kezirian EJ, et al. Drug-induced sleep endoscopy in persistent pediatric sleep-disordered breathing after adenotonsillectomy. Arch Otolaryngol Head Neck Surg 2012;138(7):638–43.

34. Fricke BL, Donnelly LF, Shott SR, et al. Comparison of lingual tonsil size as depicted on MR imaging between children with obstructive sleep apnea despite previous tonsillectomy and adenoidectomy and normal controls. Pediatr Radiol 2006;36(6):518–23.

35. Prager JD, Hopkins BS, Propst EJ, et al. Oropharyngeal stenosis: a complication of multilevel, single-stage upper airway surgery in children. Arch Otolaryngol Head Neck Surg 2010;136(11):1111–5.

36. Wootten CT, Chinnadurai S, Goudy SL. Beyond adenotonsillectomy: outcomes of sleep endoscopy-directed treatments in pediatric obstructive sleep apnea. Int J Pediatr Otorhinolaryngol 2014;78(7):1158–62.

37. Wootten CT, Shott SR. Evolving therapies to treat retroglossal and base-of-tongue obstruction in pediatric obstructive sleep apnea. Arch Otolaryngol Head Neck Surg 2010;136(10):983–7.

38. Resnick CM, Calabrese CE, Sahdev R, et al. Is tongue-lip adhesion or mandibular distraction more effective in relieving obstructive apnea in infants with robin sequence? J Oral Maxillofac Surg 2019;77(3):591–600.

39. Song SA, Wei JM, Buttram J, et al. Hyoid surgery alone for obstructive sleep apnea: a systematic review and meta-analysis. Laryngoscope 2016;126(7):1702–8.

40. Woodson BT, Soose RJ, Gillespie MB, et al. Three-year outcomes of cranial nerve stimulation for obstructive sleep apnea: the STAR trial. Otolaryngol Head Neck Surg 2016;154(1):181–8.

41. Diercks GR, Keamy D, Kinane TB, et al. Hypoglossal nerve stimulator implantation in an adolescent with down syndrome and sleep apnea. Pediatrics 2016; 137(5) [pii:e20153663].

42. Diercks GR, Wentland C, Keamy D, et al. Hypoglossal nerve stimulation in adolescents with down syndrome and obstructive sleep apnea. JAMA Otolaryngol Head Neck Surg 2017. https://doi.org/10.1001/jamaoto.2017.1871.

43. Com G, Carroll JL, Tang X, et al. Characteristics and surgical and clinical outcomes of severely obese children with obstructive sleep apnea. J Clin Sleep Med 2015;11(4):467–74.

44. Wiet GJ, Bower C, Seibert R, et al. Surgical correction of obstructive sleep apnea in the complicated pediatric patient documented by polysomnography. Int J Pediatr Otorhinolaryngol 1997;41(2):133–43.

45. Pang KP, Woodson BT. Expansion sphincter pharyngoplasty: a new technique for the treatment of obstructive sleep apnea. Otolaryngol Head Neck Surg 2007; 137(1):110–4.

46. Ulualp SO. Modified expansion sphincter pharyngoplasty for treatment of children with obstructive sleep apnea. JAMA Otolaryngol Head Neck Surg 2014; 140(9):817–22.

47. Camacho M, Dunn B, Torre C, et al. Supraglottoplasty for laryngomalacia with obstructive sleep apnea: a systematic review and meta-analysis. Laryngoscope 2016;126(5):1246–55.

48. Ishii L, Roxbury C, Godoy A, et al. Does nasal surgery improve OSA in patients with nasal obstruction and OSA? a meta-analysis. Otolaryngol Head Neck Surg 2015;153(3):326–33.

49. Poirier J, George C, Rotenberg B. The effect of nasal surgery on nasal continuous positive airway pressure compliance. Laryngoscope 2014;124(1):317–9.

50. Mickelson SA. Nasal surgery for obstructive sleep apnea syndrome. Otolaryngol Clin North Am 2016;49(6):1373–81.

51. Cheng PW, Fang KM, Su HW, et al. Improved objective outcomes and quality of life after adenotonsillectomy with inferior turbinate reduction in pediatric obstructive sleep apnea with inferior turbinate hypertrophy. Laryngoscope 2012;122(12): 2850–4.

52. Liu CM, Tan CD, Lee FP, et al. Microdebrider-assisted versus radiofrequency-assisted inferior turbinoplasty. Laryngoscope 2009;119(2):414–8.

53. Acevedo JL, Camacho M, Brietzke SE. Radiofrequency ablation turbinoplasty versus microdebrider-assisted turbinoplasty: a systematic review and meta-analysis. Otolaryngol Head Neck Surg 2015;153(6):951–6.

54. Chen YL, Tan CT, Huang HM. Long-term efficacy of microdebrider-assisted inferior turbinoplasty with lateralization for hypertrophic inferior turbinates in patients with perennial allergic rhinitis. Laryngoscope 2008;118(7):1270–4.

55. Sulman CG. Pediatric sleep surgery. Front Pediatr 2014;2:51.

56. Pandian V, Garg V, Antar R, et al. Discharge education and caregiver coping of pediatric patients with a tracheostomy: systematic review [review]. ORL Head Neck Nurs 2016;34(1):17–8, 20-7.
57. Camacho M, Certal V, Abdullatif J, et al. Myofunctional therapy to treat obstructive sleep apnea: a systematic review and meta-analysis. Sleep 2015;38(5):669–75.
58. Villa MP, Brasili L, Ferretti A, et al. Oropharyngeal exercises to reduce symptoms of OSA after AT. Sleep Breath 2015;19(1):281–9.
59. Guilleminault C, Huang YS, Monteyrol PJ, et al. Critical role of myofascial reeducation in pediatric sleep-disordered breathing. Sleep Med 2013;14(6):518–25.
60. von Lukowicz M, Herzog N, Ruthardt S, et al. Effect of a 1-week intense myofunctional training on obstructive sleep apnoea in children with Down syndrome. Arch Dis Child 2019;104(3):275–9.
61. Hoffstein V. Review of oral appliances for treatment of sleep-disordered breathing. Sleep Breath 2007;11(1):1–22.
62. Cozza P, Polimeni A, Ballanti F. A modified monobloc for the treatment of obstructive sleep apnoea in paediatric patients. Eur J Orthod 2004;26(5):523–30.
63. Padmanabhan V, Kavitha PR, Hegde AM. Sleep disordered breathing in children– a review and the role of a pediatric dentist. J Clin Pediatr Dent 2010;35(1):15–21.
64. Capua M, Ahmadi N, Shapiro C. Overview of obstructive sleep apnea in children: exploring the role of dentists in diagnosis and treatment. J Can Dent Assoc 2009; 75(4):285–9.
65. Schessl J, Rose E, Korinthenberg R, et al. Severe obstructive sleep apnea alleviated by oral appliance in a three-year-old boy. Respiration 2008;76(1):112–6.
66. Policy on obstructive sleep apnea. Pediatr Dent 2017;39(6):96–8.

Craniofacial Interventions in Children

Brandon Hopkins, MD[a],*, Kelly Dean, MD[b], Swathi Appachi, MD[c],
Amelia F. Drake, MD[d]

KEYWORDS

- Craniofacial • Cleft lip • Cleft palate • Microtia • Mandibular distraction
- Free tissue transfer

KEY POINTS

- Craniofacial interventions are common in the field of otolaryngology and extend beyond cleft lip and cleft palate repair.
- Surgical advances continue in the management of micrognathia, macroglossia, midface hypoplasia, hearing loss, facial nerve palsy, hemifacial microsomia, and microtia.
- Three-dimensional printing, nasoalveolar molding digital modeling, and free tissue reconstruction for pediatrics are all emerging fields with otolaryngologists at the forefront.
- Complex upper airway obstruction, mandibular advancement, and technologies including hypoglossal nerve stimulators have the potential to impact patients with craniofacial disorders.

INTRODUCTION

Children presenting with craniofacial conditions are common in otolaryngology and caring for them requires diverse procedures and a team approach. Craniofacial conditions can be isolated or associated with syndromes or sequences of anomalies. Orofacial clefting has traditionally been the focus of many of these interventions; however, with advances and new techniques, the scope of what can be done expands.

Disclosure Statement: The authors have no disclosures.
[a] Pediatric Otolaryngology, Pediatric Center for Airway Voice and Swallowing, Cleveland Clinic, 9500 Euclid Avenue, 7th Floor Crile Building, Cleveland, OH 44195, USA; [b] Department of Otolaryngology/Head and Neck Surgery, UNC Hospitals, University of North Carolina, 170 Manning Drive, CB# 7070, Chapel Hill, NC 27599-7070, USA; [c] Cleveland Clinic Head and Neck Institute, Cleveland Clinic, 9500 Euclid Avenue, 7th Floor Crile Building, Cleveland, OH 44195, USA; [d] Department of Otolaryngology/Head and Neck Surgery, UNC Hospitals, Craniofacial Center, University of North Carolina, 170 Manning Drive, CB# 7070, Chapel Hill, NC 27599-7070, USA
* Corresponding author.
E-mail address: hopkinb@ccf.org

Otolaryngol Clin N Am 52 (2019) 903–922
https://doi.org/10.1016/j.otc.2019.06.002
0030-6665/19/© 2019 Elsevier Inc. All rights reserved.

For instance, craniofacial issues encompass micrognathia, macroglossia, midface hypoplasia, hearing loss, facial nerve palsy, hemifacial microsomia, and microtia. A unifying theme for many of these conditions is complex upper airway obstruction.

The object of this article was to highlight the craniofacial interventions available and to provide an update on any related trends. The individualized care for each specific condition is beyond the scope of this article, as is craniosynostosis and cranioplasty.

CLEFT CARE

Many craniofacial interventions are related to orofacial clefting, with more than 400 syndromes associated.[1] Clefts can be found in 1 of 700 live births, with diverse and multifactorial causes and a variety of classification systems.[2]

UNILATERAL CLEFT LIP REPAIR

The goals of unilateral cleft lip (CL) repair remain consistent: creating symmetric length, leveling Cupid's bow, leaving adequate vermilion thickness and an inconspicuous scar, restoring muscle continuity, and addressing nasal deformity.[3]

Straight-line closure grew from work done by Carl Ferdinand von Graefe, Husson, Rose, and Thompson.[3] These pioneers demonstrate lengthening via concave excisions.[4]

Early approaches obtained length for closure at the expense of incisions at odds with the vertical philtral column.[5,6] These techniques were refined to take advantage of added length while camouflaging scar lines.[7,8]

The rotation advancement flap of Millard[3] is considered by many to be a mainstay of surgical repair. This was complemented through Mohler's[9] addition of a small piece of tissue taken from the columellar base (columellar flap), creating a scar more symmetric with the normal philtral column.

BILATERAL CLEFT LIP

Bilateral repairs have no normal side for comparison. Thus proper prolabial creation, the median tubercle, positioning of the alar cartilages, and columellar length must be considered.[10,11]

A modified Millard technique is common with presurgical nasoalveolar molding (NAM).[2,12] Philtral size is important when designing incisions and is based on age-matched population norms.[13,14]

Some of the technique modifications over time include the management of prolabial mucosa.[15] Premaxillary osteotomies are also less common, as significant midfacial growth restriction and premaxillary necrosis can occur.[2,10]

PALATOPLASTY

Palatoplasty techniques often involve a 2-flap palatoplasty (**Fig. 1**) and can be modified for complete, incomplete, or bilateral cleft palates (CPs).[16]

Recreating the muscular levator sling is frequently performed and can be accomplished via an intravelar veloplasty or a Furlow (double-opposing Z-plasty) (**Fig. 2**), which has been shown to improve speech outcomes in most studies.[17,18] These 2 techniques also can be combined creating a 6-flap palatoplasty.[19]

Other approaches used by some include closure of the palate in a 2-stage approach.[20] The goals of this approach are early soft palate closure optimizing speech with closure of the hard palate between 18 and 36 months, maximizing midfacial and dental arch growth.[21,22]

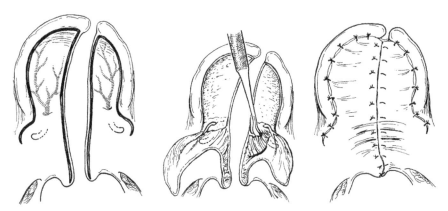

Fig. 1. Two-flap palatoplasty. (*From* Senders CW, Sykes JM. Advances in palatoplasty. *Arch Otolaryngol Head Neck Surg.* 1993;119(4):375-7; with permission.)

Variability remains in the management of the hamulus and can include fracture, blunt or sharp dissection of the tensor veli palatini, or tensor tenopexy. It has been shown that transection of this muscle or fracture may lead to worsened middle ear ventilation, but may aid in primary closure.[23–25]

NASOALVEOLAR MOLDING

Nonsyndromic CL/CP is a common craniofacial defect that may have significant and detrimental consequences including dental issues.[26] Updates with regard to dental issues include improvements in hygiene, prevention, and orthodontic advances, such as NAM (**Fig. 3**).

The concept of early management of CL and CP has changed over time, with more investigators emphasizing NAM before lip repair. NAM has gained wide acceptance and reported evidence of success.[27,28] Benefits associated with this are that it promotes better anatomic bony framework, narrows the cleft, and improves nasal symmetry, improving surgical outcomes.[29]

Recently, with the incorporation of new digital technologies, professionals can achieve successful results, while reducing the time and burden of care, that is[29]

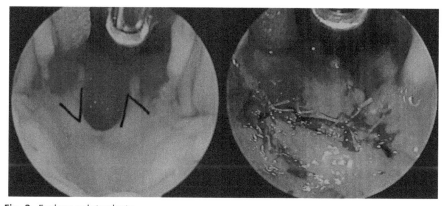

Fig. 2. Furlow palatoplasty.

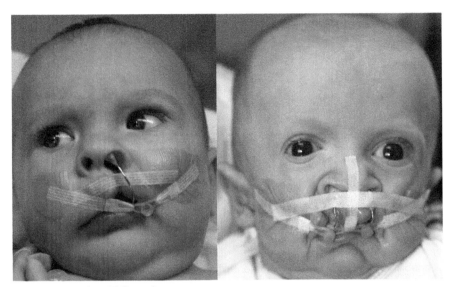

Fig. 3. Unilateral and bilateral NAM.

computer-based NAM (**Fig. 4**) allows a customized design of nasoalveolar molding, with better control of the magnitude and direction of the force. In addition, 3-dimensional (3-D) printing to fabricate complete sets of intraoral molding devices in advance of treatment can minimize the time-consuming impression-taking and the production of working plaster models, resulting in standardized and predictable outcomes.[30,31] Applications of this modification of an accepted technique are in progress.

ALVEOLAR BONE GRAFTING

The goals of alveolar bone grafting include improved maxillary dentition, improved orthodontic or prosthodontic rehabilitation, reestablishment of maxillary contour, and prevention of oroantral fistula.[32] This can be accomplished primarily during palatoplasty, as secondary bone grafting during mixed dentition, or as tertiary bone grafting

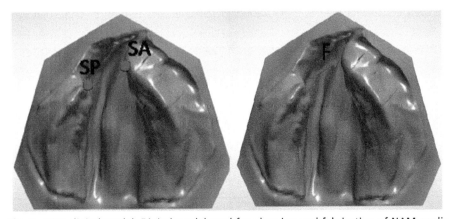

Fig. 4. NAM digital model. Digital model used for planning and fabrication of NAM appliances. SP, anterior point of the lesser segment; SA, anterior point of the greater segment; and F distance between points SA and SF representing the width of the cleft.

after permanent dentition.[33] Primary grafting has shown some risk of facial growth restriction[34–36]; however, it can result in sufficient alveolar bone development allowing eruption of primary and permanent dentition and may avoid secondary grafting.[2] Prior research indicates that early secondary grafting, that is, grafting performed before canine eruption, is optimal, as this allows for increased graft take once the canines do erupt.[34,37]

Iliac crest is often used for grafting. Advantages include ease of harvest and the ability to simultaneously prepare the alveolar cleft, but disadvantages include postoperative pain, claudication, and possible graft resorption.[38] Other sites of bone harvest include the cranium, mandibular symphysis, or tibia; these may have less donor site morbidity and decreased rates of absorption.[34,39] Bone substitute includes recombinant human bone morphogenetic protein-2, with studies showing comparable results.[32,38]

Pain can be significant at the harvest site and bupivacaine, a long-acting local anesthetic, can be used. In addition to injecting locally, placement of bupivacaine-soaked Gelfoam into the wound has shown decreased postoperative pain, length of stay, and time to ambulation.[40] Alternatively, a bupivacaine infusion pump can be used, decreasing hospital stay and pain scores.[41,42] A randomized controlled study comparing a femoral nerve block, boluses via an indwelling catheter, and a single intraoperative dose at the donor site showed that the indwelling catheter group had the most improved pain relief with the quickest return to function.[43] Ultimately, liposomal bupivacaine injection may find a future role in this procedure for long-acting pain relief, as it has been effective for procedures such as palatoplasty.[44]

AUDIOLOGY

Hearing loss and otologic problems are frequent issues in an otolaryngology practice and are found in those with CP.[45] Studies have shown that 28% of patients with CP fail their newborn hearing screen.[46] Most commonly, this is due to middle ear effusion and conductive hearing loss (CHL) due to eustachian tube dysfunction (ETD), which is near universal.[17,47] Historically, pressure equalization (PE) tubes were routinely placed early to mitigate CHL and promote speech and language development.[48,49] These can be placed at the time of lip repair, as an independent procedure near 3 months, or during palatoplasty. However, a more selective approach can be used.[17] A recent systematic review concluded that there is insufficient evidence to support routine placement of PE tubes.[50] In fact, one study demonstrated an increase in otologic complications in patients with CP who received routine PE tubes.[51] The 2013 consensus statement put forth by the American Academy of Otolaryngology reflects these studies and advocates for individualized discussion with caregivers, offering the option for hearing aid (HA) consideration.[52]

As ETD is known to improve, the use of HA has been reviewed as a way to avoid PE tubes. Studies have demonstrated improvement in hearing with an HA without the morbidity of PE tubes.[53,54] This being said, PE tube placement is still the most common means of alleviating CHL, and a survey of caregivers for patients with CP demonstrated a preference for PE tubes due to perceived simplicity of the procedure.[55] However, as emphasis on avoiding elective surgical procedures becomes more common, the use of HAs may become more attractive.

In addition to conventional HAs, surgical options for CHL have emerged. For example, osseointegrated bone conduction implants, such as bone-anchored HAs consist of an implantable abutment and external processor, are approved for children older than 5. This provides great hearing, but complications can include infections of the abutment, loss of osseointegration, and revision surgery.[56] Another implantable option that was just recently approved for children older than 12 is the Bonebridge system by Med-El (Innsbruck, Austria).[57] Instead of a percutaneous abutment, a bone conduction unit is placed under the skin, to which an external processor transmits signals.[57] A systematic review has demonstrated improved hearing thresholds and speech recognition compared with the unaided condition and decreased complications compared with percutaneous systems.[58]

Surgical options are not feasible in children younger than 5 years due to bone thickness. Fortunately, nonsurgical transcutaneous options allow for early hearing rehabilitation. One such option is the BAHA Softband, which consists of a headband with a sound processor, allowing for transcutaneous transmission of sound.[59,60] A study examining this device in patients with craniofacial abnormalities demonstrated improved aided soundfield thresholds and speech audibility.[59] A new option is a nonsurgical bone conduction option known as AdHear. This consists of an adhesive that is applied behind the ear. The sound processor then attaches to this adhesive, eliminating the need for a headband.[61] A study comparing the 2 devices did not show any statistically significant differences in hearing thresholds and speech recognition.[62] In general a transcutaneous device is a good option for patients but has more attenuation as compared with an osseointegrated device.

MICROTIA

Microtia occurs in approximately 1 to 10 per 10,000 births and is often associated with aural atresia necessitating hearing rehabilitation.[63] Microtia repair leads to decreased psychosocial stressors and can aid in the use of HA and glasses.[64,65] If repair is pursued, there are several options; these include auricular prostheses, reconstruction with an alloplastic implant, or reconstruction with autologous rib cartilage.[64]

Auricular prostheses have greatly evolved, especially with the advent of 3-D printing and further development of silicone materials.[66] Prostheses offer simplicity and no donor site morbidity as compared with autologous rib harvest, but negatives include maintenance of the prosthesis, the need for renewal every few years, and color mismatch over time.[64,66] Prostheses can be temporary, used if reconstructive surgery fails, or as definitive treatment. If definitive, osseointegrated implants can placed for securement.[66,67]

Use of alloplastic, porous polyethylene (PPE), implants for microtia repair is also an option. Advantages include single-stage surgery, smaller surgical learning curve, and less donor site morbidity as compared with rib harvest, the biggest negative being that the implant is foreign.[64] The PPE is molded to replicate the shape of the contralateral ear, and is a nonreactive material with good biocompatibility and infection resistance.[68] Placement is under a temporoparietal flap (TPF) with skin grafts as needed, and allows earlier reconstruction.[64,68] When initially described, implant fractures and exposures were noted. However, modifications to the technique, such as incorporating a large TPF and raising the subgaleal fascia, have reduced these complications to rates less than 10%.[69] Furthermore, implanted 3-D printed bioresorbable polycaprolactone scaffolds have been recently shown to promote soft tissue growth in vivo in porcine models, providing an exciting new venue for microtia reconstruction (**Fig. 5**).[70]

Finally, microtia reconstruction with autologous rib cartilage is the oldest method described and is considered the gold standard. Its advantages include autologous material and minimal maintenance once healed, whereas disadvantages include pneumothorax, multiple surgeries, steeper learning curve, and an older age at reconstruction.[64] Currently, the 2 most popular methods are the Brent or Nagata.[71] The Brent method is a 3-stage to 4-stage technique using less cartilage that can be

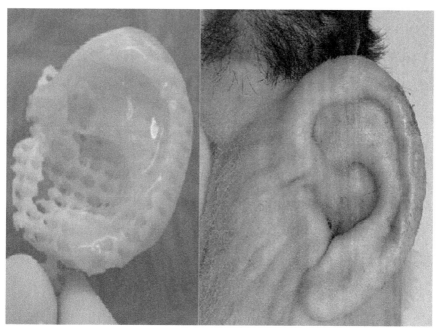

Fig. 5. Three-dimensional printed microtia scaffold. (*Courtesy of* D. Zopf, MD, Ann Arbor, MI.)

performed at age 5 to 8.[72,73] The Nagata method is a 2-stage method requiring more costal cartilage and is performed at approximately age 10.[71]

In the Brent technique, the contralateral eighth rib and the sixth/seventh rib synchondrosis are harvested.[71–73] The cartilage is then carved and placed into a skin pocket over suction drains. At a second stage, the earlobe is transposed into its normal anatomic location. In the third stage, the framework is elevated off the mastoid bone with previously banked cartilage. The fourth stage is creation of a tragus from the contralateral concha cymba.

In contrast, the Nagata method uses ribs 6 to 9.[71,74] The body of the ear again is carved from the synchondrosis, whereas the eighth/ninth are used to fashion the superior and inferior crus and antihelix. Lobule transposition and creation of the tragus are accomplished during this stage. The lobule is split to create a deep and more natural-appearing concha cavity differing from Brent.[75] A pocket is created and the framework placed over suction drains with a TPF to cover exposed mastoid. Elevation again is at a second stage. Multiple modifications have been published for various types of microtia.[76–78] The results of both methods, when healed well, create a durable reconstruction resistant to trauma.[73]

With the advent of 3-D printing and continued development in tissue engineering, future advances in microtia reconstruction may minimize the learning curve, continue to reduce the number of surgeries, and allow for earlier repair.[70,79]

VELOPHARYNGEAL DYSFUNCTION

Management of velopharyngeal dysfunction (VPD) is frequent in the otolaryngology population, whether after cleft repair or as part of a syndrome such as 22Q deletion. Its evaluation is best done in collaboration with a speech language pathologist to

rule out functional causes and should routinely involve nasal endoscopy. It is important to assess the coronal and sagittal closure patterns including the contribution of
movement from the posterior pharyngeal wall (Passavants ridge) (**Fig. 6**).[80] The
Golding-Kushner Scale can be used to grade these movements and guide one's surgical choice.

There are several techniques, including a Furlow; often used when closure gap is
coronal after a 2-flap palatoplasty, but may also be used after a prior Furlow.[81] A
sphincter pharyngoplasty is a second option when coronal closure is identified.
With good lateral wall movement, sagittal or circular closure, or large gaps, a superiorly based pharyngeal flap can be considered, but may predispose to sleep apnea.[17]
Large gaps also can be addressed via a combined Furlow and sphincter palatoplasty.[82] For smaller or more isolated gaps, an injection pharyngoplasty or posterior
wall augmentation may be considered. This can be done with various autologous or
exogenous materials with proper patient selection.[83]

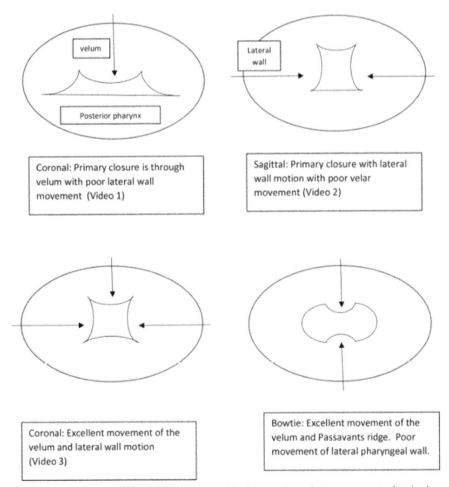

Fig. 6. Closure patterns. (*From* Glade RS, Deal R. Diagnosis and Management of Velopharyngeal Dysfunction. *Oral Maxillofac Surg Clin North Am.* 2016;28(2):181-8; with permission.)

RHINOPLASTY

Rhinoplasty continues to be a common pediatric procedure. This may be used as a primary tip rhinoplasty during lip repair to improve alar symmetry, centralize the columellar base, create nostrils of equal diameter, release the ala from the piriform rim, and for advancement of the lateral crus anteriomedially. If performed, secondary rhinoplasty is typically done between age 5 and 7.[17] This can be combined with a lip revision and can improve nasal symmetry and hooding. For a bilateral cleft this may involve columellar lengthening with techniques described including Cronin bipedicled flaps and Millard banked forked-flaps (both of which can cause a nasolabial crease) or a V to Y advancement.[10] Trends are to avoid the need for lengthening by using NAM with modified nasal stents before lip repair.[84] Primary rhinoplasty is typically performed after full growth.

FREE TISSUE TRANSFER

Minimally invasive free tissue transfers (FTT) have become more common as a pediatric craniofacial intervention. They are used for reconstruction after malignancy, palate repair, and facial nerve disorders.

Examples of use include large tissue defects seen with malignancy that can be readily addressed with FTT with limited donor site morbidity (**Fig. 7**). Alternatively, they can be used for large palatal defects which traditionally have been managed with obturators due to a deficiency in loco-regional tissue. The use of anterior lateral thigh fascia lata grafting or other FTT provides an option with low morbidity and a reliable recovery (**Fig. 8**).[85] In addition, FTT has increased the opportunities for facial nerve reanimation outside of static procedures. This is often accomplished with either a gracilis or latissimus dorsi muscle transfer with coaption to recipient site nerves.[86]

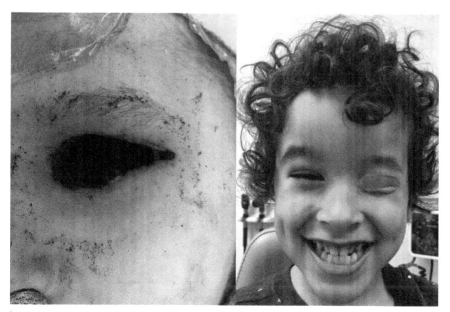

Fig. 7. Free tissue transfer after malignancy. Orbital exenteration with anterior lateral thigh free flap reconstruction.

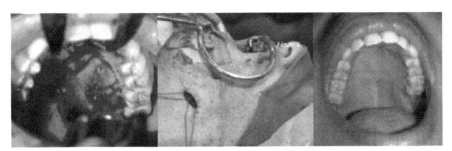

Fig. 8. Free tissue transfer for palatal defect. Palatal reconstruction with anterior lateral thigh free flap reconstruction. (*From* Fritz MA. Setting a New Standard for Complex Palate Repair. Advances in Otolaryngology & Dentistry. Available at: www.clevelandclinic.org/OtoAdvances1718. Accessed January 27, 2019; with permission.)

SLEEP APNEA IN CLEFT AND CRANIOFACIAL PATIENTS

The incidence of sleep-disordered breathing (SDB) and obstructive sleep apnea (OSA) is elevated in children with craniofacial syndromes compared with the general population. It is estimated that the risk of SDB in children with CL/CP is 22% to 65%.[87] The incidence of OSA in children with other craniofacial syndromes is between 40% and 68%, whereas it is estimated that up to 85% of infants with Pierre Robin sequence (PRS) have OSA.[88–90]

Typically, a formal workup by an otolaryngologist is necessary, along with a polysomnogram (PSG) to evaluate the extent of OSA. There are several interventions to be considered for OSA in the craniofacial population, as their upper airway obstruction is often multilevel.

The gold standard for diagnosing OSA in children is PSG, but the use of computed-topography (CT) or MRI has become common. These can show lymphoid hypertrophy and other soft tissue obstruction. More recently, cone-beam CT has been used for evaluating the skeletal and soft tissue anatomy.[91] MRI has been shown to be effective in evaluating the total volume of the upper airway in pediatric patients with OSA, and has the advantage of limiting exposure to radiation.[92] Both MRI and CT may necessitate general anesthesia in young children.

MEDICAL MANAGEMENT OF OBSTRUCTIVE SLEEP APNEA

Early in life, patients with syndromes such as PRS may benefit from a nasopharyngeal airway (NPA) bypassing obstruction.[93] An NPA is selected such that it is an appropriate size allowing its distal end to sit immediately superior to the epiglottis and inferior to the base of tongue.

A second nonsurgical intervention for OSA is high-flow nasal cannula (HFNC), which delivers warm humidified air to the bilateral nasal cavities, allowing positive pressure ventilation. This displaces the tongue anteriorly, overcoming negative inspiratory pressure. Studies show decreased OSA symptoms and overall increased compliance compared with other modalities.[94]

Maxillary expansion may also aid patients with a narrow high arched palate. Over a period of weeks, it widens the palate and expands the nasal floor. It has shown benefit in improving obstruction in properly identified patients (**Fig. 9**).[95]

Finally, continuous positive airway pressure ventilation can be considered for pediatric patients with refractory OSA. It functions in a similar manner to HFNC, and has been shown to improve OSA but is complicated by poor tolerance.[94]

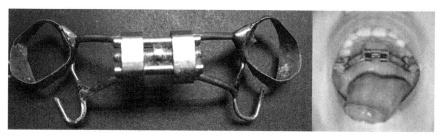

Fig. 9. Palatal expander.

SURGICAL MANAGEMENT OF OBSTRUCTIVE SLEEP APNEA
Tongue-Lip Adhesion

Tongue-lip adhesion (TLA), initially described in the 1940s and most often in patients with PRS, is a glossopexy procedure that can be performed with subperiosteal release of the floor of mouth and circum-mandibular suturing of the tongue, improving OSA.[96–98] Successful outcomes have been reported anywhere from 71% to 89%, but it is not used much anymore except in selected patients.[99,100]

Mandibular Distraction Osteogenesis

Mandibular distraction osteogenesis (MDO) is associated with more favorable feeding outcomes and successful relief of severe airway obstruction than prior options, such as TLA.[101]

In MDO, the mandible is advanced anteriorly, improving tongue-base obstruction (**Fig. 10**). An initial osteotomy is made in the mandible and a short latency period follows. Then, distraction begins and segments are slowly separated, allowing for the formation of new bone as the surrounding soft tissue elongates. A consolidation phase follows in which the newly formed bone remodels to become mature over a course of 4 to 6 weeks after which the distraction hardware is removed.

Studies have shown that up to 97% of children with craniofacial syndromes and OSA improve after MDO.[102] It has been associated with a significant decrease in the apnea-hypopnea index (AHI), and an improvement in oxygen saturation and airway volumes.[100,101,103] Long-term morbidity has not been well described, but dental trauma has been seen, as has the need for repeat procedures.

Hypoglossal Neurostimulation

Recent advancements in the treatment of OSA have led to the development of hypoglossal nerve stimulators (HGNS), implantable devices that send impulses to the hypoglossal nerve during inspiration, leading to the protrusion of the tongue musculature relieving tongue-base obstruction. The sensing electrode is placed between intercostal muscles, which senses timing of inspiration and subsequently delivers the impulse to the anterior branches of the hypoglossal nerve, stimulating the protrusor muscles of the tongue. HGNS has been studied in adults and outcomes have shown a reduction in AHI as well as improvement in quality of life measures.[104]

A study of pediatric patients with Down syndrome and refractory OSA who underwent HGNS implantation showed a reduction in AHI by 56% to 85%.[105] Further research is needed to study a broader population of children and adolescents with craniofacial anomalies and long-term efficacy of HGNS.

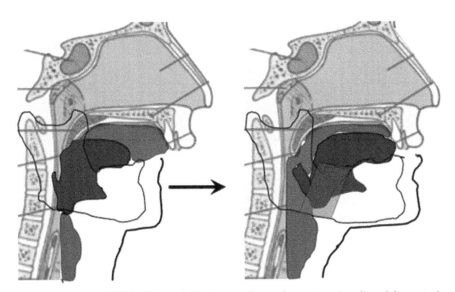

Fig. 10. Concept of MDO. Supraglottic tongue-base obstruction is relieved by anterior advancement of the hypoplastic mandible. (*From* Scott AR, Tibesar RJ, Sidman JD. Pierre Robin Sequence: evaluation, management, indications for surgery, and pitfalls. *Otolaryngol Clin North Am.* 2012;45(3):695-710, ix; with permission.)

Tonsillectomy and Adenoidectomy

In the general population, adenotonsillectomy is the first-line treatment for children with OSA. Patients with craniofacial anomalies often have multilevel airway obstruction, thus adenotonsillectomy may not completely resolve their OSA. Patients with CL/CP are also at risk of postoperative hypernasality; a superior adenoidectomy should be considered to lessen the risk of velopharyngeal insufficiency.[106,107]

Tracheostomy Decannulation

Tracheostomy is a common method for securing an airway in children with craniofacial anomalies as it bypasses many levels of obstruction, but a subsequent goal is decannulation.[98] The multilevel obstruction may require various surgeries and endoscopic evaluations via microlaryngoscopy and bronchoscopy. Several procedures discussed, including MDO and HGNS can be useful toward this goal (**Fig. 11**). Polysomnography and end-tidal CO_2 can be used to help predict successful decannulation.[108]

Mission Trips

It has been estimated that 4.8 million people lack access to surgical care globally.[109] Given that CL/CP is one of the most common anomalies, unrepaired children worldwide may undergo a lifetime of physical, psychological, and economic difficulties.[110] Studies have demonstrated that repairing CL/CP in low-income and middle-income countries is cost-effective, and surgical mission trips are an option to address the paucity of surgical access.[102,109,111] Otolaryngologists actively participate in these trips providing craniofacial care.

Although many assume that surgical mission trips are inherently beneficial, there remains controversy. For example, there is concern that quantity over quality is emphasized, these trips disrupt the host facility, and outcomes may be no better than those of local surgeons.[102,109,112] Moreover, follow-up is typically low, as seen in an analysis

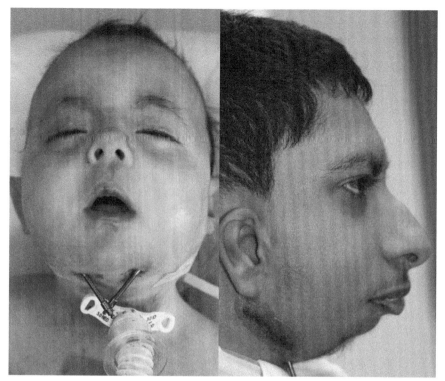

Fig. 11. MDO used for decannulation. Adolescent and infant requiring MDO before successful decannulation.

of Operation Smile rates of 36.67%.[113] Long-term, outcomes research is sparse due to difficulty in collecting data and the short-term nature of trips.[114]

Planning for a surgical trip occurs months in advance. A team consisting of otolaryngologists and other experienced CL/CP surgeons, anesthesiologists, and nurses is assembled.[102] The inclusion of surgical residents is debated; available research demonstrates benefit for trainees but may compromise the educational opportunity for local surgeons.[115,116] This should be weighed against the idea that inclusion of residents with appropriate supervision propagates future humanitarian outreach.[102] If possible, it is beneficial to work with local surgeons and providers to increase their comfort with CL/CP care. In addition, it is important to work with a host facility to determine availability of equipment and resources.

Once the team has arrived, surgical candidate screening is completed and surgeries prioritized based on maximizing benefit, and minimizing harm.[102] Children should undergo examination by either a pediatrician or anesthesiologist for preoperative clearance. After surgery, postoperative care should be provided and a follow-up plan with a local partnering provider is recommended. However, teleconferencing has made post-mission follow-up feasible. A goal of surgical missions, although often difficult to achieve, should be to empower and teach local providers how to transition to autonomous care for their own population.

SUMMARY

Otolaryngology providers commonly perform craniofacial interventions and the surgical options continue to grow, offered within the context of team care. Throughout a child's life the focus of interventions may change from airway management to speech, hearing, and language optimization, and finally to decannulation and procedures aimed at social integration and self-esteem. As otolaryngologists, we provide high-quality care in this arena and continue to expand what can be done for our patients. We aim to model a culture of communication, centered on the patient and can help address the hearing, the airway, and the cleft abnormality itself in a collaborative fashion.

REFERENCES

1. Gorlin RJ. Orofacial clefting syndromes: general aspects. In: Gorlin RJ, Cohen MM, Hennekam RCM, editors. Syndromes of the head and neck. 4th edition. New York: Oxford University Press, Inc; 2001. p. 850–76.
2. Arosarena OA. Cleft lip and palate. Otolaryngol Clin North Am 2007;40(1): 27–60, vi.
3. Millard DR. Volume I: the unilateral deformity. In: Millard DR, editor. Cleft craft: the evolution of its surgery. 1st edition. Boston: Little Brown and Company; 1976. p. 88–121.
4. Tse R. Unilateral cleft lip: principles and practice of surgical management. Semin Plast Surg 2012;26(4):145–55.
5. Tennison CW. The repair of the unilateral cleft lip by the stencil method. Plast Reconstr Surg (1946) 1952;9(2):115–20.
6. Randall P. A triangular flap operation for the primary repair of unilateral clefts of the lip. Plast Reconstr Surg Transplant Bull 1959;23(4):331–47.
7. Noordhoff MS. The surgical technique for the unilateral cleft lip-nasal deformity. Taipei (China): Noordhoff Craniofacial Foundation; 1997.
8. Fisher DM. Unilateral cleft lip repair: an anatomical subunit approximation technique. Plast Reconstr Surg 2005;116(1):61–71.
9. Mohler LR. Unilateral cleft lip repair. Plast Reconstr Surg 1987;80(4):511–7.
10. Mulliken JB. Primary repair of bilateral cleft lip and nasal deformity. Plast Reconstr Surg 2001;108(1):181–94.
11. Ghali GE, Ringeman JL. Primary bilateral cleft lip/nose repair using a modified Millard technique. Atlas Oral Maxillofac Surg Clin North Am 2009;17(2):117–24.
12. Millard DR. Volume II: bilateral and rare deformities. In: Millard DR, editor. Cleft craft: the evolution of its surgery. 1st edition. Boston: Little Brown and Company; 1977. p. 307–78.
13. Tollefson TT, Senders CW. Cleft lip repair: bilateral. In: Goudy SL, Tollefson TT, editors. Complete cleft care: cleft and velopharyngeal insufficiency treatment in children. New York: Thieme Medical Publishers, Inc.; 2015. p. 63–85.
14. Mulliken JB, Burvin R, Farkas LG. Repair of bilateral complete cleft lip: intraoperative nasolabial anthropometry. Plast Reconstr Surg 2001;107(2):307–14.
15. Manchester WM. The repair of bilateral cleft lip and palate. Br J Surg 1965; 52(11):878–82.
16. Senders CW, Sykes JM. Advances in palatoplasty. Arch Otolaryngol Head Neck Surg 1993;119(4):375–7.
17. Hartzell LD, Kilpatrick LA. Diagnosis and management of patients with clefts: a comprehensive and interdisciplinary approach. Otolaryngol Clin North Am 2014;47(5):821–52.
18. Furlow LT. Cleft palate repair by double opposing Z-plasty. Plast Reconstr Surg 1986;78(6):724–38.

19. Gage-white L. Furlow palatoplasty: double opposing Z-plasty. Facial Plast Surg 1993;9(3):181–3.

20. Schweckendiek W, Doz P. Primary veloplasty: long-term results without maxillary deformity. a twenty-five year report. Cleft Palate J 1978;15(3):268–74.

21. Gundlach KK, Bardach J, Filippow D, et al. Two-stage palatoplasty, is it still a valuable treatment protocol for patients with a cleft of lip, alveolus, and palate? J Craniomaxillofac Surg 2013;41(1):62–70.

22. Liao YF, Yang IY, Wang R, et al. Two-stage palate repair with delayed hard palate closure is related to favorable maxillary growth in unilateral cleft lip and palate. Plast Reconstr Surg 2010;125(5):1503–10.

23. Kane AA, Lo LJ, Yen BD, et al. The effect of hamulus fracture on the outcome of palatoplasty: a preliminary report of a prospective, alternating study. Cleft Palate Craniofac J 2000;37(5):506–11.

24. Noone RB, Randall P, Stool SE, et al. The effect on middle ear disease of fracture of the pterygoid hamulus during palatoplasty. Cleft Palate J 1973;10:23–33.

25. Flores RL, Jones BL, Bernstein J, et al. Tensor veli palatini preservation, transection, and transection with tensor tenopexy during cleft palate repair and its effects on eustachian tube function. Plast Reconstr Surg 2010;125(1):282–9.

26. Hosseini HR, Kaklamanos EG, Athanasiou AE. Treatment outcomes of presurgical infant orthopedics in patients with non-syndromic cleft lip and/or palate: a systematic review and meta-analysis of randomized controlled trials. PLoS One 2017;12(7):e0181768.

27. Uzel A, Alparslan ZN. Long-term effects of presurgical infant orthopedics in patients with cleft lip and palate: a systematic review. Cleft Palate Craniofac J 2011;48(5):587–95.

28. Rau A, Ritschl LM, Mücke T, et al. Nasoalveolar molding in cleft care–experience in 40 patients from a single centre in Germany. PLoS One 2015;10(3):e0118103.

29. Maillard S, Retrouvey JM, Ahmed MK, et al. Correlation between nasoalveolar molding and surgical, aesthetic, functional and socioeconomic outcomes following primary repair surgery: a systematic review. J Oral Maxillofac Res 2017;8(3):e2.

30. Yu Q, Gong X, Wang GM, et al. A novel technique for presurgical nasoalveolar molding using computer-aided reverse engineering and rapid prototyping. J Craniofac Surg 2011;22(1):142–6.

31. Bauer FX, Güll FD, Roth M, et al. A prospective longitudinal study of postnatal dentoalveolar and palatal growth: the anatomical basis for CAD/CAM-assisted production of cleft-lip-palate feeding plates. Clin Anat 2017;30(7):846–54.

32. Guo J, Li C, Zhang Q, et al. Secondary bone grafting for alveolar cleft in children with cleft lip or cleft lip and palate. Cochrane Database Syst Rev 2011;(6):CD008050.

33. Stellmach R. Historical development and current status of osteoplasty of lip-jaw-palate clefts. Fortschr Kiefer Gesichtschir 1993;38:11–4 [in German].

34. Weissler EH, Paine KM, Ahmed MK, et al. Alveolar bone grafting and cleft lip and palate: a review. Plast Reconstr Surg 2016;138(6):1287–95.

35. Hopper RA, Al-mufarrej F. Gingivoperiosteoplasty. Clin Plast Surg 2014;41(2):233–40.

36. Wang YC, Liao YF, Chen PK. Outcome of gingivoperiosteoplasty for the treatment of alveolar clefts in patients with unilateral cleft lip and palate. Br J Oral Maxillofac Surg 2013;51(7):650–5.

37. Newlands LC. Secondary alveolar bone grafting in cleft lip and palate patients. Br J Oral Maxillofac Surg 2000;38(5):488–91.

38. Wu C, Pan W, Feng C, et al. Grafting materials for alveolar cleft reconstruction: a systematic review and best-evidence synthesis. Int J Oral Maxillofac Surg 2018; 47(3):345–56.

39. Rawashdeh MA, Telfah H. Secondary alveolar bone grafting: the dilemma of donor site selection and morbidity. Br J Oral Maxillofac Surg 2008;46(8):665–70.

40. Dashow JE, Lewis CW, Hopper RA, et al. Bupivacaine administration and post-operative pain following anterior iliac crest bone graft for alveolar cleft repair. Cleft Palate Craniofac J 2009;46(2):173–8.

41. Sbitany H, Koltz PF, Waldman J, et al. Continuous bupivacaine infusion in iliac bone graft donor sites to minimize pain and hospitalization. Cleft Palate Craniofac J 2010;47(3):293–6.

42. Meara DJ, Livingston NR, Sittitavornwong S, et al. Continuous infusion of bupivacaine for pain control after anterior iliac crest bone grafting for alveolar cleft repair in children. Cleft Palate Craniofac J 2011;48(6):690–4.

43. Kumar Raja D, Anantanarayanan P, Christabel A, et al. Donor site analgesia after anterior iliac bone grafting in paediatric population: a prospective, triple-blind, randomized clinical trial. Int J Oral Maxillofac Surg 2014;43(4):422–7.

44. Day KM, Nair NM, Sargent LA. Extended release liposomal bupivacaine injection (exparel) for early postoperative pain control following palatoplasty. J Craniofac Surg 2018;29(5):e525–8.

45. Goudy S, Lott D, Canady J, et al. Conductive hearing loss and otopathology in cleft palate patients. Otolaryngol Head Neck Surg 2006;134(6):946–8.

46. Chen JL, Messner AH, Curtin G. Newborn hearing screening in infants with cleft palates. Otol Neurotol 2008;29(6):812–5.

47. Flynn T, Möller C, Jönsson R, et al. The high prevalence of otitis media with effusion in children with cleft lip and palate as compared to children without clefts. Int J Pediatr Otorhinolaryngol 2009;73(10):1441–6.

48. Paradise JL. Management of middle ear effusions in infants with cleft palate. Ann Otol Rhinol Laryngol 1976;85(2 Suppl 25 Pt 2):285–8.

49. Gould HJ. Hearing loss and cleft palate: the perspective of time. Cleft Palate J 1990;27(1):36–9.

50. Ponduri S, Bradley R, Ellis PE, et al. The management of otitis media with early routine insertion of grommets in children with cleft palate—a systematic review. Cleft Palate Craniofac J 2009;46(1):30–8.

51. Phua YS, Salkeld LJ, De chalain TM. Middle ear disease in children with cleft palate: protocols for management. Int J Pediatr Otorhinolaryngol 2009;73(2): 307–13.

52. Rosenfeld RM, Schwartz SR, Pynnonen MA, et al. Clinical practice guideline: tympanostomy tubes in children. Otolaryngol Head Neck Surg 2013;149(1 Suppl):S1–35.

53. Gani B, Kinshuck AJ, Sharma R. A review of hearing loss in cleft palate patients. Int J Otolaryngol 2012;2012:548698.

54. Maheshwar AA, Milling M a P, Kumar M, et al. Use of hearing aids in the management of children with cleft palate. Int J Pediatr Otorhinolaryngol 2002;66(1): 55–62.

55. Tierney S, O'brien K, Harman NL, et al. Risks and benefits of ventilation tubes and hearing aids from the perspective of parents of children with cleft palate. Int J Pediatr Otorhinolaryngol 2013;77(10):1742–8.

56. Badran K, Arya AK, Bunstone D, et al. Long-term complications of bone-anchored hearing aids: a 14-year experience. J Laryngol Otol 2009;123(2): 170–6.

57. MED-EL USA Obtains FDA De Novo Clearance for BONEBRIDGETM Bone Conduction Implant System. BusinessWire. Available at: https://www.businesswire.com/news/home/20180724005634/en/MED-EL-USA-Obtains-FDA-De-Novo-Clearance.   Accessed December 24, 2018.

58. Sprinzl GM, Wolf-Magele A. The Bonebridge Bone Conduction Hearing Implant: indication criteria, surgery and a systematic review of the literature. Clin Otolaryngol 2016;41(2):131–43.

59. Nicholson N, Christensen L, Dornhoffer J, et al. Verification of speech spectrum audibility for pediatric Baha Softband users with craniofacial anomalies. Cleft Palate Craniofac J 2011;48(1):56–65.

60. Hol MKS, Cremers CWRJ, Coppens-Schellekens W, et al. The BAHA Softband. A new treatment for young children with bilateral congenital aural atresia. Int J Pediatr Otorhinolaryngol 2005;69(7):973–80.

61. MED-EL. ADHEAR: stick. Click. Hear. Available at: https://blog.medel.pro/adhear-hearing-system/. Accessed December 24, 2018.

62. Gawliczek T, Munzinger F, Anschuetz L, et al. Unilateral and bilateral audiological benefit with an adhesively attached, noninvasive bone conduction hearing system. Otol Neurotol 2018;39(8):1025–30.

63. Mastroiacovo P, Corchia C, Botto LD, et al. Epidemiology and genetics of microtia-anotia: a registry based study on over one million births. J Med Genet 1995;32(6):453–7.

64. Bly RA, Bhrany AD, Murakami CS, et al. Microtia reconstruction. Facial Plast Surg Clin North Am 2016;24(4):577–91.

65. Johns AL, Lucash RE, Im DD, et al. Pre and post-operative psychological functioning in younger and older children with microtia. J Plast Reconstr Aesthet Surg 2015;68(4):492–7.

66. Federspil PA. Auricular prostheses in microtia. Facial Plast Surg Clin North Am 2018;26(1):97–104.

67. Granström G, Bergström K, Odersjö M, et al. Osseointegrated implants in children: experience from our first 100 patients. Otolaryngol Head Neck Surg 2001; 125(1):85–92.

68. Reinisch J. Ear reconstruction in young children. Facial Plast Surg 2015;31(6): 600–3.

69. Reinisch JF, Lewin S. Ear reconstruction using a porous polyethylene framework and temporoparietal fascia flap. Facial Plast Surg 2009;25(3):181–9.

70. Zopf DA, Mitsak AG, Flanagan CL, et al. Computer aided-designed, 3-dimensionally printed porous tissue bioscaffolds for craniofacial soft tissue reconstruction. Otolaryngol Head Neck Surg 2015;152(1):57–62.

71. Cabin JA, Bassiri-Tehrani M, Sclafani AP, et al. Microtia reconstruction: autologous rib and alloplast techniques. Facial Plast Surg Clin North Am 2014; 22(4):623–38.

72. Brent B. The correction of microtia with autogenous cartilage grafts: I. The classic deformity.? Plast Reconstr Surg 1980;66(1):1–12.

73. Brent B. Technical advances in ear reconstruction with autogenous rib cartilage grafts: personal experience with 1200 cases. Plast Reconstr Surg 1999;104(2): 319–34, 335-338.

74. Nagata S. A new method of total reconstruction of the auricle for microtia. Plast Reconstr Surg 1993;92(2):187–201.

75. Yamada A. Autologous rib microtia construction: nagata technique. Facial Plast Surg Clin North Am 2018;26(1):41–55.

76. Nagata S. Modification of the stages in total reconstruction of the auricle: part I. Grafting the three-dimensional costal cartilage framework for lobule-type microtia. Plast Reconstr Surg 1994;93(2):221–30, 267-268.

77. Nagata S. Modification of the stages in total reconstruction of the auricle: part II. Grafting the three-dimensional costal cartilage framework for concha-type microtia. Plast Reconstr Surg 1994;93(2):231–42, 267-268.

78. Nagata S. Modification of the stages in total reconstruction of the auricle: part III. Grafting the three-dimensional costal cartilage framework for small concha-type microtia. Plast Reconstr Surg 1994;93(2):243–53, 267-268.

79. Zopf DA, Flanagan CL, Mitsak AG, et al. Pore architecture effects on chondrogenic potential of patient-specific 3-dimensionally printed porous tissue bioscaffolds for auricular tissue engineering. Int J Pediatr Otorhinolaryngol 2018; 114:170–4.

80. Bliss M, Muntz H. Nasal endoscopy: new tools and technology for accurate assessment. Adv Otorhinolaryngol 2015;76:18–26.

81. Hsu PJ, Wang SH, Yun C, et al. Redo double-opposing Z-plasty is effective for correction of marginal velopharyngeal insufficiency. J Plast Reconstr Aesthet Surg 2015;68(9):1215–20.

82. Gosain AK, Arneja JS. Management of the black hole in velopharyngeal incompetence: combined use of a Furlow palatoplasty and sphincter pharyngoplasty. Plast Reconstr Surg 2007;119(5):1538–45.

83. Brigger MT, Ashland JE, Hartnick CJ. Injection pharyngoplasty with calcium hydroxylapatite for velopharyngeal insufficiency: patient selection and technique. Arch Otolaryngol Head Neck Surg 2010;136(7):666–70.

84. Patil PG, Nimbalkar-patil SP. Modified activation technique for nasal stent of nasoalveolar molding appliance for columellar lengthening in bilateral cleft lip/palate. J Prosthodont 2018;27(1):94–7.

85. Fritz MA. Setting a new standard for complex palate repair. Advances in otolaryngology & dentistry 2017. Available at: www.clevelandclinic.org/OtoAdvances1718. Accessed January 27, 2019.

86. Elledge R, Parmar S. Free flaps for head and neck cancer in paediatric and neonatal patients. Curr Opin Otolaryngol Head Neck Surg 2018;26(2):127–33.

87. MacLean JE, Hayward P, Fitzgerald DA, et al. Cleft lip and/or palate and breathing during sleep. Sleep Med Rev 2009;13:345–54.

88. Hoeve LJ, Pijpers M, Joosten KF. OSAS in craniofacial syndromes: an unsolved problem. Int J Pediatr Otorhinolaryngol 2003;67(Suppl 1):S111–3.

89. Driessen C, Joosten KF, Bannink N, et al. How does obstructive sleep apnea evolve in syndromic craniosynostosis? A prospective cohort study. Arch Dis Child 2013;98:538–43.

90. Anderson IC, Sedaghat AR, McGinley BM, et al. Prevalence and severity of obstructive sleep apnea and snoring in infants with Pierre Robin sequence. Cleft Palate Craniofac J 2011;48:614–8.

91. Alsufyani NA, Noga ML, Witmans M, et al. Using cone beam CT to assess the upper airway after surgery in children with sleep disordered breathing symptoms and maxillary-mandibular disproportions: a clinical pilot. J Otolaryngol Head Neck Surg 2017;46(1):31.

92. Patini R, Arrica M, Di stasio E, et al. The use of magnetic resonance imaging in the evaluation of upper airway structures in paediatric obstructive sleep apnoea syndrome: a systematic review and meta-analysis. Dentomaxillofac Radiol 2016;45(7):20160136.

93. Tan HL, Kheirandish-gozal L, Abel F, et al. Craniofacial syndromes and sleep-related breathing disorders. Sleep Med Rev 2016;27:74–88.
94. Whitla L, Lennon P. Non-surgical management of obstructive sleep apnoea: a review. Paediatr Int Child Health 2017;37(1):1–5.
95. Buccheri A, Chinè F, Fratto G, et al. Rapid maxillary expansion in obstructive sleep apnea in young patients: cardio-respiratory monitoring. J Clin Pediatr Dent 2017;41(4):312–6.
96. Douglas B. The treatment of micrognathia associated with obstruction by a plastic procedure. Plast Reconstr Surg (1946) 1946;1:300–8.
97. Camacho M, Noller MW, Zaghi S, et al. Tongue-lip adhesion and tongue repositioning for obstructive sleep apnoea in Pierre Robin sequence: a systematic review and meta-analysis. J Laryngol Otol 2017;131(5):378–83.
98. Scott AR, Tibesar RJ, Sidman JD. Pierre Robin Sequence: evaluation, management, indications for surgery, and pitfalls. Otolaryngol Clin North Am 2012;45(3): 695–710, ix.
99. Huang F, Lo LJ, Chen YR, et al. Tongue-lip adhesion in the management of Pierre Robin sequence with airway obstruction: technique and outcome. Chang Gung Med J 2005;28(2):90–6.
100. Flores RL, Tholpady SS, Sati S, et al. The surgical correction of Pierre Robin sequence: mandibular distraction osteogenesis versus tongue-lip adhesion. Plast Reconstr Surg 2014;133(6):1433–9.
101. Tibesar RJ, Scott AR, McNamara C, et al. Distraction osteogenesis of the mandible for airway obstruction in children: long-term results. Otolaryngol Head Neck Surg 2010;143(1):90–6.
102. Lyford-Pike S, Byrne P. Humanitarian missions. In: Goudy S, Tollefson T, editors. Complete cleft care: cleft and velopharyngeal insufficiency treatment in children. New York: Thieme Medical Publishers; 2015. p. 196–204.
103. Ow AT, Cheung LK. Meta-analysis of mandibular distraction osteogenesis: clinical applications and functional outcomes. Plast Reconstr Surg 2008;121: 54e–69e.
104. Strollo PJ, Soose RJ, Maurer JT, et al. Upper-airway stimulation for obstructive sleep apnea. N Engl J Med 2014;370:139–49.
105. Ishman SL, Chang KW, Kennedy AA. Techniques for evaluation and management of tongue-base obstruction in pediatric obstructive sleep apnea. Curr Opin Otolaryngol Head Neck Surg 2018;26(6):409–16.
106. Saunders NC, Hartley BE, Sell D, et al. Velopharyngeal insufficiency following adenoidectomy. Clin Otolaryngol Allied Sci 2004;29(6):686–8.
107. Tweedie DJ, Skilbeck CJ, Wyatt ME, et al. Partial adenoidectomy by suction diathermy in children with cleft palate, to avoid velopharyngeal insufficiency. Int J Pediatr Otorhinolaryngol 2009;73(11):1594–7.
108. Gurbani N, Promyothin U, Rutter M, et al. Using polysomnography and airway evaluation to predict successful decannulation in children. Otolaryngol Head Neck Surg 2015;153(4):649–55.
109. Bergmark RW, Shaye DA, Shrime MG. Surgical care and otolaryngology in global health. Otolaryngol Clin North Am 2018;51(3):501–13.
110. Magee WP, Vander Burg R, Hatcher KW. Cleft lip and palate as a cost-effective health care treatment in the developing world. World J Surg 2010;34(3):420–7.
111. Alkire B, Hughes CD, Nash K, et al. Potential economic benefit of cleft lip and palate repair in sub-Saharan Africa. World J Surg 2011;35(6):1194–201.
112. Maine RG, Hoffman WY, Palacios-Martinez JH, et al. Comparison of fistula rates after palatoplasty for international and local surgeons on surgical missions in

Ecuador with rates at a craniofacial center in the United States. Plast Reconstr Surg 2012;129(2):319e–26e.

113. Bermudez L, Carter V, Magee W, et al. Surgical outcomes auditing systems in humanitarian organizations. World J Surg 2010;34(3):403–10.

114. Sharp HM, Canady JW, Ligot FAC, et al. Caregiver and patient reported outcomes after repair of cleft lip and/or palate in the Philippines. Cleft Palate Craniofac J 2008;45(2):163–71.

115. Jafari A, Tringale KR, Campbell BH, et al. Impact of humanitarian experiences on otolaryngology trainees: a follow-up study of travel grant recipients. Otolaryngol Head Neck Surg 2017;156(6):1084–7.

116. Yeow VKL, Lee S-TT, Lambrecht TJ, et al. International task force on volunteer cleft missions. J Craniofac Surg 2002;13(1):18–25.

Innovations in Airway Surgery

Amy Manning, MD[a], Daniel J. Wehrmann, MD[b], Catherine K. Hart, MD, MS[c],*,
Glenn E. Green, MD[b]

KEYWORDS

- Airway stenosis • Tracheobronchomalacia • Stents • Scaffolds • Balloon dilation
- Endoscopic • Tissue replacement

KEY POINTS

- Airway stents can be used to support postoperative healing following airway reconstruction. Stents may also play a temporizing role in cases of malacia, compression, or stenosis not immediately amenable to surgical correction.
- Endoscopic balloon dilation is an effective, efficient approach to management of airway stenosis in many patients. It can be a primary treatment method or an adjuvant following airway reconstruction.
- External scaffolding and airway splints, both permanent and resorbable, are active areas of research that may significantly advance the management of tracheobronchomalacia.
- Management of large tracheal defects remains a challenge; however, advances in tissue engineering and tracheal transplant/replacement provide more hope for improved management options.

INTRODUCTION

The management of airway stenosis has evolved considerably over time. In the 1800s, dilation with or without stenting was the mainstay of airway management. At that time the equipment was rudimentary and the outcomes disappointing. In the 1900s, open airway surgery was introduced and rapidly expanded to include procedures to expand the cricoid framework expansion, resection procedures, and the slide tracheoplasty.

Disclosure Statement: G.E. Green has a patent for a 3D Printed Airway splint that has been licensed to Materialise. The rest of the authors have nothing to disclose.
[a] Pediatric Otolaryngology, Cincinnati Children's Hospital Medical Center, 3333 Burnet Avenue, MLC 2018, Cincinnati, OH 45229, USA; [b] Pediatric Otolaryngology, Department of Otolaryngology–Head and Neck Surgery, University of Michigan, CW-5702 (SPC 4241), 1540 East Hospital Drive, Ann Arbor, MI 48109-4241, USA; [c] Pediatric Otolaryngology, Cincinnati Children's Hospital Medical Center, University of Cincinnati College of Medicine, 3333 Burnet Avenue, MLC 2018, Cincinnati, OH 45229, USA
* Corresponding author.
E-mail address: Catherine.hart@cchmc.org

More recently, there has been a resurgence in the use of endoscopic interventions and balloon dilation along with advances in endoscopic procedures and stenting. The use of external scaffolds and tissue engineering for airway replacement are rapidly being incorporated in the management of pediatric airway surgery.

External Scaffolds

Tracheobronchomalacia is compression or collapse of the trachea and/or bronchus that is characteristically worse on expiration. Mild forms present with coughing, wheezing, or recurrent pneumonias. Severe forms may require tracheostomy and long-term positive pressure ventilation. The most severe forms may additionally require sedation and paralytics in an intensive care setting. Mortality is high for severe forms. Tracheobronchomalacia is associated with prematurity, cartilaginous disorders, congenital cardiovascular anomalies, and tracheoesophageal fistulae. In particular, enlarged pulmonary arteries, a dilated aorta, a double aortic arch, or a high-riding innominate artery may cause compression and collapse of the trachea and/or bronchi.[1,2] Similar to more distal tracheobronchomalacia, peristomal tracheal collapse associated with a tracheostomy tube may result in inability to decannulate or even phonate.

Tracheobronchomalacia continues to be a clinical challenge. Management has varied from optimizing airway clearance with medications, pneumatic splinting with positive pressure, long-term ventilation via tracheostomy, cardiovascular interventions, internal stenting of the airway, and more recently, use of externally implanted airway splints.[2-6]

External scaffolding, or airway splinting, treats tracheobronchomalacia by providing a rigid structure from which the airway can be suspended. The first external scaffolds were made of autologous rib grafts.[7] More recently, splints have been made from a variety of materials.

Bioabsorbable Airway Splints

Tracheobronchomalacia of infancy will normally resolve with airway growth after 2 to 3 years.[1,2] An optimal airway splint will support the airway while still allowing growth during this time, after which the device is no longer needed. Bioresorbable airway splints (and degradable internal airway stents) are ideally suited for the growing child with tracheobronchomalacia.

Commercially available facial fracture plates made of L-lactide-co-glycolide have been used by Javia and Zur to support airway malacia associated with a tracheostomy with short-term follow-up (but with 3-year follow-up in one patient).[8] Gorostidi and colleagues[9] describe promising results with off-label use of L-lactide-co-glycolide facial fracture plates. Their 7-patient case series had 6 to 24 months follow-up. Hsueh and Li used polylactic acid plates also designed for facial fracture plating to treat peristomal collapse and enable extubation.[10] Only short-term follow-up is noted. Each of these plates starts to lose strength rapidly after 9 months.[11]

The newest advance designed to be an improved solution is custom-manufactured bioresorbable airway splints. The splints are manufactured with 3-dimensional (3D) printing based on computed tomography of the airway (**Fig. 1**). Microdesign elements create mechanical properties specifically allowing for airway growth while maintaining strength for 2 years after which the splints resorb. These splints are manufactured from 96% polycaprolactone/4% hydroxyapatite via laser sintering and sterilized via ethylene oxide. These splints are not commercially available and have been manufactured only in research laboratories. Initial human use was reported in 2013 and the first 3 cases reported in 2015.[12,13] After a median sternotomy and subsequent dissection,

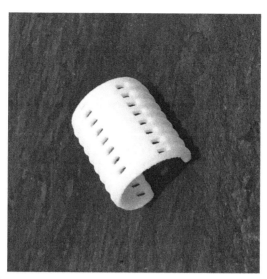

Fig. 1. 3D-printed airway splint.

the splints are sutured over the malacic portion of the airway such that the airway is suspended from the splint. Intraoperative bronchoscopy is performed before, during, and after splint placement to confirm patency of the malacic area. More than 15 patients have been implanted with good long-term results with more than 6 years follow-up.

The development of airway splints continues to be an active area of research with new advances being rapidly translated into human use.

Permanent External Airway Splinting

For children in whom significant airway growth and remodeling is expected, a bioresorbable option is generally preferable. However, because of a lack of a readily available splint with ideal bioresorption properties, permanent materials have been used to treat severe cases of tracheomalacia. Ando and colleagues[14] have used polytetrafluoroethylene in a recently published series of 98 patients with long-term follow-up. Significant complications were noted, including a high rate of revision surgery, erosion, and need for explantation.

In contradistinction, tracheal collapse that develops in older children and adults is not amenable to the use of bioresorbable tracheal splints, because these patients are not expected to outgrow their malacia. A permanent splint created from a permanent biocompatible material is needed rather than repeated placement of bioresorbable splints.

Johnston first used autologous rib grafting to externally stent malacic segments of the airway in 2 patients who had severe tracheobronchomalacia who were subsequently decannulated.[7] In 2007, Göbel and colleagues[15] published a review looking at 12 patients who underwent permanent splinting for tracheobronchomalacia with ceramic rings; 17-year follow-up showed improvement in malacia without major complications.

In 2017, Morrison and colleagues[5] described the creation of a patient-specific permanent splint using computed tomography of the airway. The splint was 3D printed out of polyetherketoneketone. Implantation was performed via a midline sternotomy approach by placing the splint around the affected trachea and suspending the trachea to the splint with polypropylene sutures. This patient was extubated 3 weeks postoperatively and subsequently discharged home. Repeat studies showed a widely patent trachea at the site of previous malacia.[5] The patient subsequently did well for 4 years until she passed away from her underlying progressive neurologic disease.

Treatment of tracheobronchomalacia in older children and adults remains an active area of research with the recent development of a variety of devices and surgical techniques.

Endoluminal Stents

The use of stenting in pediatric laryngotracheal stenosis is multifaceted, and stents play an integral role in the surgical management of these patients. The indication, level, and length of airway pathology help to determine the most appropriate type of stent used. In general, stents are most useful as a temporary option to provide a semirigid framework for postsurgical healing of the airway or as a temporizing measure to a more definitive therapy.

Laryngeal stenting

Laryngeal stents are primarily used for postoperative purposes in laryngotracheal reconstruction (LTR) procedures performed in a "double-stage" fashion. At the time of reconstruction, the stent is sutured in place in the subglottis and provides a semi-rigid framework around which the cartilage grafts heal, maintaining patency of the reconstructed area.[16] The stent is typically removed endoscopically 2 to 8 weeks following reconstruction.[17] A variety of materials exist, including the Teflon Aboulker stents and soft silicone stents (such as a cut end of a Montgomery T-tube or a Rutter stent) (**Fig. 2**). In a randomized controlled trial, Preciado[18] compared surgical outcomes in patients with grade III subglottic stenosis treated by double-stage LTR, using either a Teflon Aboulker stent or a cut Montgomery T-tube silastic stent with the superior end sutured closed. He reported a longer time to decannulation and increased granulation tissue formation in the silastic stent group but less dysphagia with the silastic stent. Silastic stents (such as the Rutter stent) are more commonly used than the Teflon stents.

Alternatively, a silicone Montgomery T-tube can be placed as a laryngeal stent. It was one of the first-described stents, first described in 1965.[19] Advantages of

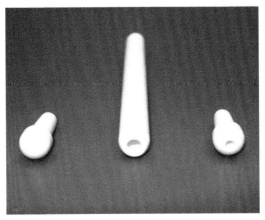

Fig. 2. Silicone suprastomal stent (Rutter stent).

T-tube use include potential for long-term stenting, voicing, and stenting at the level of a tracheostomy stoma, as the T-tube acts as both a stent and a tracheostomy tube. The length of the T-tube can be modified intraoperatively to the desired length. Disadvantages include the need for meticulous care and potential for mucous plugging or obstruction with granulation tissue, and they cannot be easily changed at home. Their propensity for mucous plugging, particularly with smaller tubes, precludes their use in children younger than 4 years of age.[20]

Tracheobronchial stenting

Severe congenital or acquired tracheal or bronchial stenosis or malacia can be a challenging dilemma for clinicians. The use of stents in these cases has been reported to lead to immediate clinical improvement; however, the long-term use of indwelling central airway stents has been fraught with complications.[16] Unlike subglottic stenting, tracheobronchial stents are not typically used as a framework to reinforce postsurgical healing, but rather to provide rigidity to a collapsible, compressed, or stenotic segment of the airway. Traditionally, 2 main types of tracheobronchial stents have been used: silicone stents and metallic stents. More recently, a variety of absorbable stents have been investigated.

In 1995, Filler and colleagues[21] reported on the first use of metallic angioplasty Palmaz stents in the airways of 7 pediatric patients; they saw immediate clinical improvement in all patients. Follow-up time ranged from 1 to 25 months, and they reported restenosis in 2 patients despite stent placement and described a mild inflammatory reaction to the stent in all patients. They noted that the stents became epithelialized and thus did not interfere with mucociliary clearance. The initial success of this approach reported by these and other investigators[16,22] led to initial widespread adaptation of their use. Reported advantages included ease of deployment and potential to accommodate growth of the airway with future stent dilation. In subsequent series of greater numbers of children treated with metallic tracheobronchial stents, with longer follow-up time, high rates of complications have been reported. In 2004, Lim and colleagues[23] presented their complications of metallic stent placement in the pediatric population. Witnessed complications of long-term indwelling metallic stents were severe and included stent fracture, stenosis/scarring at stent site, granulation tissue often requiring emergent and difficult stent removal, and stent erosion into neighboring structures of the mediastinum. Their resultant recommendation was to limit the use of tracheal or bronchial stenting to patients in whom alternative options have failed or are contraindicated and that they be used as a temporizing bridge for a limited duration.

In contrast to metallic stents, silicone stents have their own benefits and drawbacks. They are easy to place and to remove; however, they disrupt mucociliary clearance, which can lead to life-threatening mucous plugging events, and are prone to migration and formation of granulation tissue, which can occlude the ends of the stent. A 2005 series of 14 children published by Fayon and colleagues[24] discussed placement of a total of 26 silicone tracheal or bronchial stents. They reported initial ventilatory improvement in all cases but eventual failure in 43% caused by migration or creasing of the stent leading to obstruction. In addition, they reported one mortality due to formation of a mucous plug in the stent. There were no cases of bleeding or erosion, and removal and replacement of the stents, if necessary, was uncomplicated. Their series included patients aged 2 months to 8 years, and duration of stenting was less than 1 day to 15 months. They recommended daily treatment with nebulized humidification and chest physiotherapy to help prevent mucous plugging and concluded that silicone stenting was a feasible short-term option in the pediatric population. Conversely, Gildea and colleagues[25] reported a 75% rate of serious complications following silicone stent placement in 12 pediatric patients for benign indications, including migration, expectoration of the stent, and mucous plugging requiring emergent bronchoscopy.

In 2015, Antón-Pacheco and colleagues[26] reported on their experience in treating a small series of 4 patients with severe tracheal or bronchial stenosis or malacia with custom bioabsorbable polydioxanone (PDS) stents. Absorbable mesh stents are an intriguing option, with the potential to, as metallic wire stents, integrate into the airway wall and preserve mucociliary clearance but without the risk for long-term erosion into neighboring structures or need for removal. Despite their small sample size of 4 patients, their experience is encouraging, with each patient experiencing both immediate and sustained symptomatic benefit with no major stent-related complications, in follow-up time ranging from 5 to 40 months. They describe the need for restenting in 2 of their patients, who required the support of the stent for longer than its 3- to 4-month period before absorption.

A 2013 series by Serio and colleagues[27] reported the group's experience with a total of 235 tracheobronchial stents in 100 patients over a period of 7 years. They used a variety of types of stents (silicone, metallic, and bioabsorbable PDS) with a median follow-up period of 41.4 months. Eighty patients showed initial clinical improvement. The most common complication in both silicone and metallic stents was granulation tissue, which required treatment with laser ablation or stent removal. Absorbable PDS stents were used in only 3 patients, one of whom required repeated stenting after the stent had resorbed, whereas the PDS stent was ineffective in the remaining 2 patients due to insufficient radial strength. Their series did not include any life-threatening stent complications.

Laryngotracheal stenting in the pediatric population serves varied goals. In patients with subglottic and glottis stenosis, temporary stents play an important role in postoperative healing to ensure patency of a reconstructed airway segment. Conversely, the use of tracheal and bronchial stents is not typically in the postoperative healing period, but rather a potential option to alleviate obstruction due to severe airway compression, collapse, or stenosis not amenable to surgical correction. Although tracheal and bronchial stents often have immediate initial clinical improvement, their long-term use is fraught with potentially severe complications that limit their use to patients in whom surgical correction of the underlying issue has failed or is contraindicated or as a temporizing measure. Bioabsorbable stents show promise as a potential solution to the typical issues facing either metallic or silicone stents. The patient population in which these stents may be applied is varied and complex, and the decision to use a stent should be guided by a multidisciplinary team and patients should be closely observed while an indwelling stent is in place.

Balloon Dilation

The concept of dilation of laryngotracheal stenosis is not new but has been recently revisited and evolved considerably with the advent of balloon dilation instruments and improvement in endoscopic visualization. Classically, dilation was performed in a rigid "bougienage" fashion; however, this was largely abandoned due to concern for mucosal shearing and further airway injury. The first reports of endoscopic balloon dilation for pediatric laryngotracheal stenosis date from the early 1990s, with Hebra and colleagues[28] using spherical angioplasty balloons in combination with intraluminal stents. Since that time, multiple studies have been published reporting on different investigators' experience with balloon dilation in the pediatric airway with relatively good success and few complications. Most of the available evidence is limited to retrospective case series.[29–32]

In 2014, Lang and Brietzke[33] published a systematic review and meta-analysis of 7 retrospective studies encompassing 150 patients treated with both primary and adjuvant (following reconstructive procedures) balloon dilation. They found no association between treatment success and patient age, sex, cause of stenosis, history of prematurity or lung disease, or subjective firmness of stenosis scar. A random effects model estimated the rate of treatment success (defined as avoiding tracheostomy or laryngotracheal reconstruction) at 65.3%. A mean of 1.6 dilations was required per patient. Gastroesophageal reflux, weight less than 5 kg, and presence of concomitant airway disorders such as laryngomalacia were associated with lower rate of success. A regression model yielded decreased odds of success with increasing severity of stenosis by Myer-Cotton grade. The investigators recognized short follow-up time as a limitation of the study; average reported follow-up time was 4.6 months.

Avelino and colleagues[34] published in 2015 a prospective descriptive study of the use of balloon dilation in pediatric subglottic stenosis at their institutions. Their study involved 48 children with an average follow-up time of 7.8 months with an overall success rate of 60%. They found that balloon dilation was significantly more successful in children with acute stenosis (present for 30 days or fewer) than more chronic, mature scar (100% vs 39%, $P<.0001$). Success of balloon dilation was also significantly associated with grade of stenosis, younger patient age, and absence of tracheostomy. Complications were uncommon, with 3 patients experiencing transient dysphagia and a single patient developing a submucosal cyst as a result of the balloon dilation. They limited their investigation to children undergoing primary dilation and those without concomitant airway comorbidities.

An appealing aspect of endoscopic balloon dilation is that it is straightforward, requires a short operative time, and does not preclude open reconstruction at a later time, if needed. The patient is kept spontaneously breathing while the airway is examined with a zero-degree Hopkins rod. The stenosis is then sized using endotracheal tubes, as described by Cotton and Myer.[35] The airway is then dilated with the balloon and sizing repeated to provide objective evidence of increasing airway cross-sectional area. Selection of balloon size is generally based on the outer diameter of the ideal size endotracheal tube for the child's age, plus an additional 1 to 2 mm.[36] Adjunctive measures such as laser or sharp scar band division and injection of steroids into the stenotic segment, as well as serial dilation, may improve success rate. Practitioners must observe patients meticulously, as it is not uncommon for stenosis to recur and for repeat dilation or more extensive surgery to become necessary, and long-term data surrounding the use of balloon dilation in this population are limited.

Balloon dilation is an effective technique that can be a primary treatment method for managing intraluminal airway stenosis. It can also be used following airway reconstruction to counter the effect of restenosis at graft sites or along an anastomosis.

Advances in Endoscopic Techniques

Since the introduction and popularization of open airway reconstruction techniques in the second half of the twentieth century, several of these techniques have been adapted to be performed endoscopically. Along with more generalized popularity of "minimally invasive" surgical approaches, endoscopic airway techniques have the potential to offer shorter operative time, shorter hospital and intensive care unit (ICU) stays, possibly fewer operative risks, and more appealing cosmetic results.

Endoscopic cricoid split

In 1980, Cotton and Seid described a novel alternative to tracheostomy for management of inability to extubate premature infants due to development of subglottic stenosis.[37] Their approach involved division of the cricoid ring, allowing for expansion, followed by intubation with a larger endotracheal tube for a period of time as a stent. More recently, this general technique has been applied endoscopically by several groups, for management of both subglottic stenosis (SGS) and bilateral vocal fold immobility (BVFI).[38–42]

The procedure is performed under general anesthesia with the patient spontaneously ventilating. The patient is placed in suspension with a vallecula laryngoscope such as the pediatric Lindholm laryngoscope. Vocal fold spreaders and an operating microscope provide adequate visualization of the larynx. The anterior and posterior aspects of the cricoid ring can then be divided vertically with either CO_2 laser or with cold steel instruments. Division of the cricoid relieves the natural spring exerted by the full ring. The subglottic area is then dilated with a noncompliant balloon inflated to burst pressure to expand the ring. The patient is then intubated with an endotracheal tube one-half size larger than an age-appropriate tube and transported to the ICU, where the child remains intubated for up to 2 weeks. The patient is brought back to the operating room on the day before planned extubation, at which time the surgical site is examined and the endotracheal tube is downsized. The patient is then extubated in the ICU the following day.

In 2010, Mirabile and colleagues[38] published their review of 18 patients with SGS grades II to IV treated via endoscopic anterior cricoid split. Postoperatively, they used either an endotracheal tube or a Montgomery T-tube for stenting. Fifteen of their patients (83%) were able to successfully avoid tracheostomy placement or were decannulated. They applied the technique both to congenital and acquired SGS, including those with cartilage involvement and firm fibrotic scar. Importantly, they limited the use of this technique to patients with adequate pulmonary status and no prior attempts at reconstruction of the subglottic area. Reported failures were due to granulation tissue formation at the surgical site, and 83% of patients required subsequent balloon dilation to maintain airway patency. In 2018, Carr and colleagues[42] reported a series of 9 patients; they reported success in all except for one patient, who had poor pulmonary reserve and required tracheostomy due to severe chronic lung disease of prematurity. Although small, these studies indicate a similar success rate to open cricoid split in a carefully chosen patient population.

Similarly, several investigators have published on the use of endoscopic cricoid split in the treatment of congenital BFVI. BVFI is uncommon but is the second most common cause of stridor in infants after laryngomalacia.[40] It is estimated that more than 50% will have spontaneous resolution of their vocal fold immobility in the first 12 months of life, thus a treatment that causes minimal long-term alteration of the larynx is appealing. Gold-standard treatment has traditionally been tracheostomy; however, this is unacceptable to many families and has significant economic burden and safety issues (a recent large national series reported 14% mortality of 885 included infants).[43] In 2018, Rutter and colleagues[40] published a multiinstitutional case series of 19 infants with BFVI treated with endoscopic anterior and posterior cricoid split. Fourteen of nineteen (73.7%) patients were able to either avoid tracheostomy or be decannulated due to the procedure. The majority (67%) did not have return of vocal fold motion in this series; however, patients in whom the surgery was successful were more likely to have return of vocal fold motion. The investigators reported a single incidence of transient aspiration postoperatively. Endoscopic cricoid split seems to be a possible alternative treatment to tracheostomy in select patients with congenital BVFI.

Endoscopic posterior cartilage graft

First described in 2002 by Inglis and colleagues,[44] endoscopic posterior cricoid division with placement of a posterior cartilage graft has become an option for treatment of SGS, posterior glottic stenosis (PGS), or BVFI. Their described technique begins similarly to that discussed earlier for endoscopic division of the posterior cricoid plate. They then carved a costal cartilage graft in a keystone shape with posterior flanges such that it "snaps" into place. The graft is not sutured in place, and the patient was not left intubated nor was a suprastomal stent placed; however, the investigators did perform a temporary tracheostomy in patients who did not already have a tracheostomy in place, for airway protection in the event of graft dislodgement in the early postoperative period. In 2017, Dahl and colleagues'[45] series included 33 patients who had undergone the procedure, with a 65.6% decannulation rate. Gerber and colleagues[46] published a multiinstitutional series of 28 patients who underwent the procedure; 25/28 patients were decannulated or avoided tracheostomy, whereas Provenzano reported on 12 children with SGS, PGS, or BVFI with a success rate of 67%.[47–56] Potential advantages of the technique include less risk to voice and vocal folds than alternative endoscopic procedures including arytenoidectomy, cordotomy, or vocal fold lateralization, because it causes no manipulation or destruction of the vocal folds or adjacent tissue. Compared with the open approach, there is less destabilization of the larynx, as no laryngofissure is required. Potential patients need to have an easily visualized larynx.

Tissue Engineering/Airway Replacement

Large tracheal defects are one of the greatest challenges for the airway surgeon. Excision and reanastomosis with intrathoracic and laryngeal releases can readily allow reconstruction for defects up to half of the trachea, but there are no good options for defects larger than this.[57,58] A similar conundrum exists for patients with loss of integrity of large portions of the airway through failed reconstruction attempts, large anastomotic dehiscence, burns, or congenital disease. Tracheal agenesis, where the bronchi come off of the esophagus, represents the greatest challenge. All of the entities are rare and largely fatal, but recent advances offer hope for the future.

An ideal method of tracheal replacement has not yet been found. Challenges include creating a structurally sound connection between the native airway and the tracheal replacement construct, avoiding granulation tissue and infection, as well as allowing for mucous clearance of the airway. Any reconstruction is at potential reconstruction of forming a fistula with nearby vasculature including the innominate artery, the aorta, and the pulmonary arteries.[59] For young children, growth of the construct is ideal but is unachievable at present. A description of various tracheal replacement techniques follows, including autologous tissue grafting, tissue allografting, tissue engineering, and synthetic scaffolding.

Composite tissue grafting for tracheal replacement
As early as 1946, composite allografts have been used to create a trachea. Long-term survival is possible. Recently, Kolb and colleagues[60] performed total replacement of the trachea in a 12-year-old girl with long-segment tracheal stenosis. A myocutaneous latissimus dorsi free flap was tubed and reinforced with costal cartilage to provide for the free flap. The reconstruction was performed around a silicone tube, which was subsequently removed. This patient was able to be decannulated and was reported to be doing well 4 years out from her free flap reconstruction. The paucity of these cases shows both the rarity and the extreme challenge of tracheal replacement surgery.

Tissue allografts
Allografting uses decellularized tissue that can be implanted and incorporated into the surrounding tissue without the need for immunosuppression.[57] This has led to its investigation in tracheal replacement surgery, to recreate the tracheal lining. However,

these tissue allografts lack structural integrity and thus require airway support through stenting as the neotrachea heals.

Aortic allografts have been used in patients requiring tracheal resection for malignancy. Makris and colleagues[61] describe a series of 6 such patients. These patients had intraluminal silicone stents placed, as well as a pedicled vascularized flap wrapped around the outer wall of the trachea to provide increased vasculature to the allograft. These patients required aggressive pulmonary physiotherapy in the perioperative period, as mucociliary clearance was affected. Four of the six patients were disease free and alive at 34 months.

Tissue engineering
Given the unique challenges that exist with tracheal replacement, there is interest in using tissue engineering to create a trachea de novo. The tissue-engineered trachea requires (1) a scaffold for structural support; (2) an epithelial lining, preferably with functional cilia; and (3) a blood supply. No tissue-engineered construct meets these criteria.[62] Scaffolds can be biodegradable (replaced with cartilage or bone over time) or permanent.

Three children have undergone tracheal replacement where stem cells were seeded into a decellularized allogenic trachea. Four-year survival was reported in one patient, whereas another died of uncertain causes after 2 weeks.[63,64]

Tissue engineering continues to push the boundaries of tracheal replacement, attempting to obtain both the integrity needed of the trachea as well as maintaining the tracheal epithelial lining and function. The authors remain optimistic that this will eventually represent an ideal long-term solution.

Synthetic scaffolds for trachealization of the esophagus
In the neonate where growth is needed and size is limited, the previously described methods for tracheal replacement prove to be inadequate. For tracheal agenesis, all patients with long-term survival have undergone trachealization of the esophagus.[65] The esophagus is separated from the alimentary track with creation of a spit fistula in the neck and gastric separation inferiorly. The proximal end of the esophagus is then brought out of the neck as an end stoma. A scaffold is placed around the esophagus, and the bronchi are marsupialized into the distal trachea. This enables the esophagus to serve as a function conduit to the bronchi. At a later date, a gastric pull-up is performed and the spit fistula is taken down. Survival past 9 years has been noted.[66] 3D-printed scaffolds have the potential to support a more elaborate design with the potential for connection to the larynx for speech and a potential for eventual decannulation; these have been used in one patient with good early results.

SUMMARY

Airway surgery is constantly evolving as previously used techniques are modified and new options for management of airway pathology are developed. Advances in external scaffolds, airway stenting, and endoscopic airway management provide new options for managing complex airway problems in the pediatric population.

REFERENCES

1. Hysinger EB, Panitch HB. Paediatric tracheomalacia. Paediatr Respir Rev 2016; 17:9–15.
2. Choi S, Lawlor C, Rahbar R, et al. Diagnosis, classification, and management of pediatric tracheobronchomalacia: a review. JAMA Otolaryngol Head Neck Surg 2018.

https://doi.org/10.1001/jamaoto.2018.3276. Available at: https://jamanetwork.com/journals/jamaotolaryngology/fullarticle/2719203. Accessed February 2, 2019.

3. Panitch HB, Allen JL, Alpert BE, et al. Effects of CPAP on lung mechanics in infants with acquired tracheobronchomalacia. Am J Respir Crit Care Med 1994; 150(5):1341–6.
4. Zopf DA, Green GE, Green GE. Bioprinting in otolaryngology and airway reconstruction. 3D Bioprinting in Regenerative Engineering. Boca Raton (FL): CRC Press; 2018 https://doi.org/10.1201/b21916-7.
5. Morrison RJ, Sengupta S, Flanangan CL, et al. Successful treatment of severe acquired tracheomalacia with a patient-specific 3D-printed permanent tracheal splint. JAMA Otolaryngol Head Neck Surg 2017;143(5):523–5.
6. McGill M, Raol N, Gipson KS, et al. Preclinical assessment of resorbable silk splints for the treatment of pediatric tracheomalacia. Laryngoscope 2018. https://doi.org/10.1002/lary.27540.
7. Johnston MR, Loeber N, Hillyer P, et al. External stent for repair of secondary tracheomalacia. Ann Thorac Surg 1980;30(3):291–6.
8. Javia LR, Zur KB. Laryngotracheal reconstruction with resorbable microplate buttressing. Laryngoscope 2012;122(4):920–4.
9. Gorostidi F, Reinhard A, Monnier P, et al. External bioresorbable airway rigidification to treat refractory localized tracheomalacia. Laryngoscope 2016;126(11): 2605–10.
10. Hsueh WD, Smith LP. External airway splint to treat tracheomalacia following laryngotracheal reconstruction. Int J Pediatr Otorhinolaryngol 2017;94:68–9.
11. Bhanot S, Alex JC, Lowlicht RA, et al. The efficacy of resorbable plates in head and neck reconstruction. Laryngoscope 2002;112(5):890–8.
12. Zopf DA, Hollister SJ, Nelson ME, et al. Bioresorbable airway splint created with a three-dimensional printer. N Engl J Med 2013;368(21):2043–5.
13. Morrison RJ, Hollister SJ, Niedner MF, et al. Mitigation of tracheobronchomalacia with 3D-printed personalized medical devices in pediatric patients. Sci Transl Med 2015;7(285):285ra64.
14. Ando M, Nagase Y, Hasegawa H, et al. External stenting: a reliable technique to relieve airway obstruction in small children. J Thorac Cardiovasc Surg 2017; 153(5):1167–77.
15. Göbel G, Karaiskaki N, Gerlinger I, et al. Tracheal ceramic rings for tracheomalacia: a review after 17 years. Laryngoscope 2007;117(10):1741–4.
16. Preciado D, Zalzal G. Laryngeal and tracheal stents in children. Curr Opin Otolaryngol Head Neck Surg 2008;16(1):83–5.
17. Smith DF, de Alarcon A, Jefferson ND, et al. Short- versus long-term stenting in children with subglottic stenosis undergoing laryngotracheal reconstruction. Otolaryngol Head Neck Surg 2018;158(2):375–80.
18. Preciado D. A randomized study of suprastomal stents in laryngotracheoplasty surgery for grade III subglottic stenosis in children. Laryngoscope 2014;124: 207–13.
19. Montgomery WW. T-tube tracheal stent. Arch Otolaryngol 1965;82:320–1.
20. Stern Y, Willging JP, Cotton RT. Use of Montgomery T-tube in laryngotracheal reconstruction in children: is it safe? Ann Otol Rhinol Laryngol 1998;107:1006–9.
21. Filler RM, Forte C, Fraga JC, et al. The use of expandable metallic stents for tracheobronchial obstruction in children. J Pediatr Surg 1995;30:1050–6.
22. Jacobs JP, Quintessenza JA, Botero LM, et al. The role of airway stents in the management of pediatric tracheal, carinal, and bronchial disease. Eur J Cardiothorac Surg 2000;18:505–12.

23. Lim LH, Cotton RT, Azizkhan RG, et al. Complications of metallic stents in the pediatric airway. Otolaryngol Head Neck Surg 2004;131:355–61.

24. Fayon M, Donato L, de Blic J, et al. French experience of silicone tracheobronchial stenting in children. Pediatr Pulmonol 2005;39:21–7.

25. Gildea TR, Murthy SC, Sahoo D, et al. Performance of a self-expanding silicone stent in palliation of benign airway conditions. Chest 2006;130:1419–23.

26. Antón-Pacheco JL, Luna C, García E, et al. Initial experience with a new biodegradable airway stent in children: is this the stent we were waiting for? Pediatr Pulmonol 2016;51(6):607–12.

27. Serio P, Fainardi V, Leone R, et al. Tracheobronchial obstruction: follow-up study of 100 children treated with airway stenting. Eur J Cardiothorac Surg 2014;45: e100–9.

28. Hebra A, Powell DD, Smith CD, et al. Balloon tracheoplasty in children: results of a 15-year experience. J Pediatr Surg 1991;26(8):957–61.

29. Hautefort C, Teissier N, Viala P, et al. Balloon dilation laryngoplasty for subglottic stenosis in children: eight years' experience. Arch Otolaryngol Head Neck Surg 2012;138:235–40.

30. Bent JP, Shah MB, Nord R, et al. Balloon dilation for recurrent stenosis after pediatric laryngotracheoplasty. Ann Otol Rhinol Laryngol 2010;119:619–27.

31. Durden F, Sobol SE. Balloon laryngoplasty as a primary treatment for subglottic stenosis. Arch Otolaryngol Head Neck Surg 2007;133:772–5.

32. Whigham AS, Howell R, Choi S, et al. Outcomes of balloon dilation in pediatric subglottic stenosis. Ann Otol Rhinol Laryngol 2012;121(7):442–8.

33. Lang M, Brietzke SE. A systematic review and meta-analysis of endoscopic balloon dilation of pediatric subglottic stenosis. Otolaryngol Head Neck Surg 2014;150:174–9.

34. Avelino M, Maunsell R, Jubé Wastowski I. Predicting outcomes of balloon laryngoplasty in children with subglottic stenosis. Int J Pediatr Otorhinolaryngol 2015; 79(4):532–6.

35. Myer CM, O'Connor DM, Cotton RT. Proposed grading system for subglottic stenosis based on endotracheal tube sizes. Ann Otol Rhinol Laryngol 1994;103: 319–23.

36. Jefferson ND, Cohen AP, Rutter MJ. Subglottic stenosis. Semin Pediatr Surg 2016;25(3):138–43.

37. Cotton RT, Seid AB. Management of the extubation problem in the premature child. Anterior cricoid split as an alternative to tracheotomy. Ann Otol Rhinol Laryngol 1980;89(6):508–11.

38. Mirabile L, Serio PP, Baggi RR, et al. Endoscopic anterior cricoid split and balloon dilation in pediatric subglottic stenosis. Int J Pediatr Otorhinolaryngol 2010; 74(12):1409–14.

39. Horn DL, Maguire RC, Simons JP, et al. Endoscopic anterior cricoid split with balloon dilation in infants with failed extubation. Laryngoscope 2012;122(1): 216–9.

40. Rutter MJ, Hart CK, Alarcon A, et al. Endoscopic anterior-posterior cricoid split for pediatric bilateral vocal fold paralysis. Laryngoscope 2018;128(1):257–63.

41. Sedaghat S, Tapia M, Fredes F, et al. Endoscopic management of bilateral vocal fold paralysis in newborns and infants. Int J Pediatr Otorhinolaryngol 2017; 97:13–7.

42. Carr S, Dritsoula A, Thevasagayam R. Endoscpic cricoid split in a tertiary referral pediatric centre. J Laryngol Otol 2018;132:753–6.

43. Lee JH, Smith PB, Quek MB, et al. Risk factors and in-hospital outcomes following tracheostomy in infants. J Pediatr 2016;173:39–44.

44. Inglis AF Jr, Perkins JA, Manning SC, et al. Endoscopic posterior cricoid split and rib grafting in 10 children. Laryngoscope 2003;113(11):2004–9.

45. Dahl JP, Purcell PL, Parikh SR, et al. Endoscopic posterior cricoid split with costal cartilage graft: a fifteen-year experience. Laryngoscope 2017;127(1):252–7.

46. Gerber ME, Modi VK, Ward RF, et al. Endoscopic posterior cricoid split and costal cartilage graft placement in children. Otolaryngol Head Neck Surg 2013;148(3): 494–502.

47. Provenzano MJ, Hulstein BA, Solomon DH, et al. Pediatric endoscopic airway management with posterior cricoid rib grafting. Laryngoscope 2011;121:1062–6.

48. Benjamin B, Inglis A. Minor congenital laryngeal clefts: diagnosis and classification. Ann Otol Rhinol Laryngol 1989;98(6):417–20.

49. Johnston DR, Watters K, Ferrari LR, et al. Laryngeal cleft: evaluation and management. Int J Pediatr Otorhinolaryngol 2014;78(6):905–11.

50. Yamashita M, Chinyanga HM, Steward DJ. Posterior laryngeal cleft - anaesthetic experiences. Can Anaesth Soc J 1979;26(6):502–5.

51. Chien W, Ashland J, Haver K, et al. Type I laryngeal cleft: establishing a functional diagnostic and management algorithm. Int J Pediatr Otorhinolaryngol 2006; 70(12):2073–9.

52. Sandu K, Monnier P. Endoscopic laryngotracheal cleft repair without tracheotomy or intubation. Laryngoscope 2006;116(4):630–4.

53. Leboulanger N, Garabédian EN. Laryngo-tracheo-oesophageal clefts. Orphanet J Rare Dis 2011;6:81.

54. Rahbar R, Rouillon I, Roger G, et al. The presentation and management of laryngeal cleft: a 10-year experience. Arch Otolaryngol Head Neck Surg 2006; 132(12):1335–41.

55. Yeung JC, Balakrishnan K, Cheng ATL, et al. International Pediatric Otolaryngology Group: consensus guidelines on the diagnosis and management of type I laryngeal clefts. Int J Pediatr Otorhinolaryngol 2017;101:51–6.

56. Koltai PJ, Morgan D, Evans JN. Endoscopic repair of supraglottic laryngeal clefts. Arch Otolaryngol Head Neck Surg 1991;117(3):273–8.

57. Belsey R. Resection and reconstruction of the intrathoracic trachea. Br J Surg 1950;38(150):200–5.

58. Etienne H, Fabre D, Caro AG, et al. Tracheal replacement. Eur Respir J 2018; 51(2):1702–11.

59. Kaye R, Green GE, Smith LP. Tracheal replacement for transplantation. In: Ruis R, editor. Encyclopedia of tissue engineering and regenerative medicine. Amsterdam, Netherlands: Elsevier; 2019. p. 281–4.

60. Kolb F, Simon F, Gaudin R, et al. 4-year follow-up in a child with a total autologous tracheal replacement. N Engl J Med 2018;378(14):1355–7.

61. Makris D, Holder-Espinasse M, Wurtz A, et al. Tracheal replacement with cryopreserved allogenic aorta. Chest 2010;137(1):60–7.

62. Law JX, Liau LL, Aminuddin BS, et al. Tissue-engineered trachea: a review. Int J Pediatr Otorhinolaryngol 2016;91:55–63.

63. Hamilton NJ, Kanani M, Roebuck DJ, et al. Tissue-engineered tracheal replacement in a child: a 4-year follow-up study. Am J Transplant 2015;15(10):2750–7.

64. Elliott MJ, Butler CR, Varanou-Jenkins A, et al. Tracheal replacement therapy with a stem cell-seeded graft: lessons from compassionate use application of a GMP-compliant tissue-engineered medicine. Stem Cells Transl Med 2017;6:1458–64.

65. Densmore JC, Oldham KT, Dominguez KM, et al. Neonatal esophageal trachealization and esophagocarinoplasty in the treatment of flow-limited Floyd II tracheal agenesis. J Thorac Cardiovasc Surg 2017;153(6):e121–5.
66. Tazuke Y, Okuyama H, Uehara S, et al. Long-term outcomes of four patients with tracheal agenesis who underwent airway and esophageal reconstruction. J Pediatr Surg 2015;50(12):2009–11.

Aerodigestive Programs Enhance Outcomes in Pediatric Patients

Christopher T. Wootten, MD, MMHC[a,b,*], Ryan Belcher, MD[a,b],
Christian K. Francom, MD[c], Jeremy D. Prager, MD, MBA[c]

KEYWORDS

- Aerodigestive • Integrated practice unit • Efficiency • Cost • Value

KEY POINTS

- Aerodigestive programs began as coordinated clinics for improving the outcomes of airway surgery.
- Modern programs function as integrated practice units, focusing on integrated specialties and procedures tailored to complex patients and disease states.
- A growing body of literature demonstrates the opportunities for increasing care value through aerodigestive programs.
- Programmatic growth across the nation, as well as national organization, has led to improved communication and direction among programs; however, challenges remain.

INTRODUCTION

Beginning in the mid-1950s, indexed reports exist that use the term aerodigestive to describe the anatomic location of inhaled or ingested foreign bodies in children. Calcaterra and Maceri[1] seem to be the first investigators to incorporate the term aerodigestive dysfunction into the title of a publication. This was in the context of

Disclosure Statement: J.D. Prager is treasurer, consultant, and cofounder of Triple Endoscopy, Inc, and a listed inventor on University of Colorado patents pending US 62/732,272, US62/680,798, US 15/853,521, US 15/887,438, CA 2,990,182, AU 2016283112, EU 16815420.1, and JP 2017 to 566710, which are related to endoscopic methods and technologies. The rest of the authors have nothing to disclose.
[a] Department of Otolaryngology, Vanderbilt University Medical Center, 2200 Children's Way, Doctor's Office Tower 7th Floor, Nashville, TN 37232, USA; [b] Pediatric Otolaryngology, Vanderbilt University Medical Center, 2200 Children's Way, Doctor's Office Tower 7th Floor, Nashville, TN 37232, USA; [c] Department of Otolaryngology, University of Colorado School of Medicine, Children's Hospital Colorado, University of Colorado, 13123 East 16th Avenue B-411, Aurora, CO 80045, USA
* Corresponding author. Monroe Carell Jr. Children's Hospital at Vanderbilt, Doctors' Office Tower, 7th Floor 2200 Children's Way, Nashville, TN 37232-9307.
E-mail address: christopher.t.wootten@vumc.org

compressive or invasive thyroid tumors affecting airway, breathing, feeding, and swallowing. Yet, by the early-1990s, considerable experience with airway reconstruction had led Cotton and colleagues[2] to hypothesize about aerodigestive dysfunction or disease in children and, in particular, to articulate the importance of a thorough assessment of the entire airway before undertaking laryngotracheal reconstruction. Host or foreign body reaction to stents and the importance of systemic and inhaled steroids to mitigate airway granulomatous reaction were being discussed as a way to reconcile success and failure for the hundreds of children who had been operated on at Cincinnati Children's Hospital over the preceding decades. In 1999, the same institution opened the first Pediatric Aerodigestive Center with the charge to colocate specialists from multiple disciplines to diagnose and manage the interrelated conditions known as aerodigestive disease. From the perspective of the otolaryngologist, the Center's multidisciplinary purpose was to diagnose and control for disease states that may have detrimental effects on surgical success rates. Controlling gastroesophageal reflux disease (GERD) was the initial multidisciplinary task; however, as experience and communication increased so did the list of aerodigestive diseases to identify and treat.

In 2002, Hartnick and colleagues[3] published a case report demonstrating the clinical value of this multidisciplinary approach. The investigators describe a young airway reconstruction patient whose preoperative workup included a normal pH study and esophageal eosinophilia on esophagogastroduodenoscopy (EGD) with biopsy. She was placed on antireflux medications but struggled to maintain an adequate airway postoperatively until she was placed on steroid therapy and demonstrated resolution of eosinophilia and improvement in her airway. This was the first published association between what the investigators called allergic esophagitis and subglottic stenosis. Although the understanding of the entity now known as eosinophilic esophagitis continues to evolve, its association with large and small airway disease states and varied clinical presentation is the subject of continued publication, requiring awareness that crosses disciplines.[4]

Through experiences such as these, and the integration of previously separate disciplines, aerodigestive programs continued to spread within individual health care organizations as well as between organizations. During the same time period, the method of delivering complex, coordinated care to particular populations began to undergo its own evolution. Pediatric multidisciplinary care as administered in the medical home model has been broadly and repeatedly endorsed by influential medical societies, including the American Academy of Pediatrics and the American Academy of Family Practice, since the mid-1960s. Likewise, the Centers for Medicare and Medicaid Services supports medical homes for children with complex health care needs in which there is a satisfaction of the triple aim: improved care, improved health, and lower costs. The concept of the medical home is sound for optimizing outcomes while lowering costs in caring for children with medical complexity.[5] There are publications that specifically address the medical home concept in the management of pediatric airway problems (see later discussion). Highlights from these publications include lower overall cost of care, fewer days in-hospital per year, and a shift of care from inpatient environments to outpatient environments.

However, the current practice of pediatric multispecialty aerodigestive care has grown in sophistication beyond the medical home concept. In 2018, Boesch and colleagues[6] published the first contemporary and multicentric assessment of the landscape of aerodigestive care as practiced across the United States. More a reflection of than a directive to aerodigestive centers, the investigators delineate the structure and functions of aerodigestive programs via the Delphi method to resolve expert opinions. What is clear from multicentric, multidisciplinary expert input is that aerodigestive care is increasingly performed in an integrated practice unit (IPU) model.[7] In the prevailing IPU model, the specific aerodigestive population, defined as the aerodigestive patient, is being diagnosed and managed by a multidisciplinary team colocated in time and space in dedicated facilities and supported by dedicated staff. The staff and providers convene regularly outside of the patient care arena to assess IPU operations, including a discussion of how health information and technologies are being leveraged to improve care and to measure the cost of that care. Ideally, throughout the aerodigestive IPU, there exists a focus on increasing care value.

Although 1 of several disorders qualify a child as an aerodigestive patient, these disorders are collectively rare. The unifying theme among the seemingly disparate aerodigestive conditions is not the primary organ system affected, a set of common embryologic errors, or a unified locoregional inflammatory response to some antigen. Rather, aerodigestive disorders are unified by a common contemporary approach to their management. The efflorescence of aerodigestive programs is not driven by an increased incidence of aerodigestive conditions. Instead, it is driven by a nationwide tendency toward care delivery models that provide integrated care.

Although the provision of integrated care through an increasing array of aerodigestive centers improves on the inefficiencies of piecemeal medicine, challenges remain. For example, as health care systems increasingly provide contemporary management of aerodigestive disease in children, it remains possible that more centers does not equal greater access. Furthermore, the authenticity of the IPU and its processes may be degraded by poor incentive alignment within and among providers, the organization, and payers, as well as insufficient community need due to IPU service area overlap. Fortunately, aerodigestive centers are communicating with each other. An international organization of pediatric aerodigestive care, the Aerodigestive Society (www.aerodigestive.us), is convening annually to promote valuable activities and to reduce unnecessary testing and intervention.[8] Where there is a deficit of guidance, expert opinion has been garnered through Delphi studies. These opinions are forming the basis of multicenter research into the data objects, outcomes, and resource utilizations that define multidisciplinary aerodigestive care. Engagement with health care providers and patients is occurring at a quickening pace through the cooperation of the Aerodigestive Society, the various allied medical subspecialty groups, and the American Academy of Pediatrics. Authentic, appropriate, and accessible aerodigestive care is the mantra moving forward.

DISCUSSION
Evolving Models of Aerodigestive Care Delivery

Integrated care is organized around the patient. However, there are several different models of multidisciplinary care that tout patient-centricity. Indeed, colocated multispecialty care represents a convenience to families of children with aerodigestive conditions. Coordinating visits helps minimize travel costs, time off work, and lost revenue. Going a step further, the patient-centered medical home (PCMH) model cares for children with complex conditions using a multidisciplinary team that hinges on a primary pediatrician. Indeed, the concept of a PCMH was initially developed in order to meet the challenges of coordinating and delivering primary care. Those goals have then been applied to more complex medical needs and populations. In these settings, the pediatrician, embedded in the team, both administers and coordinates care for the patient to ensure patient-centricity, minimize waste, and maximize clinical effectiveness. Medical homes lean on a primary care provider in a care coordination role to shepherd the patient to appropriate services integral to the patient's treatment. These services include medical services; surgical services; social work; physical, occupational, and speech therapy; and community resources, to name a few. In the PCMH, the core primary care provider integrates and organizes the recommendations from the various medical home team members for the benefit of the patient in a way that is easy for the family to understand and to follow. Effective medical homes have open lines of communication among team members and through the primary care provider.[9] Casey and colleagues[10] describe their experience with a hospital-based multidisciplinary clinic for medically complex children. In the investigators' experience, their medical home resulted in a significant decrease in Medicaid costs to provide care. Since that writing, the tertiary care-based medical home has been proposed as viable for pediatric aerodigestive care.[11]

The IPU does not feature a core health care provider tasked with coordinating and integrating multidisciplinary care. Rather, the IPU cares for children through a dedicated, multidisciplinary team of clinicians who devote a significant portion of their time to the medical condition. In this model, providers see themselves as part of a common organizational unit. The team takes responsibility for the full cycle of care for the condition. Exactly how care is integrated is a key distinction between the PCMH and the IPU. The IPU also mandates effective communication. Indeed, education, engagement, and follow-up are managed by the IPU's single scheduling and administrative structure. In the IPU, the value of the administrative structure, that is, the extent to which it has managed costs, achieved meaningful patient-reported outcomes, and leveraged the information platform, is the subject of deliberate self-scrutiny.

Enhanced Outcomes

An integrated care model offers many opportunities to improve the value of care. Using a rudimentary understanding of value (ie, value= [quality/cost]), aerodigestive programs have steadily added to the literature, demonstrating how they accomplish this goal. A sampling of this literature follows, many examples of which address both the numerator and denominator of this value equation.

Reducing unnecessary testing

Hart and colleagues[12] reviewed patients who underwent pH multichannel intraluminal impedance (pH-MII) probe testing before airway reconstruction to determine if the results of pH-MII were associated with surgical outcomes. The investigators noted that fewer patients than anticipated (17.5%) had their management adjusted based on pH-MII results, particularly those patients with a prior history of fundoplication. For those patients without a history of fundoplication, pH-MII remained a valuable tool in decision-making for the investigators. DeBoer and colleagues[13] evaluated the yield of gastrointestinal testing in pediatric patients in an aerodigestive clinic. For all comers over a 3-year period, 144 of 193 pH-MII were normal (74.6%). EGD with biopsy was negative for histologic abnormalities in 188 of 295 patients (63.7%). Upper gastrointestinal fluoroscopy (UGI) was normal in 47 of 54 patients (87%). Children with feeding difficulty, tracheoesophageal fistula or esophageal atresia, and asthma were most likely to have an abnormal EGD or pH-MII. Although many of the patients were on acid suppression medication at the time of testing, the low yield of pH-MII testing demonstrates a gap between the current state of clinical diagnosis and test result. Given the growing concerns regarding overuse and risk of acid suppression medication, the investigators modified their protocol for aerodigestive patients, removing pH-MII from routine use. In addition, the investigators comment that their investigation allowed for discontinuation of medication in those who did not need it. Data did support ongoing EGD and UGI use in this study.

Wentland and colleagues[14] reviewed their patients' experience undergoing videofluoroscopic swallow study (VFSS) after laryngeal cleft repair. The investigators' multidisciplinary group reviewed the available literature and their own experience, leading to a modification of their previously published algorithm for swallow evaluation after cleft repair and a reduction in the number of VFSSs per patient. Though there was a small number of patients in this study, multidisciplinary discussion led to modification of an algorithm and a reduction in VFSS charges and radiation exposure.

Reducing charges and costs, risk, and time to diagnosis while maintaining viability

As aerodigestive programs have grown and spread, publications regarding their inherent efficiency, charge, and cost-reduction have increased in number. Collaco and colleagues[15] described the potential opportunity for reduction in cost for families, as well as the potential reduction in anesthetic exposures and procedural charges due to enrollment in an aerodigestive program. In 2016, Skinner and colleagues[16] demonstrated a shift from inpatient to outpatient care and a subsequent reduction in charges after enrollment in an aerodigestive program.

A 2017 retrospective examination of a single aerodigestive center revealed that after enrollment in the program there was a decrease in inpatient days and direct costs, extrapolated from an average for the state.[17] The study had several limitations, including that an overall shift from inpatient to outpatient care has been occurring, as well as that the patients may have been clinically improving or may have been seen at other institutions.

A recent single institution study examined patient and family experience before and after the creation of an aerodigestive program.[18] Patients with similar diseases achieved a reduction in time to diagnosis (6 vs 150 days) with fewer required specialist consultations (5 vs 11) compared with those seen in the same institution before creation of the aerodigestive program. These patients also underwent fewer radiology studies and anesthetic exposures. Charges for evaluations were also reduced from a median of $10,374 to $6055.

Although these studies focus on charges to the payer, cost to the institution to deliver care is also reduced. Costs for time-dependent resources (operating rooms, supplies, medications) were reduced approximately 40% when procedures were combined into 1 anesthetic event versus separated into 3 customary procedures (flexible bronchoscopy, rigid laryngoscopy and bronchoscopy, EGD).[19] Charges were similarly reduced. These effects can be achieved while maintaining a positive revenue stream when the program is defined as the sum of the clinic encounter and the endoscopic procedures.[20]

Developing new techniques

Medical innovation occurs by many different methods, among which is colocating multiple specialties and techniques. Colocation and sharing of ideas and techniques, when applied to aerodigestive diseases, can have significant impacts on care value. Unsedated transnasal esophagoscopy (TNE) with biopsy for pediatric eosinophilic esophagitis was discussed, then piloted, through the efforts of providers within the aerodigestive program.[21] After demonstrating that mucosal biopsies were appropriate for diagnosis when obtained in this manner, patients and parents were surveyed about their experience of TNE. All parents and 76.2% of subjects would undergo the TNE again. TNE was preferred over EGD by 85.7% of parents and 52.4% of subjects.

Charges associated with TNE were 60.1% lower than for previous EGD. A follow-up study of 294 TNE demonstrated a consistent reduction in charges, no adverse events, and 71 minutes average check-in to check-out compared with 3 hours for EGD.[22] Charge reduction occurred largely through the absence of anesthesia and facility fee. Risk reduction is obvious given the absence of anesthetic exposure.

Tracheopexy for tracheomalacia is yet another example of new techniques being applied through aerodigestive program care delivery methodology. First described as a treatment of tracheomalacia in 2015, the technique has been applied to those patients with congenital tracheomalacia most commonly due to tracheoesophageal fistula or esophageal atresia.[23] The investigators describe a multidisciplinary team of pediatric surgeons, pediatric cardiothoracic surgeons, and pediatric pulmonologists primarily driven by pediatric surgeons. Publication and communication regarding this technique coalesced with an increasing commitment among aerodigestive programs to better treat the population of patients with severe tracheobronchomalacia. As a result, multiple groups have adapted this surgical method through the use of a thoracoscopic approach.[24,25]

The number of aerodigestive IPUs has grown, and coordinated care is taking place across a broader geography.

Over the past decade, the number of identifiable aerodigestive teams providing care to children has increased. A recent publication noted 34 programs, 31 in the United States, most of which had been in existence for 5 years or less.[26] A separate study by the first 2 authors of the present work, based on an Internet survey of aerodigestive programs in each state (search term aerodigestive followed by a state name) and their dates of establishment (Christopher Wootten, 2019, unpublished work), demonstrates the broad geographic distribution of these programs. Paralleling the high population density in the New England and mid-Atlantic regions, those same areas demonstrate the highest concentration of aerodigestive teams. The pattern of growth is demonstrated by comparing program density in 2007, 2010, 2013, and 2016 (**Figs. 1–4**).

The question arises, does an increasing number and geographic distribution of aerodigestive centers correspond to a commensurate increase in airway reconstructive operations? To attempt to answer this question, the Pediatric Health Information System (PHIS) was interrogated (www.childrenshospitals.org/phis) by the first 2 authors of the present study. The PHIS database is an administrative database that contains inpatient, emergency department, ambulatory surgery, and observation encounter–level data from more than 45 not-for-profit, tertiary care pediatric hospitals in the United States.

The PHIS database was queried for pediatric patients 18 years or younger who had undergone airway reconstruction surgery between 2007 and 2016 using coding that contains groups of *International Statistical Classification of Diseases and Related Health Problems*, 10th revision, procedural coding system codes and current procedural terminology codes. The frequency of the airway reconstruction surgeries in each year were evaluated. The data were placed in a United States heat map format for the following years: 2007, 2010, 2013, and 2016 (see **Figs. 1–4**). The PHIS data are not provider-generated, so it is not possible to establish a 1-to-1 correlation between PHIS data points and specific types of airway reconstruction. However, over the decade spanning 2007 to 2016, the efflorescence and geographic dissemination of airway cases as detected by PHIS suggests that aerodigestive centers' growth parallels growth in PHIS-reported case volume.

With a broadening geographic distribution of airway cases being performed over the past decade, one might assume improved access to care. The quality of that care is less known. For certain operations, the center's experience and even the surgeon's

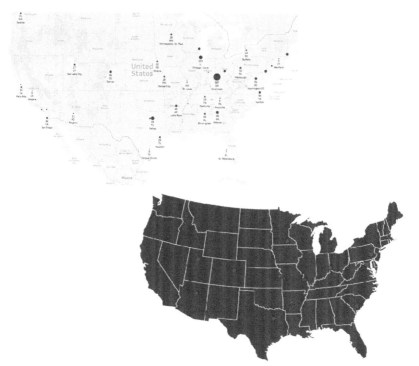

Fig. 1. Pediatric Health Information System (PHIS) heat map data indicating the number and geographic locations of unique patients with laryngotracheal surgical interventions in calendar year 2007 (*upper*) and the contemporaneous geographic distribution of aerodigestive centers (*stars*) that were verifiable by Internet query (*lower*).

individual experience with an intervention has been correlated with outcomes.[27–29] It is imperative that surgeons and centers study their outcomes for complex airway reconstructions. Further, communication between aerodigestive programs should include a frank disclosure of best practices that seem to yield improved outcomes, as well as a disclosure of practices that are best avoided to soften the learning curve in airway surgery. Professional societies facilitate this communication and benchmarking.

THE IMPORTANCE OF PROFESSIONAL SOCIETIES IN THE MAINTENANCE OF QUALITY AND THE CREATION OF FOCUS

The elevation of evidence-based medicine over the past 4 decades has shown that, even among the best institutions and physicians, there has been significant unexplained variation in the quality and volume of care.[30] In the midst of this evolution of medicine toward focusing on patient-centered experiences, the clinical effectiveness of interventions, meaningful outcomes, and efficient health care delivery, IPUs have been developed and shown to provide patient-centered care.[31]

IPU and PCMH providers have made great strides in improved care for their patients, especially for patients with complex medical problems and comorbidities. Communication and association between disease-specific IPUs across the country has created collaborative improvement networks. These networks, often uniting as medical societies, can serve as catalysts to advance knowledge through meetings, communications, and research initiatives, which allows IPUs to share best practices,

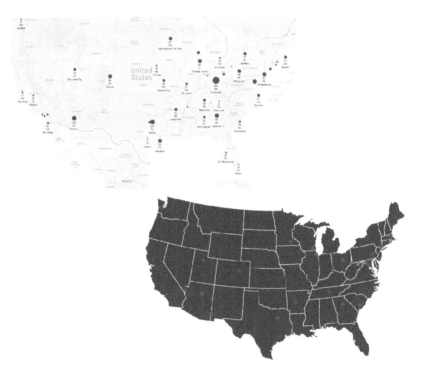

Fig. 2. PHIS heat map data indicating the number and geographic locations of unique patients with laryngotracheal surgical interventions in calendar year 2010 (*upper*) and the contemporaneous geographic distribution of aerodigestive centers (*stars*) that were verifiable by Internet query (*lower*).

advocate for recognition in academic and training programs, focus research efforts, raise money, and engage patient populations for improved patient-centered care. Increasingly, medical societies may become a source for medical research funding for their own members' research initiatives because the National Institutes Health funding is at an historic low and continues to decrease.[32]

An often-cited example of treatment advances and improvement of morbidity and mortality due to medical society collaboration, benchmarking, and implementation of patient registries is found in the cystic fibrosis (CF) population. A national patient registry for CF patients in the United States was initially established in the mid-1960s. In the 1990s, epidemiologists started appreciating the registry's usefulness to evaluate risk factors for disease progression. The CF Foundation has also long supported a benchmarking program that identifies CF centers that have excellent outcomes according to their registry data, then studies these CF centers' exceptional organizational and structural features that contribute to these findings. This has ultimately led to less variation in the spread of effective treatment strategies for the CF population.[33]

In the realm of pediatric aerodigestive care, integrated care teams voted, in 2014, to organize as the Aerodigestive Society. However, the impetus for this organization was not patient-driven as in the case of the CF Foundation; instead, it was provider-driven. Unlike CF, which is a discrete, genetically linked multiorgan condition, aerodigestive conditions are many disorders with many etiologic factors. What links them are the common integrated care teams that have formed nationwide to help patients and populations realize value in the treatment of aerodigestive disease.

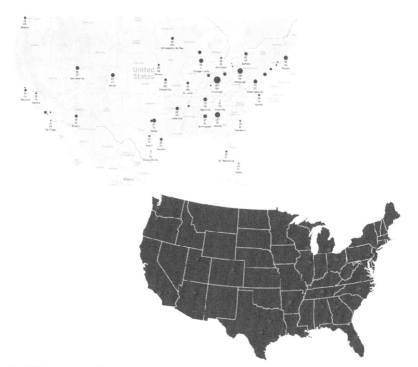

Fig. 3. PHIS heat map data indicating the number and geographic locations of unique patients with laryngotracheal surgical interventions in calendar year 2013 (*upper*) and the contemporaneous geographic distribution of aerodigestive centers (*stars*) that were verifiable by Internet query (*lower*).

THE FUTURE OF AERODIGESTIVE CARE

The Aerodigestive Society has benefited from Delphi projects that defined the structure and function of aerodigestive teams and the airway outcomes they seek from laryngotracheal operations. The Society will continue to use Delphi methodology to assess and focus expert opinion on intake practices, diagnostic practices, interventions, clinical outcomes, and patient-reported outcomes. These agreed-on data objects will form the basis for an aerodigestive collaborative database that is multicentric and powered to answer nuanced questions about the inherently rare aerodigestive diseases and their treatments.

Certainly, the Aerodigestive Society is not the only professional organization that will help shape the quality and availability of care for children with aerodigestive conditions. National and international organizations within otolaryngology, pulmonology, gastroenterology, speech pathology, occupational therapy, esophageal atresia–tracheoesophageal fistula, and other fields have created sections and/or committees that educate their membership on the contemporary landscape of pediatric aerodigestive care. The journals affiliated with these allied professional organizations will continue to be the most appropriate venue for publishing original research into aerodigestive disorders.

Finally, the nature of aerodigestive research will not be restricted to clinical inquiry. Already, considerable work has been done on the economic logic underpinning integrated care delivery for aerodigestive disease. A 4-center value-based health care

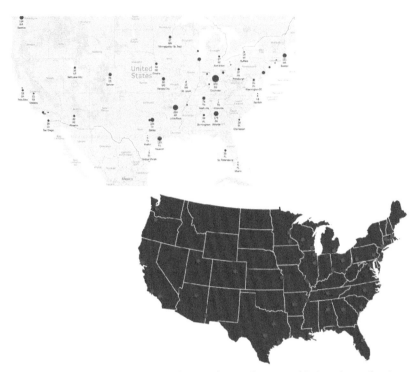

Fig. 4. PHIS heat map data indicating the number and geographic locations of unique patients with laryngotracheal surgical interventions in calendar year 2016 (*upper*) and the contemporaneous geographic distribution of aerodigestive centers (*stars*) that were verifiable by Internet query (*lower*).

analysis in the management of oropharyngeal dysphagia is underway. What is clear from such health care business studies is the importance of leveraging emerging technologies such as nationally visible electronic medical records, telehealth, and automated patient-reported outcomes and biometrics that continually recenter the aerodigestive care delivery model on the patient.

SUMMARY

Aerodigestive programs fit into the modern medical trend of incorporating disparate disciplines into 1 location and team in order to provide more comprehensive, family-centered and patient-centered care in an efficient and cost-effective manner. Combining disciplines, by its nature, leads to improved communication and the development of improvements and innovation in care delivery. By deconstructing the siloed approach to care delivery, these programs and others may function as IPUs for disease states and populations, tracking outcomes that may include both clinical quality measurements and other metrics of care value (eg, cost of care delivery, time to diagnosis, reduction in unnecessary testing). Time will tell whether or not aerodigestive programs continue to develop and thrive. The external pressures that helped create the environment in which these programs have developed are subject to change from political and economic forces that may reinforce program development or serve to dissuade organizations, payers, and providers from coalescing into IPUs.

ACKNOWLEDGMENTS

The authors wish to thank Ajit Munjuluru, Business Intelligence, Department of Biostatistics, Vanderbilt University Medical Center, for querying the PHIS database.

REFERENCES

1. Calcaterra TC, Maceri DR. Aerodigestive dysfunction secondary to thyroid tumors. Laryngoscope 1981;91(5):701–7.
2. Cotton RT, Myer CM 3rd, O'Connor DM. Innovations in pediatric laryngotracheal reconstruction. J Pediatr Surg 1992;27(2):196–200.
3. Hartnick CJ, Liu JH, Cotton RT, et al. Subglottic stenosis complicated by allergic esophagitis: case report. Ann Otol Rhinol Laryngol 2002;111(1):57–60.
4. Rubinstein E, Rosen RL. Respiratory symptoms associated with eosinophilic esophagitis. Pediatr Pulmonol 2018;53(11):1587–91.
5. Mosquera RA, Avritscher EB, Samuels CL, et al. Effect of an enhanced medical home on serious illness and cost of care among high-risk children with chronic illness: a randomized clinical trial. JAMA 2014;312(24):2640–8.
6. Boesch RP, Balakrishnan K, Acra S, et al. Structure and functions of pediatric aerodigestive programs: a consensus statement. Pediatrics 2018; 141(3) [pii:e20171701].
7. Porter ME, Lee TH. The strategy that will fix healthcare. Harv Bus Rev 2013.
8. The Aerodigestive Society. Available at: https://aerodigestive.us/. Accessed January 1, 2019.
9. Bannister SL, Wickenheiser HM, Keegan DA. Key elements of highly effective teams. Pediatrics 2014;133(2):184–6.
10. Casey PH, Lyle RE, Bird TM, et al. Effect of hospital-based comprehensive care clinic on health costs for Medicaid-insured medically complex children. Arch Pediatr Adolesc Med 2011;165(5):392–8.
11. Galligan MM, Bamat TW, Hogan AK, et al. The pediatric aerodigestive center as a tertiary care-based medical home: a proposed model. Curr Probl Pediatr Adolesc Health Care 2018;48(4):104–10.
12. Hart CK, de Alarcon A, Tabangin ME, et al. Impedance probe testing prior to pediatric airway reconstruction. Ann Otol Rhinol Laryngol 2014;123(9):641–6.
13. DeBoer EM, Kinder S, Duggar A, et al. Evaluating the yield of gastrointestinal testing in pediatric patients in aerodigestive clinic. Pediatr Pulmonol 2018; 53(11):1517–24.
14. Wentland C, Hersh C, Sally S, et al. Modified best-practice algorithm to reduce the number of postoperative videofluoroscopic swallow studies in patients with Type 1 Laryngeal Cleft Repair. JAMA Otolaryngol Head Neck Surg 2016; 142(9):851–6.
15. Collaco JM, Aherrera AD, Au Yeung KJ, et al. Interdisciplinary pediatric aerodigestive care and reduction in health care costs and burden. JAMA Otolaryngol Head Neck Surg 2015;141(2):101–5.
16. Skinner ML, Lee SK, Collaco JM, et al. Financial and health impacts of multidisciplinary aerodigestive care. Otolaryngol Head Neck Surg 2016;154(6):1064–7.
17. Appachi S, Banas A, Feinberg L, et al. Association of enrollment in an aerodigestive clinic with reduced hospital stay for children with special health care needs. JAMA Otolaryngol Head Neck Surg 2017;143(11):1117–21.
18. Boesch RP, Balakrishnan K, Grothe RM, et al. Interdisciplinary aerodigestive care model improves risk, cost, and efficiency. Int J Pediatr Otorhinolaryngol 2018; 113:119–23.

19. Ruiz AG, Bhatt JM, DeBoer EM, et al. Demonstrating the benefits of a multidisciplinary aerodigestive program. Accepted by Laryngoscope 2/27/19. Presented at ASPO. Austin, TX, May 20, 2017.

20. Mudd PA, Silva AL, Callicott SS, et al. Cost analysis of a multidisciplinary aerodigestive clinic: are such clinics financially feasible? Ann Otol Rhinol Larygnol 2017;126(5):401–6.

21. Friedlander JA, DeBoer EM, Soden JS, et al. Unsedated transnasal esophagoscopy for monitoring therapy in pediatric eosinophilic esophagitis. Gastrointest Endosc 2016;83(2):299–306.

22. Nguyen N, Lavery WJ, Capocelli KE, et al. Transnasal endoscopy in unsedated children with eosinophilic esophagitis using virtual reality video goggles. Clin Gastroenterol Hepatol 2019. https://doi.org/10.1016/j.cgh.2019.01.023.

23. Bairdain S, Smithers CJ, Hamilton TE, et al. Direct tracheobronchopexy to correct airway collapse due to severe tracheobronchomalacia: short-term outcomes in a series of 20 patients. J Pediatr Surg 2015;50(6):972–7.

24. Polites SF, Kotagal M, Wilcox LJ, et al. Thoracoscopic posterior tracheopexy for tracheomalacia: a minimally invasive technique. J Pediatr Surg 2018;53(11): 2357–60.

25. Masaracchia MM, Polaner DM, Prager JD, et al. Pediatric tracheomalacia and the perioperative anesthetic management of thoracoscopic posterior tracheopexy. Paediatr Anaesth 2018;28(9):768–73.

26. Gumer L, Rosen R, Gold BD, et al. Size and prevalence of pediatric aerodigestive programs in 2017. J Pediatr Gastroenterol Nutr 2019. https://doi.org/10.1097/MPG.0000000000002268.

27. Hannen EL, Racz M, Kavey RE, et al. Pediatric cardiac surgery: the effect of hospital and surgeon volume on in-hospital mortality. Pediatrics 1998;101(6):963–9.

28. Javid PJ, Jaksic T, Skarsgard ED, et al. Survival rate in congenital diaphragmatic hernia the experience of the Canadian Neonatal Network. J Pediatr Sugr 2004; 39(5):657–60.

29. Johnston LE, Tracci MC, Kern JA. Surgeon, not institution, case volume is associated with limb outcomes after lower extremity bypass for critical limb ischemia in the Vascular Quality Initiative. J Vasc Surg 2017;66(5):1457–63.

30. Miles PV, Conway PH, Pawlson LG. Physician professionalism and accountability: the role of collaborative improvement networks. Pediatrics 2013;131(Suppl 4): S204–9.

31. Novikov Z, Glover WJ, Trepman PC, et al. How do integrative practices influence patient-centered care?: an exploratory study comparing diabetes and mental health care. Health Care Manage Rev 2016;41(2):113–26.

32. Hromas R, Abkowitz JL, Keating A. Facing the NIH funding crisis: how professional societies can help. JAMA 2012;308(22):2343–4.

33. Schechter MS. Benchmarking to improve the quality of cystic fibrosis care. Curr Opin Pulm Med 2012;18:596–601.

Beyond Nodules—Diagnostic and Treatment Options in Pediatric Voice Disorders

Anne Hseu, MD[a],*, Julina Ongkasuwan, MD[b]

KEYWORDS

- Pediatric voice • Dysphonia • Laryngeal • Benign vocal fold lesions
- Vocal fold immobility • Posterior glottic insufficiency

KEY POINTS

- Pediatric dysphonia is common; vocal pathologies are varied and not necessarily due to nodules.
- Multidisciplinary care is recommended for optimal treatment of voice disorders in children.
- Benign true vocal fold lesions in children may require voice therapy and/or surgical management.
- Several medialization procedures are available for children with vocal fold movement impairment.
- Posterior glottic insufficiency can be a diagnostic and management challenge.

INTRODUCTION

Pediatric dysphonia is common, with prevalence rates cited as high as 38% in the United States.[1,2] Etiologies are diverse and include congenital, infectious, iatrogenic, and phonotraumatic causes. Voice disorders can have significant impact on communication and quality of life, with influences on self-esteem and perceptions of children by adults and peers.[3–6] It is, therefore, necessary for an otolaryngologist to pursue a thorough and timely work-up of pediatric dysphonia to rule out any worrisome pathology and minimize negative impacts to a child's development.

DIAGNOSIS AND MANAGEMENT

Voice evaluation and laryngeal assessment in the pediatric population can be challenging, because patient participation and cooperation can be limiting. Thus,

J. Ongkasuwan has a royalty agreement with Springer.
[a] Boston Children's Hospital, 300 Longwood Avenue, BCH 3129, Boston, MA 02115, USA;
[b] Baylor College of Medicine, Texas Children's Hospital, 6701 Fannin, Suite 640, Houston, TX 77030, USA
* Corresponding author.
E-mail address: anne.hseu@childrens.harvard.edu

comprehensive evaluations, including acoustic, aerodynamic, endoscopic, perceptual, and voice handicapping assessments, are important to obtaining accurate diagnoses and guiding treatment. Multiple validated quality-of-life assessments, modified from the adult literature, are available to track a child's progress. These include the Pediatric Voice Outcome Survey (PVOS), the Pediatric Voice-Related Quality-of-Life (PVRQOL) survey, and the pediatric Voice Handicap Index (pVHI). The PVOS is composed of 3 questions and is best used to document global changes in the voice preoperatively and postoperatively. The PVRQOL is a 10-item questionnaire designed to capture social-emotional subdomains. The pVHI is longer, 21 questions, and is also designed to reflect function, physical, and emotional elements of voice quality of life. Clinicians should be aware that these questionnaires are by parental proxy and there may be differences in perceived vocal handicaps by a child versus a parent.[1,7]

Laryngeal endoscopy, however, is the mainstay of diagnostic evaluation. Nearly all children can be evaluated with a pediatric flexible fiberoptic endoscope, which can be as small as 2.1 mm in diameter. Distal chip videostroboscopy also can be performed, which can provide improved images and important details regarding the mucosal wave. These endoscopes are available in pediatric sizes (3.1 mm or 3.2 mm) and provide images comparable to standard adult stroboscopes. Transoral rigid videostroboscopy is surprisingly well tolerated in younger children as well.[8] In contrast to adults, the pediatric larynx is situated high in the neck with the cricoid cartilage at the level of C4.[9] Given this, transoral rigid examinations in children often can be performed without oropharyngeal anesthetic, which can be the limiting factor to a successful examination. In most children, evaluation of the larynx can be completed in a clinic and does not require examination under anesthesia. The prospect of a scope examination, however, can be frightening to a child and requires patience on the part of the clinician. Thorough child and parental education prior to the examination can be helpful. In the uncommon situation in which a child cannot tolerate laryngoscopy, laryngeal ultrasound may provide important information on vocal fold lesions and mobility.[10–13] Laryngeal ultrasound typically is performed transcervically with a 10-MHz to 15-MHz linear probe, with minimal patient discomfort.

Caring for a child with a voice disorder requires a collaborative approach involving the expertise of multiple health care and educational professionals. This team may be composed of a pediatric otolaryngologist and a speech language pathologist with experience in the assessment and treatment of voice problems in children. Many young children have coexistent language, articulation, and voice problems. A skilled speech language pathologist can help tease out which of these elements is most impairing intelligibility in order to prioritize therapy and educate caregivers.

Although surgical versus medical management depends on the etiology of dysphonia, voice therapy for children can play an important role both preoperatively and postoperatively. At times, preoperative voice therapy can aid in pointing to a diagnosis. In some children, adequate view of the larynx is difficult when there is compensatory muscle tension dysphonia. A short course of therapy, therefore, can help to improve exposure of the larynx during the laryngeal examination. Postoperatively, voice therapy can be critical in optimizing vocal outcomes after the laryngeal structure has been altered.

Etiologies of pediatric dysphonia are vast and management depends on an accurate diagnosis. This article focuses on a few pathologies that have been traditionally more challenging to treat in the pediatric population.

BENIGN TRUE VOCAL FOLD LESIONS

Nodules are the most common benign laryngeal finding in dysphonic children, occurring in up to 60% of pediatric patients presenting with hoarseness.[2,14] Less is known about the true prevalence of benign lesions (also known as not nodules) in children. Diagnoses, such as vocal fold polyps, cysts, and fibrous masses, may be more difficult to evaluate in children, because they are less likely to tolerate videostroboscopy (**Fig. 1**). Similar to those in adults, these lesions tend to be asymmetric, more anterior, or more posterior to the midmembranous true vocal fold or have a deeper disruption to the mucosal wave. These findings thus are more difficult to assess with laryngoscopy alone. Prior studies have pointed to a high incidence of non-nodule pathologies in children initially diagnosed with nodules.[15]

There is no set algorithm for the management of benign true vocal fold lesions in children. Treatment involves both voice therapy and surgical excision. Timing and extent of surgical excision depend largely on family preference and a patient's ability to meet vocal demands. In almost all circumstances, preoperative therapy can be invaluable both in aiding with an accurate diagnosis and in treatment. In some children, therapy alone can be sufficient in optimizing voice for a child's needs. In other children, lack of response to therapy may point to an alternate diagnosis, such as fold polyps, cysts, or fibrous masses (not nodule). For this reason, it is important to follow children diagnosed with nodules, particularly in those that do not respond to therapy alone, because repeat laryngoscopy or videostroboscopy can help confirm or rule out the diagnosis.

Factors that may prompt more aggressive surgical treatment include frequent aphonia, painful speaking, and difficulties communicating at school and home. Timing of surgery also may be influenced by adequate true vocal fold exposure for microflap excisions. Removal of benign true vocal fold lesions often is limited to 1 side to limit the risk of postoperative scarring. This may leave a contralateral reactive lesion, which resolves over time or with therapy. Parents need to be carefully counseled to manage their expectations for immediate postoperative voice improvement.

UNILATERAL VOCAL FOLD MOVEMENT IMPAIRMENT

Unilateral vocal fold movement impairment (VFMI) in children may be a result of congenital, idiopathic, or, most commonly, iatrogenic causes. The intimate association of the recurrent laryngeal nerve (RLN) to the great vessels and esophagus makes the RLN particularly vulnerable to injury during surgeries in infancy. Reported rates of VFMI after congenital heart surgery range from 9% to 58.7%,[16–18] patent ductus arteriosus ligation from 8.8% to 52%,[19–22] and tracheoesophageal fistula repair from 5% to 6%.[23,24]

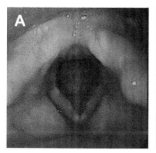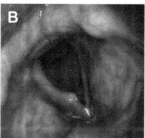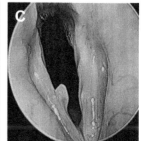

Fig. 1. Benign vocal fold lesion. (A) Bilateral true vocal fold nodules. (B) Right true vocal fold cyst. (C) Right true vocal fold polyp.

Infants with unilateral VFMI often present with an asthenic (weak) and or breathy cry, feeding difficulties, and occasionally stridor.[16–19,22,25–27] Older children may use compensatory strategies, such as supraglottic phonation or a high head voice. The dysphonia and difficulty being heard can result in embarrassment and social withdrawal.[5,28]

In infancy, swallowing and feeding are the focus of medical management. Because children have greater language skills in their toddler and preschool years, voice quality becomes the focus for children with VFMI. Treatments for unilateral VFMI include voice therapy to maximize voicing efficiency and compensation.[29] If the voice quality remains a barrier to communication, surgical medialization can be considered. Medialization techniques can be divided into 3 groups: injection laryngoplasty, framework surgery, and reinnervation. Unfortunately, there are no widely available treatments at present that restore dynamic mobility of the vocal folds.

Injection Laryngoplasty

Injection laryngoplasty in children typically is performed transorally under general anesthesia[30,31]; however, some older children may be candidates for an awake transcervical approach. Injection materials include carboxymethyl cellose, collagen, hyaluronic acid, and autologous fat. Other materials, such as calcium hydroxylapatite have an inflammatory potential, which is concerning in the immature vocal fold.[32] Unfortunately, none of the currently available injectable materials is permanent, thus potentially requiring multiple anesthetic procedures. Duration of effect from injection laryngoplasty can be from 1 month, in the case of carboxymethyl cellulose gel, up to a year for calcium hydroxylapatite. Autologous fat has a less predictable rate of resorption, with some sources reporting persistence for years.[33] In the case of VFMI, the injection is begun posteriorly, just lateral to the vocal process, to encourage medial rotation of the vocal process. with additional injection in the midfold region if needed. An additional potential benefit of vocal fold medialization is improvement in pulmonary toilet, especially in individuals after cardiothoracic surgery. Although common in the adult postcardiothoracic surgery population,[34] early postoperative injection laryngoplasty in infants and children after congenital heart surgery is currently being explored.[35] Care must be taken in the infant larynx not to cause airway compromise.

Laryngeal Framework Surgery

Laryngeal framework surgery, such as type 1 thyroplasty with or without arytenoid adduction, is the mainstay of permanent vocal fold medialization in adults. Classically, a silastic wedge or polytetrafluoroethylene (ePTFE; Gore-Tex) ribbon is placed through a window in the thyroid cartilage with the patient awake or lightly sedated but vocalizing to optimize implant size and position. In addition, an arytenoid adduction may be needed to medialize the posterior glottis. Modifications of the technique for use in children have been described using a laryngeal mask airway and flexible scope to determine implant placement.[36] Although thyroplasty implants are permanent, the problem remains that the implant potentially requires revision as the child grows. There also is a rare risk of extrusion, displacement, or infection with any foreign implanted material.[37]

Nonselective Laryngeal Reinnervation

Many variations of laryngeal reinnervation have been described , including direct implantation of a neuromuscular pedicle into the thyroarytenoid muscle, selective adductor reinnervation, and hypoglossal nerve reinnervation.[38] Nonselective laryngeal reinnervation (NSLR) with end-to-end anastomoses of the ansa cervicalis to the RLN has become more popular for medialization of pediatric unilateral neuronal VFMI.[39]

The procedure provides durable bulk and tone to the vocal fold and also allows for closure of the posterior glottis. Preoperative confirmation of neuronal injury can be obtained with laryngeal electromyography of the posterior cricoarytenoid muscles using a spontaneous tubeless ventilation anesthetic technique. NSLR should be performed only once an adequate amount of time has elapsed to allow for spontaneous recovery of vocal fold movement. In children with RLN injury during infancy, waiting 2 years to 3 years before performed NSLR is appropriate. Deferring medialization until the child is older can also assuage concerns about the effects of prolonged anesthesia on neurocognitive development.[40] Concurrent injection laryngoplasty often also is done at the time of NSLR. It takes 4 months to 6 months to hear a change in the voice after NSLR and the final voice result occurs at 1 years to 2 years postoperatively.[41] Successful NSLR can be performed many years after initial injury.[42,43] Several studies have demonstrated that NSLR can improve voice[43,44]; however, the surgery is not perfect. The goal now is to try to identify which factors may predict a better voice outcome. Voice therapy is a useful adjunct in many cases to help patients develop consistency and comfort with their new voice. Importantly, NSLR does not preclude the ability to perform injection laryngoplasty or type 1 thyroplasty should the reinnervation fail to achieve the desired voice result.

POSTERIOR GLOTTIC INSUFFICIENCY

Prolonged intubation can also cause pressure erosion of the posterior glottic structures resulting in posterior glottic insufficiency (PGI).[45] One of the hallmarks of PGI is voice quality that is worse than expected on awake in-office laryngoscopy. The arytenoids can obscure the view of the posterior glottis making the diagnosis difficult to make.[46] Direct laryngoscopy and careful inspection of the larynx often reveal an endotracheal tube-shaped deficiency in the posterior glottis. The vocal processes may appear eroded and the membranous vocal folds atrophic (**Fig. 2**).

PGI is not only a diagnostic challenge but also a management challenge. Bilateral injection laryngoplasty into the membranous vocal folds can help close the anterior portion of the glottis and improve volume. The mucosa of the posterior glottis, however, is typically tightly adherent to the underlying cartilage and does not elevate well with injection, resulting in persistent air escape and limited improvement. The posterior glottis can be reapproximated using an endoscopic posterior cricoid reduction laryngoplasty.[47,48] Other endoscopic management techniques for reconstituting

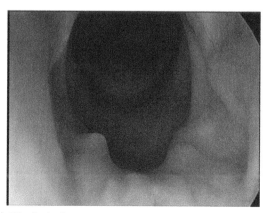

Fig. 2. Posterior glottic diastasis.

the deficient tissue include aryepiglottic and arytenoid rotation flaps[47] and buccal mucosa grafts.[49]

Children can have both VFMI and PGI. It is the smallest premature infants who require both a patent ductus arteriosus ligation and prolonged intubation. If a surgeon only addresses one of the problems, the voice will remain suboptimal.

SUMMARY

Children can have dysphonia for myriad reasons. Not all hoarseness is due to vocal fold nodules and children do not always just grow out of it. Careful inspection of the larynx is essential for accurate diagnosis to guide voice therapy and surgical treatment.

REFERENCES

1. Carding PN, Roulstone S, Northstone K, ALSPAC Study Team. The prevalence of childhood dysphonia: a cross-sectional study. J Voice 2006;20(4):623–30.
2. Martins RHG, Hidalgo Ribeiro CB, Fernandes de Mello BMZ, et al. Dysphonia in children. J Voice 2012;26(5):674.e17-20.
3. Sajisevi M, Cohen S, Raynor E. Pediatrician approach to dysphonia. Int J Pediatr Otorhinolaryngol 2014;78(8):1365–7.
4. Lass NJ, Ruscello DM, Bradshaw KH, et al. Adolescents' perceptions of normal and voice-disordered children. J Commun Disord 1991;24(4):267–74.
5. Connor NP, Cohen SB, Theis SM, et al. Attitudes of children with dysphonia. J Voice 2008;22(2):197–209.
6. Ma EP-M, Yu CH-Y. Listeners' attitudes toward children with voice problems. J Speech Lang Hear Res 2013;56(5):1409.
7. Cohen W, Wynne DMG. Parent and child responses to the pediatric voice-related quality-of-life questionnaire. J Voice 2015;29(3):299–303.
8. Ongkasuwan J, Devore D, Hollas S, et al. Transoral rigid 70-degree laryngoscopy in a pediatric voice clinic. Laryngoscope 2018;27706. https://doi.org/10.1002/lary.27706.
9. Sulica L. Voice: anatomy, physiology, and clinical evaluation. In: Johnson J, editor. Bailey's head and neck surgery. 5th edition. Philadelphia: Lippincott Williams & Wilkins; 2013. p. 952.
10. Friedman EM. Role of ultrasound in the assessment of vocal cord function in infants and children. Ann Otol Rhinol Laryngol 1997;106(3):199–209. Available at: http://www.embase.com/search/results?subaction=viewrecord&from=export&id=L27123210.
11. Wang LM, Zhu Q, Ma T, et al. Value of ultrasonography in diagnosis of pediatric vocal fold paralysis. Int J Pediatr Otorhinolaryngol 2011. https://doi.org/10.1016/j.ijporl.2011.06.017.
12. Ongkasuwan J, Ocampo E, Tran B. Laryngeal ultrasound and vocal fold movement in the pediatric cardiovascular intensive care unit. Laryngoscope 2017. https://doi.org/10.1002/lary.26051.
13. Ongkasuwan J, Devore D, Hollas S, et al. Laryngeal ultrasound and pediatric vocal fold nodules. Laryngoscope 2017. https://doi.org/10.1002/lary.26209.
14. Akif Kiliç M, Okur E, Yildirim I, et al. The prevalence of vocal fold nodules in school age children. Int J Pediatr Otorhinolaryngol 2004;68(4):409–12.
15. Mortensen M, Schaberg M, Woo P. Diagnostic contributions of videolaryngostroboscopy in the pediatric population. Arch Otolaryngol Head Neck Surg 2010;136(1):75–9.

16. Dewan K, Cephus C, Owczarzak V, et al. Incidence and implication of vocal fold paresis following neonatal cardiac surgery. Laryngoscope 2012. https://doi.org/10.1002/lary.23575.

17. Skinner ML, Halstead LA, Rubinstein CS, et al. Laryngopharyngeal dysfunction after the Norwood procedure. J Thorac Cardiovasc Surg 2005. https://doi.org/10.1016/j.jtcvs.2005.07.013.

18. Averin K, Uzark K, Beekman RH, et al. Postoperative assessment of laryngopharyngeal dysfunction in neonates after Norwood operation. Ann Thorac Surg 2012. https://doi.org/10.1016/j.athoracsur.2012.01.009.

19. Pereira KD, Webb BD, Blakely ML, et al. Sequelae of recurrent laryngeal nerve injury after patent ductus arteriosus ligation. Int J Pediatr Otorhinolaryngol 2006. https://doi.org/10.1016/j.ijporl.2006.05.001.

20. Benjamin JR, Smith PB, Cotten CM, et al. Long-term morbidities associated with vocal cord paralysis after surgical closure of a patent ductus arteriosus in extremely low birth weight infants. J Perinatol 2010. https://doi.org/10.1038/jp.2009.124.

21. Zbar RIS, Chen AH, Behrendt DM, et al. Incidence of vocal fold paralysis in infants undergoing ligation of patent ductus arteriosus. Ann Thorac Surg 1996. https://doi.org/10.1016/0003-4975(95)01152-8.

22. Clement WA, El-Hakim H, Phillipos EZ, et al. Unilateral vocal cord paralysis following patent ductus arteriosus ligation in extremely low-birth-weight infants. Arch Otolaryngol Head Neck Surg 2008;134(1):28–33. Available at: http://archotol.jamanetwork.com/.

23. Lal DR, Gadepalli SK, Downard CD, et al. Challenging surgical dogma in the management of proximal esophageal atresia with distal tracheoesophageal fistula: outcomes from the Midwest Pediatric Surgery Consortium. J Pediatr Surg 2018;53(7):1267–72.

24. Kovesi T, Porcaro F, Petreschi F, et al. Vocal cord paralysis appears to be an acquired lesion in children with repaired esophageal atresia/tracheoesophageal fistula. Int J Pediatr Otorhinolaryngol 2018;112:45–7.

25. Sachdeva R, Hussain E, Moss MM, et al. Vocal cord dysfunction and feeding difficulties after pediatric cardiovascular surgery. J Pediatr 2007. https://doi.org/10.1016/j.jpeds.2007.03.014.

26. Truong MT, Messner AH, Kerschner JE, et al. Pediatric vocal fold paralysis after cardiac surgery: rate of recovery and sequelae. Otolaryngol Head Neck Surg 2007. https://doi.org/10.1016/j.otohns.2007.07.028.

27. Carpes LF, Kozak FK, Leblanc JG, et al. Assessment of vocal fold mobility before and after cardiothoracic surgery in children. Arch Otolaryngol Head Neck Surg 2011. https://doi.org/10.1001/archoto.2011.84.

28. Mornet E, Coulombeau B, Fayoux P, et al. Assessment of chronic childhood dysphonia. Euro Ann Otorhinolaryngol Head Neck Dis 2014;131(5):309–12.

29. Schindler A, Bottero A, Capaccio P, et al. Vocal improvement after voice therapy in unilateral vocal fold paralysis. J Voice 2008;22(1):113–8.

30. Cohen MS, Mehta DK, Maguire RC, et al. Injection medialization laryngoplasty in children. Arch Otolaryngol Head Neck Surg 2011;137(3):264–8.

31. Hseu A, Choi S. When should you perform injection medialization for pediatric unilateral vocal fold immobility? Laryngoscope 2018;128(6):1259–60.

32. DeFatta RA, Chowdhury F, Sataloff R. Complications of injection laryngoplasty using calcium hydroxylapatite. J Voice 2012;26(5):614–8.

33. Pagano R, Morsomme D, Camby S, et al. Long-term results of 18 fat injections in unilateral vocal fold paralysis. J Voice 2017;31(4):505.e1-e9.

34. Fullmer T, Wang DC, Price MD, et al. Incidence and treatment outcomes of vocal fold movement impairment after total arch replacement 2019;129(3):699–703.
35. Bertelsen C, Jacobson L, Osterbauer B, et al. Safety and efficacy of early injection laryngoplasty in pediatric patients. Laryngoscope 2018. https://doi.org/10.1002/lary.27436.
36. Sipp JA, Kerschner JE, Braune N, et al. Vocal fold medialization in children. Arch Otolaryngol Head Neck Surg 2007;133(8):767.
37. Watanabe K, Hirano A, Honkura Y, et al. Complications of using Gore-Tex in medialization laryngoplasty: case series and literature review. Eur Arch Otorhinolaryngol 2019;276(3):255–61.
38. Aynehchi BB, McCoul ED, Sundaram K. Systematic review of laryngeal reinnervation techniques. Otolaryngol Head Neck Surg 2010;143(6):749–59.
39. Bouhabel S, Hartnick CJ. Current trends in practices in the treatment of pediatric unilateral vocal fold immobility: a survey on injections, thyroplasty and nerve reinnervation. Int J Pediatr Otorhinolaryngol 2018;109(March):115–8.
40. Sun L. Early childhood general anaesthesia exposure and neurocognitive development. Br J Anaesth 2010;105(Suppl 1):i61–8.
41. Smith ME, Roy N, Houtz D. Laryngeal reinnervation for paralytic dysphonia in children younger than 10 years. Arch Otolaryngol Head Neck Surg 2012;138(12):1161–6.
42. Smith ME, Roy N, Stoddard K. Ansa-RLN reinnervation for unilateral vocal fold paralysis in adolescents and young adults. Int J Pediatr Otorhinolaryngol 2008;72(9):1311–6.
43. Smith ME, Houtz DR. Outcomes of laryngeal reinnervation for unilateral vocal fold paralysis in children: Associations with age and time since injury. Ann Otol Rhinol Laryngol 2016;125(5):433–8.
44. Zur KB, Carroll LM. Recurrent laryngeal nerve reinnervation in children: acoustic and endoscopic characteristics pre-intervention and post-intervention. A comparison of treatment options. Laryngoscope 2015;125:S1–15.
45. Benjamin B. Prolonged intubation injuries of the larynx: endoscopic diagnosis, classification, and treatment. Ann Otol Rhinol Laryngol 2018;127(8):492–507.
46. Zeitels SM, De Alarcon A, Burns JA, et al. Posterior glottic diastasis: mechanically deceptive and often overlooked. Ann Otol Rhinol Laryngol 2011;120(2):71–80.
47. Sidell DRR, Zacharias S, Balakrishnan K, et al. Surgical management of posterior glottic diastasis in children. Ann Otol Rhinol Laryngol 2015;124(1):72–8.
48. Padia R, Smith ME. Posterior glottic insufficiency in children: a unique cause of dysphonia and challenge to identify and treat. Ann Otol Rhinol Laryngol 2017;126(4):268–73.
49. Helman SNN, Karle W, Pitman MJJ. Management of posterior glottal insufficiency with use of a buccal graft. Ann Otol Rhinol Laryngol 2016;126(2):159–62.

Assessment and Management of Thyroid Disease in Children

Amy L. Dimachkieh, MD[a], Ken Kazahaya, MD, MBA[b], Daniel C. Chelius Jr, MD[a],*

KEYWORDS

- Thyroid • Hyperthyroidism • Thyroid nodule • Thyroid cancer • Pediatric

KEY POINTS

- Graves disease is the most common cause of hyperthyroidism in children and can be treated effectively with antithyroid medical therapy, radioactive iodine ablation, or total thyroidectomy.
- Thyroid nodules are uncommon in children but are associated with 25% chance of malignancy and warrant thorough and complete examination with imaging and fine-needle aspiration if indicated.
- Thyroid patients should be evaluated and treated by an experienced multidisciplinary thyroid team and high-volume thyroid surgeon to minimize risk of recurrence and perioperative complications.
- Risk stratification of children with pediatric thyroid cancer is performed postoperatively to determine utility of adjuvant treatment with radioactive iodine, but further research needs to be done for consensus regarding ^{131}I dosimetry and which patients clearly benefit from adjuvant therapy.

INTRODUCTION

Assessment and management of thyroid disease in children are difficult due to the inherent biochemical differences between the pediatric and adult thyroid gland and the long life expectancy of children. For example, the pediatric thyroid gland is more sensitive to radiation than the adult thyroid gland, and pediatric thyroid cancer is more likely to present with advanced disease at the time of diagnosis. There is a paucity of literature regarding the surgical management of pediatric thyroid disease, and recommendations are historically based on studies from the adult population. The medical and surgical treatment of thyroid disease in children

Disclosure: The authors having nothing to disclose except that each is part of a multidisciplinary thyroid surgery program at their respective institutions.
[a] Department of Otolaryngology–Head and Neck Surgery, Pediatric Thyroid Tumor Program and Pediatric Head and Neck Tumor Program, Baylor College of Medicine, Texas Children's Hospital, 6701 Fannin Street, Suite D0420, Houston, TX 77030, USA; [b] Division of Pediatric Otolaryngology, University of Pennsylvania, Pediatric Thyroid Center, Children's Hospital of Philadelphia, 3401 Civic Center Boulevard, Philadephia, PA 19104, USA
* Corresponding author.
E-mail address: dccheliu@texaschildrens.org

Otolaryngol Clin N Am 52 (2019) 957–967
https://doi.org/10.1016/j.otc.2019.06.009
0030-6665/19/© 2019 Elsevier Inc. All rights reserved.

oto.theclinics.com

has lifelong benefits and consequences, and careful consideration should be taken when treating children and adolescents with benign or malignant thyroid disease.

HYPERTHYROIDISM

Graves disease is the most common cause of hyperthyroidism in children, with an incidence of 0.1/100,000 person-years in children and 3/100,000 person years in adolescents.[1] It is more common in girls than boys, but both more severe and without gender predilection under age 4.[1] Children with hyperthyroidism may present with goiter, tachycardia, palpitations, weight loss, headaches, sleep disturbances, anxiety, and heat intolerance.[1] The diagnosis is typically made based on symptoms, laboratory findings (suppressed thyroid-stimulating hormone [TSH] level combined with elevated free T4 level), and the presence of TSH-receptor antibodies. Imaging with radioactive iodine uptake (RAIU) scans are occasionally used if the diagnosis is unclear. Thyroid ultrasound also is common if there is concern for nodules or compressive symptoms.

Options for therapy in children include antithyroid medical therapy, surgery, and radioactive iodine (RAI). Antithyroid medical therapy is limited to methimazole in children. Although it is generally well tolerated, adverse drug reactions, such as rash, edema, arthralgias, and immunosuppression, are more common in children than in adults.[2] Propylthiouracil is not used in children due to severe hepatotoxicity. Other medical therapies include β-blockade for symptom management. Long-term remission rates with antithyroid drugs are low, only 40% to 60%.[2–4] Patients with thyrotoxicosis, adverse drug reactions, poor compliance, or failure achieve remission with antithyroid drugs are candidates for definitive therapy with RAI or surgery (total thyroidectomy).

The utility of RAI ablation for the treatment of Graves disease depends on the gland uptake (RAIU), goiter size (<80 g), and risk of recurrence. Age is also a major consideration, with younger children being poor candidates. The age cutoff is controversial; however, with the American Thyroid Association (ATA) recommending no RAI ablation in children under age 5 and others limiting this option to children over 10 years old.[5] A single therapeutic dose RAI usually is successful. In 10% of cases, repeat doses are required to achieve gland suppression. RAI is easy to administer and has few side effects. There is little agreement on the secondary risks of RAI; however, short-term side effects have been reported, including nausea/emesis, radiation thyroiditis, sialadenitis, dry mouth, and transient bone marrow suppression while rarely reported long-term side effects have included permanent salivary gland dysfunction, permanent bone marrow suppression, pulmonary fibrosis, second malignancies, and fertility alterations.[6] RAI is contraindicated in pregnancy and patients should avoid pregnancy for 6 months after treatment.

Surgery with total thyroidectomy may be used in patients with large thyroid goiter, age under 5 years, severe Graves orbitopathy, low RAIU, patients who are interested in immediate symptom resolution, and those with high risk of recurrence.[7] Preoperatively, patients should be treated with antithyroid medications until euthyroid with use of methimazole, β-blockers, inorganic iodine, and steroids to minimize intraoperative bleeding and risk of thyrotoxicosis. Postoperatively, patients begin thyroid hormone replacement immediately and should be monitored for transient hypoparathyroidism and subsequent hypocalcemia. Thyrotoxic patients are at increased risk for hungry bone syndrome or a disturbance in the calcium homeostasis in the immediate postsurgical period.[8] There are several safe options for the treatment of hyperthyroidism in children, but the treatment selection should be tailored carefully to the patient with careful considerations to patient age, gland size, RAIU, and risk of recurrence.

THYROID NODULES AND CANCER

Pediatric patients with thyroid nodules require experienced multidisciplinary evaluation with pediatric thyroid surgeons, endocrinology, radiology, and genetics. Some teams also incorporate dedicated oncologists, interventional radiologists, and pathologists to facilitate robust decision making in more complex cases. The evaluation and diagnostic approach to pediatric thyroid nodules differ from adults due to the increased risk of malignancy regardless of size. The ATA guidelines for pediatric thyroid nodules are summarized in **Fig. 1**.

Thyroid cancer in children is rare, representing less than 1% of all childhood cancers. The incidence of thyroid cancer is increasing in children and adolescents and is 5-times more common in girls than boys, albeit with an excellent prognosis when diagnosed early.[9] Differentiated thyroid cancer most commonly presents as a thyroid nodule. There is an increased incidence of thyroid tumors of all sizes, indicating that this trend may not be attributed to increased and improved diagnostic evaluation.[10] There is a 3-times increased risk of thyroid cancer in patients with Hashimoto thyroiditis.[11] Additional risk factors for pediatric thyroid cancer include diagnostic, therapeutic, or environmental radiation; iodine deficiency; and genetic predisposition syndromes. A family history of thyroid cancer confers a much higher risk of developing differentiated thyroid cancer and has been designated familial nonmedullary thyroid cancer. Although the genetic causes of familial nonmedullary thyroid cancer continue to be investigated, it seems to be a "polygenic disorder with variable penetrance" that causes thyroid cancer at a younger age and with a more aggressive presentation (multifocality and metastasis) than nonfamilial, sporadic cancers.[12] There also are several specific genetic syndromes that may increase risk for differentiated thyroid cancer, with the most common, including

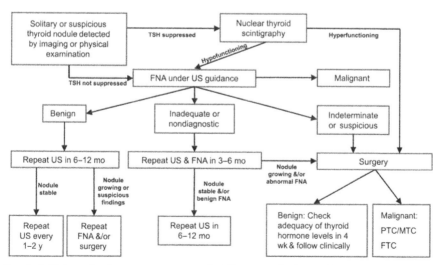

Fig. 1. Initial evaluation, treatment, and follow-up of the pediatric thyroid nodule. FTC, follicular thyroid cancer; PTC/MTC, papillary thyroid cancer/medullary thyroid cancer. (*From* Francis G, Waguespack S, Bauer A, et al. ATA Guidelines Task Force. Management guidelines for children with thyroid nodules and differentiated thyroid cancer. Thyroid. 2015;25:716–59; with permission.)

- APC-associated polyposis (familial adenomatous polyposis, Gardner syndrome, and Turcot syndrome); gene APC (5q21-q22)
- Carney complex; gene PRKAR1A (17q24.2), CNC2 (2p16)
- DICER1 syndrome; gene DICER1 (14q32.13)
- PTEN hamartoma tumor syndrome (Cowden syndrome); gene PTEN (10q23)
- Werner syndrome; gene WRN (8p12)

Other less common genetic syndromes associated with differentiated thyroid cancer include Beckwith-Wiedemann syndrome, familial paraganglioma syndromes, Li-Fraumeni Syndrome, McCune-Albright syndrome, and Peutz-Jeghers syndrome. Rearrangements of the RET/PTC protooncogene are the most common molecular abnormalities in pediatric papillary thyroid cancer. This is in contrast to the BRAF mutations that account for most of adult PTC.[13] Due to this molecular difference, pediatric PTC behaves very differently and is more locoregionally aggressive, is less responsive to ^{131}I, and has different treatment targets.

Medullary and follicular thyroid cancers account for less than 10% of pediatric thyroid cancer. Medullary thyroid cancer may be sporadic or familial, and most pediatric cases are associated with multiple endocrine neoplasia syndromes (multiple endocrine neoplasia types 2A and 2B). Most cases are associated with germline RET mutations and patients should undergo genetics evaluation. Patients are stratified by risk category depending on mutation and those with highest-risk mutation should undergo prophylactic thyroidectomy in the first year of life. Those with high-risk mutations should undergo thyroidectomy prior to 5 years of age, and those with moderate to low-risk mutations should be screened with serum calcitonin levels.[14]

The ATA recommends that pediatric thyroid surgery be performed by a pediatric thyroid surgeon who performs more than 30 cervical endocrine procedures per year in order to reduce complications, duration of stay, and cost.[15]

THYROID SURGERY
Preoperative Considerations

A complete history should be performed with a focus on any thyroid-related symptoms, palpitations, weight loss or gain, skin or hair changes, heat and cold intolerance, compressive symptoms, voice changes, and family history of thyroid-related diseases. The Pediatric Voice-Related Quality-of-Life survey has been validated for use in pediatric voice disorders and may be considered in assessing preoperative and postoperative pediatric voice.[16] A complete head and neck physical examination should be performed, with particular attention to thyroid size, trachea location, and regional lymphadenopathy. In particular, a fixed thyroid gland as well as bulky and fixed regional lymphadenopathy increases concern for malignancy. In-office laryngoscopy should be performed in patients with preoperative voice complaints, recent changes in voice quality, or a high-risk primary tumor, such as one that encases the area of the recurrent laryngeal nerve (RLN) or is fixed to surrounding structures.

Preoperative imaging in all patients with benign and malignant disease includes a complete thyroid ultrasound. Thyroid nodules should be characterized on ultrasound according to the 2015 ATA guidelines and risk stratified accordingly for consideration of fine-needle aspiration (FNA) biopsy.[15,17] In the setting of known or suspected thyroid cancer, ultrasound also should carefully assess the central and lateral nodal basins with mapping of suspicious lymph nodes.[15] This is best performed by someone experienced with thyroid and cervical ultrasound, whether a dedicated ultrasound technician, radiologist, or member of the multidisciplinary thyroid team. Biopsy with

FNA is recommended for any suspicious lymph nodes and cytopathology stratified according to the Bethesda system for reporting thyroid cytopathology:

a. Nondiagnostic (fewer than 6 follicular groups of 10–15 cells each, absent follicular cells, or poor fixation)
b. Benign
c. Atypia or follicular lesion of undetermined significance
d. Follicular neoplasm or suspicious for follicular neoplasm
e. Suggestive of malignancy
f. Malignant

Molecular genetic studies with FNA also may be considered when the cytologic result is indeterminate. This testing evaluates specimens for RAS, BRAF, RET/PTC, and PAX8/PPAR gamma genetic mutations to increase positive predictive value.[18]

Preoperative axial anatomic imaging with MRI or CT is used in patients with large or fixed thyroid masses, vocal fold paralysis, or bulky regional metastatic lymphadenopathy. Additional chest imaging with radiograph or CT should be used in patients with extensive regional lymphadenopathy to evaluate for pulmonary metastases. Pediatric differentiated thyroid cancer has a high incidence of cervical node metastases, and preoperative planning should be complete to ensure that the patient undergoes thoughtfully planned surgery. This minimizes the risk of tumor recurrence and the risk of revision surgery, even if postoperative RAI therapy is delayed due to CT contrast washout.[15]

Preoperative thyroid function tests typically are evaluated to document thyroid functional status (TSH) as well as preoperative calcium and vitamin D levels. An intact parathyroid hormone level (Intact PTH) is typically ordered immediately prior to total thyroidectomy to facilitate postoperative calcium management. Additionally, a thyroglobulin level is routinely ordered in patients with differentiated thyroid cancer and calcitonin in cases of medullary thyroid cancer.[19] (**Table 1**).

Extent of Primary Thyroid Surgery

Once surgery is elected in the management of pediatric thyroid disease, the extent of surgery must be considered carefully and differs from recommendations in similar adult thyroid diseases. For autoimmune hyperthyroidism, ablation of all native thyroid function with a total thyroidectomy or near-total thyroidectomy is favored over the historical subtotal thyroidectomy with functional preservation due to similar risks to the RLN and parathyroid glands, with much higher cure and lower recurrence rates.[20] A total thyroidectomy is also recommended for known differentiated pediatric thyroid cancer. Although lobectomy is considered in some cases of adult thyroid cancer, there

Table 1
Preoperative laboratory tests

Test	Timing	Indication
TSH	Routine	Thyroid functional status
Calcium, vitamin D	Routine	Baseline
Anti-thyroperoxidase antibodies	If indicated	Suspected or confirmed hyperthyroidism
PTH intact	Routine, immediately preoperative	Baseline
Thyroglobulin	Depends	Differentiated thyroid cancer
Calcitonin	Depends	Medullary thyroid cancer

is a higher risk of multifocal disease in pediatric patients, with a significantly higher risk of locoregional recurrence for lobectomy alone.[15,21] In children, a lobectomy may be considered for follicular neoplasms or for nodules suspicious for malignancy but indeterminate on pathology. A lobectomy also may be offered for nodules with troublesome clinical correlates, such as compressive symptoms, cosmetic changes, size greater than 4 cm, rapid or continuous growth, or patient preference for definitive diagnosis rather than serial imaging and observation.[15] Although ethanol ablation and RAI are considered for autonomically hyperfunctioning nodules in adults, children with a hot nodule should undergo at least thyroid lobectomy due to increased risk of incidental thyroid cancer in the nodule.[15]

Extent of Neck Dissection

Because regional metastases are already present in up to 50% of pediatric patients at the time of diagnosis in cases of well-differentiated thyroid cancer, preoperative and intraoperative assessment of the central and lateral neck compartments, as described previously, is critical.[22] The benefits of neck dissection are to

- Decrease locoregional recurrence and the need for further surgery
- Stratify patient risk for consideration of adjuvant therapy
- Theoretically improve the efficacy of adjuvant RAI therapy in intermediate and high-risk patients

When there is histopathologically confirmed nodal metastasis, a level-based selective neck dissection should be completed rather than a berry-picking nodal excision.[15] In the central neck, this should include a bilateral level VI dissection, sparing the parathyroid glands and recurrent laryngeal nerves. The ATA guidelines on pediatric thyroid nodules and thyroid cancer advocate for a prophylactic central neck dissection for

- Large primary tumors with extrathyroidal extension
- Confirmed metastasis to levels II to V

The recommendations are less clear in the absence of these factors and defer to surgeon experience, noting the higher risk of complications in children undergoing central neck dissection.[15] Furthermore, the ATA recommends ipsilateral central neck dissection in the case of an isolated thyroid nodule based on adult studies of regional metastatic spread. This may not be relevant in children, however, where there is a higher risk of multifocal primary disease. Further studies are warranted to clarify this question.

In the lateral neck, the number of adjacent levels dissected also remains controversial. Some surgeons adopt a standard approach of levels IIA to 5B, excluding IIB and 5A, for any FNA-positive lateral neck disease, and others support a radiographically determined extent of dissection once there has been any histopathologic confirmation. There is a paucity of evidence to clarify this question in children, but limited literature supports a dissection extensive enough to result in a positive nodal yield of less than 45% (lymph node ratio) of all excised nodes to decrease the possibility of recurrence.[23]

Use of Intraoperative Recurrent Laryngeal Nerve Monitoring

Intraoperative monitoring of the RLN (IMRLN) during thyroid surgery has been controversial even in adults where there is a much more robust literature than in children. IMRLN has been suggested to be safe in children and to facilitate identification of the RLN.[24] It has not been shown to decrease the incidence of RLN injury or vocal outcomes in adults or children.[25] The ATA currently recommends use of IMRLN in children under 10, children with preoperative vocal changes, and children undergoing revision surgery.[15] The authors have found it useful as well in cases of bulky or posteriorly invasive primary disease. There are commercially available nerve-monitoring endotracheal tubes, currently as small as 5.0 cuffed. For patients requiring a smaller tube, electrodes may be directly inserted into the laryngeal musculature during laryngoscopy or taped onto a smaller endotracheal tube.

Other Intraoperative Considerations

There are no specific guidelines regarding intraoperative antibiotics for pediatric thyroidectomy, and general perioperative care guidelines for cervical surgery in children vary with regard to antibiotic recommendations. Similarly, there are no specific guidelines on postoperative closed suction drains in pediatric thyroidectomy. Postoperative hematoma and seroma, theoretically preventable with drain usage, are such rare events that it would be difficult to demonstrate efficacy in children. The authors do not routinely use postoperative drains except in cases of unusual blood loss or preoperative infected surgical field (**Box 1**).

POSTOPERATIVE MANAGEMENT
Postoperative Calcium Monitoring

Other than monitoring for routine complications of pediatric cervical surgeries, such as bleeding or hematoma, the most important aspect of postoperative care after pediatric thyroidectomy is surveillance of parathyroid function and calcium homeostasis. As with many aspects of pediatric thyroid care, most of the literature utilized in guideline development for perioperative calcium management is based on adult thyroid care.[15] Pediatric thyroidectomy is particularly different in this regard, with a much higher risk of significant morbidity from the transient hypoparathyroidism and associated hypocalcemia that occur in 20% to 40% of patients.[26,27] Permanent hypocalcemia is a life-altering and potentially life-threatening complication requiring lifelong calcium monitoring and supplementation. Although early reports of permanent hypocalcemia were as high as 20%, more recent data from high-volume pediatric thyroid surgery centers give a rate of 0.4% to 0.6%.[27] Younger age, concomitant lymphadenectomy, and hyperthyroidism increased the risk of transient and permanent hypocalcemia in several series.[19,28] Large-scale analysis of postoperative hypocalcemia in children is complicated by a lack of standard definition, with some studies referencing various calcium and parathyroid hormone levels across a multitude of time points. Multiple centers have publicized or presented perioperative calcium management protocols

---

Box 1
Summary of recommendations to reduce perioperative and intraoperative risk in pediatric thyroid surgery

Decision making by a coordinated, multidisciplinary team

High-volume pediatric thyroid surgeon (>30 cases per year)

Tedious dissection to spare parathyroid function

Reimplantation of devitalized parathyroid tissue

Systematic postoperative monitoring of intact parathyroid hormone, calcium, and phosphorus levels

Intraoperative RLN monitoring at minimum:
- Patients under 10 years old
- Patients with recurrent or bulky primary disease
- Patients undergoing central neck dissection
- Patients with preoperative vocal changes

but few in peer-reviewed literature. Some protocols include routine preoperative calcium and vitamin D supplementation with others advocate routine postoperative calcium, calcitriol, or both. There have been multiple adult algorithms proposed around postoperative parathyroid hormone measurements, but the cutoffs have not adequately predicted the severity of hypocalcemia risk in children.[28] Within the purview of multidisciplinary thyroid programs, standardized local protocols should be implemented that anticipate and decrease the risk of symptomatic postoperative hypocalcemia and need for intravenous calcium usage with its significant potential complications. Protocols also should consider outpatient calcium wean as quickly as safely feasible. Monitoring of transient and permanent hypoparathyroid rates within a program is critical to demonstrate surgical quality, and higher-than-expected hypoparathyroidism rates should trigger a critical review of surgical management.

Postoperative Risk Stratification and Adjuvant Treatment

Children with papillary thyroid cancer are stratified according to low, intermediate, and high-risk groups to facilitate postoperative management, follow-up, and additional treatments with RAI. Risk stratification is performed within 12 weeks after surgery using the American Joint Committee on Cancer TNM classification system for differentiated thyroid cancer. There is a maximum delay of 12 weeks after surgery before staging to allow for adequate surgical recovery and still avoid delaying additional therapy with RAI when indicated. There is still research needed to determine the utility of risk stratification in pediatric thyroid patients because these data are extrapolated from the authors' adult patients (**Table 2**).

Adjunctive RAI iodine is used in select cases to improve disease-free survival in children with papillary thyroid cancer.[131]I should be used selectively, however, because it is not without risks to young patients and the prognosis of pediatric differentiated thyroid cancer is favorable without additional therapies.[29] There is no current consensus in the literature regarding the utility of RAI for remnant thyroid ablation and treatment of known residual disease to decrease locoregional recurrence, distant metastases, and overall survival. Additionally, therapeutic RAI treatment is recommended for children with iodine-avid unresectable local and regional disease and in some children with small-volume pulmonary metastases.

There is no current consensus on empiric dosing of ^{131}I versus whole-body dosimetry for the treatment of children and this should be performed by a radiologist

Table 2		
Risk stratification of pediatric differentiated thyroid cancer		
American Thyroid Association Pediatric Risk Level	**Thyroid Disease**	**Regional Disease**
ATA pediatric low risk	Disease <4 cm and confined to thyroid	Nx, N0, or incidental N1a metastases
ATA pediatric intermediate risk	Disease >4 cm limited to the thyroid with minimal extrathyroidal extension	Extensive N1a or minimal N1b disease
ATA pediatric high risk	Locally invasive disease with or without distant metastasis	Regionally extensive disease N1b

Nx, regional lymph nodes not assessed; N0, no regional lymph node metastasis; N1a, metastasis to level VI (pretracheal, paratracheal, prelaryngeal/Delphian lymph nodes); N1b, metastasis to ipselateral, contralateral, or bilateral cervical levels I-V, superior mediastinal level VII, or retropharyngeal lymph nodes.

Table 3
Short-term and long-term risks of ^{131}I therapy

Short Term	Long Term
Sialadenitis, xerostomia, dental caries, stomatitis, ocular dryness, nasolacrimal duct obstruction	Lifelong xerostomia, dental caries, salivary gland malignancy
Gonadal injury, transient amenorrhea, and menstrual irregularities	Increase in infertility, miscarriage, birth defects
Acute bone marrow suppression	Rare long-term bone marrow suppression
	Increased risk of secondary malignancy, increased mortality Pulmonary fibrosis

experienced in dosing pediatric patients.[15] RAI has short-term and long-term risks and those risks should be disclosed with the family when considering adjunctive ^{131}I therapy (**Table 3**).

Recommendations for Treatment of Persistent or Recurrent Disease

The management of persistent or recurrent papillary thyroid cancer in children should be personalized to the patient, location and size of disease, surgical and ^{131}I treatment history, and iodine avidity of the disease. Small (<1-cm) cervical lymph node disease can be observed safely given the excellent prognosis of PTC in children and the very low risk to clinically significant progression. In these cases, the use of therapeutic ^{131}I is unfavorable. Patients with larger (>1-cm) persistent or recurrent disease may be considered for surgery by a high-volume thyroid surgeon. Recurrences and persistent disease should be confirmed with imaging (US or cross-sectional) and pathologic examination by FNA. For the very rare cases of recurrent and advanced locoregional or metastatic disease, the new generation of tyrosine kinase inhibitors may have a role in children as they have in adults who have failed ^{131}I therapy. There are ongoing phase II trials of tyrosine kinase inhibitors for these patients. In the most advanced locally recurrent disease, external beam radiotherapy may have a limited role in palliation or disease stabilization, although these cases are exceptionally rare.

SUMMARY

The management of pediatric thyroid disease requires a nuanced approach by a consistent, multidisciplinary team that is as familiar with the relevant guidelines and literature as with the significant controversies specific to children. Future research will help resolve care controversies but must rely on standardized definitions of complications, staging, and risk assessment facilitated by interinstitutional collaborations. The pediatric thyroid surgeon plays a major role in disease management but should take steps to minimize the risk of surgical complications and to ensure oncologically sound decision making with regard to timing and extent of surgery. Complications and outcomes must be monitored and compared with published standards with a low threshold for critical surgical review in the event of deviation.

REFERENCES

1. Okawa E, Grant F, Smith J. Pediatric Graves' disease: decisions regarding therapy. Curr Opin Pediatr 2015;27:442–7.

2. Rabon S, Burton A, White P. Graves' disease in children: long-term outcomes of medical therapy. Clin Endocinol (Oxf) 2016;85:632–5.

3. Leger J. Graves' disease in children. Endocr Dev 2014;26:171–82.

4. Ohye H, Minagawa A, Noh J, et al. Antithyroid drug treatment for graves' disease in children: a long-term retrospective study at a single institution. Thyroid 2014; 24:200–7.

5. Ross D, Burch HB, Cooper DS, et al. 2016 American Thyroid Association guidelines for diagnosis and management of hyperthyroidism and other causes of thyrotoxicosis. Thyroid 2016;26:1343–421.

6. Albano D, Bertagna F, Panarotto MB, et al. Early and late adverse effects of radioiodine for pediatric differentiated thyroid cancer. Pediatr Blood Cancer 2017;64: e26595.

7. Wu V, Lorenzen A, Beck A, et al. Comparative analysis of radioactive iodine versus thyroidectomy for the definitive treatment of Graves disease. Surgery 2017;16:147–55.

8. Dembinski TC, Yatscoff RW, Blandford DE. Thyrotoxicosis and hungry bone syndrome–a cause of posttreatment hypocalcemia. Clin Biochem 1994;27(1): 69–74.

9. Dermody S, Walls A, Harley E. Pediatric thyroid cancer: an update from the SEER database 2007-2012. Int J Pediatr Otorhinolaryngol 2016;89:121–6.

10. Vergamini L, Frazier A, Abrantes F, et al. Increase in the incidence of differentiated thyroid carcinoma in children, adolescents and young adults: a population-based study. J Pediatr 2014;164:1481–5.

11. Larson SD, Jackson LN, Riall TS, et al. Increased incidence of well-differentiated thyroid cancer associated with Hashimoto thyroiditis and the role of the PI3k/Akt pathway. J Am Coll Surg 2007;204(5):764–73.

12. Bauer A. Clinical behavior and genetics of nonsyndromic, familial nonmedullary thyroid cancer. Front Horm Res 2013;41:141–8.

13. Chan C, Young J, Prager J, et al. Pediatric thyroid cancer. Adv Pediatr 2017;64: 171–90.

14. Wells SA Jr, Pacini F, Robinson BG, et al. Multiple endocrine neoplasia type 2 and familial medullary thyroid carcinoma: an update. J Clin Endocrinol Metab 2013; 98(8):3149–64.

15. Francis G, Waguespack S, Bauer A, et al, ATA Guidelines Task Force. Management guidelines for children with thyroid nodules and differentiated thyroid cancer. Thyroid 2015;25:716–59.

16. Boseley M, Cunningham M, Volk M, et al. Validation of the pediatric voice-related quality-of-life survey. Arch Otolaryngol Head Neck Surg 2006;132:717–20.

17. Lim-Dunham JE, Erdem T, Alsabban K, et al. Ultrasound risk stratification for malignancy using the 2015 American Thyroid Association Management guidelines for children with thyroid nodules and differentiated thyroid cancer. Pediatr Radiol 2017;47:429–36.

18. Guille J, Opoku-Boateng A, Thibeault S, et al. Evaluation and management of the pediatric thyroid nodule. Oncologist 2015;20:19–27.

19. Chen Y, Masiakos P, Gaz R, et al. Pediatric thyroidectomy in a high volume thyroid surgery center: Risk factors for postoperative hypocalcemia. J Pediatr Surg 2015; 50:1316–9.

20. Genovese BM, Noureldine SI, Gleeson EM, et al. What is the best definitive treatment for Graves' disease? A systematic review of the existing literature. Ann Surg Oncol 2013;20:660–7.

21. Jazab B, Handkiewicz Junak D, Wloch J, et al. Multivariate analysis of prognostic factors for differentiated thyroid carcinoma in children. Eur J Nucl Med 2000;27: 833–41.
22. Spinelli C, Tognetti F, Strambi S, et al. Cervical lymph node metastases of papillary thyroid carcinoma in the central and lateral compartments in children and adolescents: predictive factors. World J Surg 2018;42:2444–53.
23. Rubenstein JC, Dinauer C, Herrick-Reynolds K, et al. Lymph node ratio predicts recurrence in pediatric papillary thyroid cancer. J Pediatr Surg 2019;54:129–32.
24. White WM, Randolph GW, Hartnick CJ, et al. Recurrent laryngeal nerve monitoring during thyroidectomy and related cervical procedures in the pediatric population. Arch Otolaryngol Head Neck Surg 2009;135:88–94.
25. Angelos P. Recurrent laryngeal nerve monitoring: state of the art, ethical and legal issues. Surg Clin North Am 2009;89:1157–69.
26. Hanba C, Svider PF, Siegel B, et al. Pediatric thyroidectomy. Otolaryngol Head Neck Surg 2017;156:360–7.
27. Baumgarten HD, Bauer AJ, Isaza A, et al. Surgical management of pediatric thyroid disease: complication rates after thyroidectomy at the Children's Hospital of Philadelphia high-volume Pediatric Thyroid Center. J Pediatr Surg 2019 [pii:S0022-3468(19)30122-30128].
28. Yu YR, Fallon SC, Carpenter JL, et al. Perioperative determinants of transient hypocalcemia after pediatric total thyroidectomy. J Pediatr Surg 2017;52:684–8.
29. Hay I, Johnson T, Kaggal S, et al. Papillary thyroid carcinoma (PTC) in children and adults: comparison of initial presentation and long-term postoperative outcome in 4432 patients consecutively treated at the Mayo Clinic during eight decades (1936-2015). World J Surg 2018;42:329–42.

Professionalism, Quality, and Safety for Pediatric Otolaryngologists

Ellen M. Friedman, MD[a], Romaine F. Johnson, MD, MPH[b],*

KEYWORDS

- Professionalism • Quality • Safety • Emotional intelligence

KEY POINTS

- Professionalism consists of behaviors that build trusting relationships.
- Developing the components of emotional intelligence can enable physicians to optimize their clinical impact and personal satisfaction throughout their careers.
- Health care quality means providing services to patients that give the desired health outcomes and are consistent with best practices.
- High-reliability organization is the holy grail of safety and quality, and its principles provide the framework for an optimal safety culture.

The means represent the ideal in the making, and the end in process.
—Martin Luther King Jr (1929–1968)

PROFESSIONALISM

What is professionalism? Although there are many attempts to define professionalism, it may be most accurate to rephrase Supreme Court Judge Potter's comments about the definition of pornography, "you know it when you see it." In truth, with professionalism, you recognize professionalism when you see it, and you also recognize it when you do not see it. Essentially, professionalism consists of behaviors that build trusting relationships.

The basic principles of professionalism have been outlined in the Physician's Charter initially published in 2002.[1] This document explains the 3 foundational principles of professionalism (**Box 1**) as well as its 10 professional responsibilities (**Box 2**). The current interest and emphasis on professionalism are further confirmed by the integration of professionalism as one of the core competencies for residency training in all programs through the Accreditation Council for Graduate Medical Education. Although

---

The authors have no conflicts of interest or disclosures to make.
[a] Center for Professionalism, Office of the Provost, Baylor College of Medicine, One Baylor Plaza, Suite 206A, Office of the Provost, Houston, TX 77030, USA; [b] Department of Otolaryngology, Head and Neck Surgery, UT Southwestern Medical Center, Dallas, TX, USA
* Corresponding author. 2350 North Stemmons Freeway, F6.207, Dallas, TX 75207.
E-mail address: Romaine.Johnson@UTSouthwestern.edu

Otolaryngol Clin N Am 52 (2019) 969–980
https://doi.org/10.1016/j.otc.2019.06.010
0030-6665/19/© 2019 Elsevier Inc. All rights reserved.

Box 1
Fundamental principles

Principle of primacy of patient welfare
The principle is based on a dedication to serving the interest of the patient. Altruism contributes to the trust that is central to the physician-patient relationship. Market forces, societal pressures, and administrative exigencies must not compromise this principle.

Principle of patient autonomy
Physicians must have respect for patient autonomy. Physicians must be honest with their patients and empower them to make informed decisions about their treatment. Patients' decisions about their care must be paramount, as long as those decisions are in keeping with ethical practice and do not lead to demands for inappropriate care.

Principle of social justice
The medical profession must promote justice in the health care system, including the fair distribution of health care resources. Physicians should work actively to eliminate discrimination in health care, whether based on race, gender, socioeconomic status, ethnicity, religion, or any other social category.

Data from The American Board of Internal Medicine Foundation (ABIM). The Physician Charter. Available at: https://abimfoundation.org/what-we-do/physician-charter; with permission.

this move documents the importance of professionalism during residency training, its role throughout one's career cannot be overemphasized.

"Although there is not one universally accepted definition of professionalism, the most important concept is that professionalism is a set of behaviors than can be learned, developed and improved with attention and determination. As with any skill, professionalism can be continually refined and strengthen over time with practice."[2] The skills include clear and respectful communication, altruism, humanism, collaboration, and empathy. With motivation and attention, everyone can improve their skill set and at the same time improve their daily clinical effectiveness, reputation, career satisfaction, patient outcomes, patient satisfaction, and quality of work life.

Emotional Intelligence and Professionalism

Many of the positive behaviors associated with professionalism are acknowledged elements of the framework of emotional intelligence. Emotional intelligence, described at length by Daniel Goleman,[3] is a skill set that enables an individual to understand and modulate reactions to emotions, ones' own and those of others. Developing the components of emotional intelligence and embodying the behaviors outlined in the Physician's Charter will enable physicians to optimize their clinical impact and personal satisfaction throughout their careers.

These skills will enable physicians to enhance the collegiality of the work environment, decrease miscommunications, improve patient safety, and decrease their risk of malpractice litigation. In addition, professionalism enables physicians to build their reputations and increase their referring network. Beyond these advantages, professionalism has an overriding positive impact on teamwork and collaboration. Teamwork is of increasing importance, because there is an increasing reliance on team medicine. It is critical for each of us to develop the ability to participate effectively on multidisciplinary teams. Otolaryngologists frequently participate in teams; demonstrating professionalism consistently will help otolaryngologists be effective leaders. This will successfully ensure a culture of patient safety and continuous quality improvement. The benefits of improved teamwork exceed purely patient-centered benefits; it also creates a more satisfying and pleasant work environment for

Box 2
A set of professional responsibilities

Commitment to professional competence
   Physicians must be committed to lifelong learning and be responsible for maintaining the
   medical knowledge and clinical and team skills necessary for the provision of quality care.
   More broadly, the profession as a whole must strive to see that all of its members are
   competent and must ensure that appropriate mechanisms are available for physicians to
   accomplish this goal.

Commitment to honesty with patients
   Physicians must ensure that patients are completely and honestly informed before the
   patient has consented to treatment and after treatment has occurred. This expectation does
   not mean that patients should be involved in every minute decision about medical care;
   rather, they must be empowered to decide on the course of therapy. Physicians should also
   acknowledge that in health care, medical errors that injure patients do sometimes occur.
   Whenever patients are injured as a consequence of medical care, patients should be
   informed promptly because failure to do so seriously compromises patient and societal trust.
   Reporting and analyzing medical mistakes provide the basis for appropriate prevention and
   improvement strategies and for appropriate compensation to injured parties.

Commitment to patient confidentiality
   Earning the trust and confidence of patients requires that appropriate confidentiality
   safeguards be applied to disclosure of patient information. This commitment extends to
   discussions with persons acting on a patient's behalf when obtaining the patient's own
   consent is not feasible. Fulfilling the commitment to confidentiality is more pressing now than
   ever before, given the widespread use of electronic information systems for compiling patient
   data and an increasing availability of genetic information. Physicians recognize, however, that
   their commitment to patient confidentiality must occasionally yield to overriding
   considerations in the public interest (for example, when patients endanger others).

Commitment to maintaining appropriate relations with patients
   Given the inherent vulnerability and dependency of patients, certain relationships between
   physicians and patients must be avoided. In particular, physicians should never exploit
   patients for any sexual advantage, personal financial gain, or other private purpose.

Commitment to improving quality of care
   Physicians must be dedicated to continuous improvement in the quality of health care. This
   commitment entails not only maintaining clinical competence but also working collaboratively
   with other professionals to reduce medical error, increase patient safety, minimize overuse of
   health care resources, and optimize the outcomes of care. Physicians must actively participate
   in the development of better measures of quality of care and the application of quality
   measures to assess routinely the performance of all individuals, institutions, and systems
   responsible for health care delivery. Physicians, individually and through their professional
   associations, must take responsibility for assisting in the creation and implementation of
   mechanisms designed to encourage continuous improvement in the quality of care.

Commitment to improving access to care
   Medical professionalism demands that the objective of all health care systems be the
   availability of a uniform and adequate standard of care. Physicians must individually and
   collectively strive to reduce barriers to equitable health care. Within each system, the
   physician should work to eliminate barriers to access based on education, laws, finances,
   geography, and social discrimination. A commitment to equity entails the promotion of
   public health and preventive medicine as well as public advocacy on the part of each
   physician, without concern for the self-interest of the physician or the profession.

Commitment to a just distribution of finite resources
   While meeting the needs of individual patients, physicians are required to provide health
   care that is based on the wise and cost-effective management of limited clinical resources.
   They should be committed to working with other physicians, hospitals, and payers to
   develop guidelines for cost-effective care. The physician's professional responsibility for
   appropriate allocation of resources requires scrupulous avoidance of superfluous tests and

procedures. The provision of unnecessary services not only exposes one's patients to avoidable harm and expense but also diminishes the resources available for others.

Commitment to scientific knowledge
Much of medicine's contract with society is based on the integrity and appropriate use of scientific knowledge and technology. Physicians have a duty to uphold scientific standards, to promote research, and to create new knowledge and ensure its appropriate use. The profession is responsible for the integrity of this knowledge, which is based on scientific evidence and physician experience.

Commitment to maintaining trust by managing conflicts of interest
Medical professionals and their organizations have many opportunities to compromise their professional responsibilities by pursuing private gain or personal advantage. Such compromises are especially threatening in the pursuit of personal or organizational interactions with for-profit industries, including medical equipment manufacturers, insurance companies, and pharmaceutical firms. Physicians have an obligation to recognize, disclose to the general public, and deal with conflicts of interest that arise in the course of their professional duties and activities. Relationships between industry and opinion leaders should be disclosed, especially when the latter determine the criteria for conducting and reporting clinical trials, writing editorials or therapeutic guidelines, or serving as editors of scientific journals.

Commitment to professional responsibilities
As members of a profession, physicians are expected to work collaboratively to maximize patient care, be respectful of one another, and participate in the processes of self-regulation, including remediation and discipline of members who have failed to meet professional standards. The profession should also define and organize the educational and standard-setting process for current and future members. Physicians have both individual and collective obligations to participate in these processes. These obligations include engaging in internal assessment and accepting external scrutiny of all aspects of their professional performance.

Data from The American Board of Internal Medicine Foundation (ABIM). The Physician Charter. Available at: https://abimfoundation.org/what-we-do/physician-charter; with permission.

physicians, which, in turn, helps to combat burnout.[4] In other words, improved communication and teamwork are not purely altruistic; one will also personally benefit by working in a more civil and enjoyable setting.

Health care organizations and patients also benefit from a culture with increased professionalism. The hospitals benefit by increasing physician retention, improving patient satisfaction, and building their national ranking.[5] This is documented by higher retention rates of physicians and lower burnout rates in organizations with higher degrees of professionalism. Perhaps most importantly, in a culture of increased professionalism, patients enjoy an increased sense of trust in their physicians and more compassionate care and experience fewer complications. Patients who trust their physicians have higher compliance with suggested treatment regimens, lower no-show rates on clinic visits, and higher patient satisfaction.[6]

Commercialism and Medicine

Although there is universal agreement that professional behavior is desirable, it can be challenging to maintain one's professionalism consistently. There are many reasons some may fall short of their own aspirational behavior. There are considerations that are inherent stresses in medicine, including caring for ill patients, dealing with complications, long hours, and unexpected outcomes. However, new challenges in the professional environment have emerged that complicate professional life. The current commercialism of medicine has brought along with it a growing cynicism among physicians and the public. Watcher has noted that "our businesslike efforts to measure and improve quality are now blocking the altruism, indeed the love, that motivates people to enter the helping professions. While we're figuring out how to get better, we need to tread more lightly in assessing the work of the professionals who practice in our most human and sacred fields."[7] These factors contribute to increasing moral distress that learners and even seasoned clinicians experience. These distractions include productivity requirements, decreased reimbursements, practice guidelines, increased bureaucracy, and the electronic medical record. The increasing business focus of medicine can cause physicians to become less engaged, cynical, or even demoralized.

In addition, increasing accessibility via e-mail, text messaging, and instant messaging has made it more difficult for physicians to set boundaries and maintain reasonable work-life integration. Physicians can feel alone in the pursuit of excellence, and at times, even victimized by the system. These feelings can create a negative work environment with mounting territorialism and excessive competitive feelings. Often these factors have contributed to an increasing amount of daily incivility that may be experienced by those working in the medical arena. The breakdown of morale of the medical staff can lead to the well-publicized epidemic of burnout.[8]

Professionalism Lapses

Although the roots of professionalism lapses may be understood, the negative impact cannot be tolerated. Wandering from the principles of professionalism jeopardizes not only our patients' safety but also our personal connection and satisfaction with our career. Some lapses in professionalism represent overtly criminal behavior, such as Medicaid fraud, sexual misconduct, and conflicts of interest in clinical practice or research. In these cases, physicians have flagrantly disregarded their commitment to society and themselves, often placing greed or personal gain above their higher missions. Fortunately, these incidences are quite uncommon.

More frequent are behaviors that are rude or disrespectful or that exhibit incivility. Physician-to-physician conflicts impact patient safety by limiting cooperation and communication among care team members. A study by the Institute of Medicine (IOM) points to poor communication and deficient teamwork as common causes of adverse patient outcomes, even more prevalent than lack of knowledge or clinical skills.[4] Poor communication results in medical and surgical errors as well as poor patient compliance with recommended treatments. Incivilities in the health care system flow in many directions, between primary care physicians and specialists, between surgeons and internal medicine physicians, and between emergency room physicians and inpatient consultants. Poor behavior can be manifest in many ways, such as becoming impatient, or being easily annoyed, argumentative, or dismissive. Common courtesy among colleagues has become less common. In fact, surveys in medical schools indicate that most medical students throughout the country acknowledge that they have witnessed faculty bad mouthing other physicians and other institutions.[9] The impact of witnessing this behavior on medical students is interesting and concerning, but equally or more important is that these conflicts threaten patient safety as well as physicians' sense of satisfaction in their careers.

Although individual resilience plays a pivotal role in professionalism, organizational and institutional culture can also place a burden on physicians. There can be conflicting demands exemplified by the dilemma balancing the commitment to the mission and to the economic margin, as reimbursements go down and costs increase. The message to place profit over purpose can create significant moral distress. The challenges are great.

QUALITY AND SAFETY

Ever since the IOM's publication, "To Err is Human,"[10] and "Crossing the Quality Chasm: A New Health System for the 21st Century,"[11] the focus on health care quality has exploded. Its interest within otolaryngology is no exception. For example, from the years 1990 to 2000, there were fewer than 100 articles indexed in PubMed under the auspices of quality improvement in otolaryngology and zero for pediatric otolaryngology. In contrast, there were more than 1200 articles published under the same subject headings during the last 10 years and close to 200 for pediatric otolaryngology. This increase in quality and safety (Q&S) manuscripts underscores the interest within the specialty and the breadth of original reporting as well.[12–15]

Why Is It Important?

To paraphrase the IOM, quality in health care is the extent that services provided to individuals and populations give rise to the probability of the wanted health outcomes and are harmonious with the current state of medical knowledge.[11] This definition provides several important take-home points and ultimately explains why the study of Q&S is essential. First, the goal is to provide quality care to individuals and populations of individuals. That is, "process" is important, but outcomes are the end game.[10] Performing preoperative tests can be a critical process, but it is linked to and judged by whether it improves the patient's outcomes. Third, establishing and adhering to "best practices" rounds out a proverbial 3-legged stool of the Q&S paradigm. Best practices can be summarized as what is considered the standard of care knowing what we know about the limitations of what we can do.

Other important topics emphasized by the IOM landmark reports are defining the domains of quality, value, and safety in health care.[11] The IOM defines the domains of quality as delivery of health care that is "safe, timely, effective, efficient, equitable, and patient-centered." Health care value is summed up by the equation "Value = Outcomes/cost."[11] A process that improves outcomes may have value even if it is expensive; alternatively, inexpensive therapies may lack value if they will not change the outcomes. Safety in health care is "the freedom from accidental injury when interacting in any health care system."[7] All of these concepts provide useful constructs to evaluate processes and outcomes in Q&S efforts.

This complexity of delivery is a principal reason the study of quality is essential.[10,11,16] A patient has to navigate the various processes to reach whatever outcome that is desired, from discussing their symptoms with various providers; to obtaining a test that may require certain behaviors in order to achieve a valid result (eg, remaining NPO for cholesterol testing); to taking medications correctly. Each step or process can lead to an adverse outcome. The same holds for providers who steer the health care system to deliver care, from making sure to consent the correct patient for the correct procedure; to understanding how the medical equipment works in order to perform the procedure; to writing appropriate discharge orders and instructions in an electronic medical record; to explaining to waiting families what surgery was performed and the expected recovery in a straightforward manner. A misstep at any point could result in adverse outcomes. Therefore, understanding the complexity of the health care system and findings way to minimize the risk inherent in these systems is essential.

Despite the importance of Q&S, there are barriers to embracing these issues, in particular, the standardization of processes.[16,17] This reluctance is due to numerous causes, which include (1) fee-for-service payment structures for patient care; (2) highly skilled labor, which increases the risk of implicit biases centering around the infallibility of their skill sets (think of the surgeon as God motif); (3) the "culture of blame" and perceiving failure as the fault of a single individual that is endemic in health care organizations.

So how does one improve Q&S? Q&S is improved by improving the processes around patient's care. Remember this adage for future reference, "standardization plus situation awareness leads to quality and safety." The processes involved in patient care: patient identification, drug administration, safe hand-offs after surgery, and so forth, have some of the most significant impacts on the outcomes. Simply, process improvement is Q&S improvement.[16] Moreover, process improvement is about using the best evidence available to standardize the approach to patient care.

The Methodologies of Quality and Safety Improvement

Q&S improvements should be continuous. Some desired outcomes cannot be achieved if poor processes are in place, and safety events (undesired outcomes) that do occur cannot be mitigated without new or improved ones. There are several methodologies available to direct these efforts. One of the most well-known is the Plan-Do-Study-Act tool.[18,19] This Q&S tool developed in the 1930s and used broadly in health care provides an outline for any quality and process improvement study.

The Planning phase includes organizing a team and identifying stakeholders, writing problem and principle aim statements, gathering initial data, and creating an intervention based on the data. For example, a project examining unplanned readmission after tracheostomy may include otolaryngologist, pulmonologist, nurse specialist, social workers, and case managers. The problem statement could be, "the unplanned 30-day readmission and revisit rates after the index discharge among the tracheostomy patients is 15% compared to 5% for the hospital average." Further study would then lead to the aim of the study, for example, "this project aims to decrease the percentage of revisits and readmission after discharge to 5%." More specifics can be added to the aim statement, like the date range for the project; why the project is essential; the project goals; as well as the financial aspects of the project. This aim can be the basis of a project charter once the details of the proposal are sufficiently detailed.[20]

The Do phase consists of carrying out the intervention, analyzing the results, and comparing them to past performance. The Study phase looks at the data and compares with the baseline or benchmark data; determines the effectiveness of the interventions; and summarizes the lessons learned from the effort. Also, finally, the Act phase broadens the process implementation if successful or involves going back to the planning phase if not successful: wash, rinse, repeat. That is, as each Q&S initiative ends, a new one begins.

Another more comprehensive methodology is the Balanced Scorecard. The Balanced Scorecard created by Kaplan and Norton[21–23] is a strategic management tool. It aligns the values and objectives of the organization around several "perspectives" to help align various stakeholders as process improvement is undertaken. The CHAMP (Children's Health Airway Management Program)[24] uses this process to improve pediatric tracheostomy outcomes. The program makes use of the following perspectives: financial strength, clinical excellence, operational excellence, and exceptional experience. Each perspective has measures that determine the success of the program. For example, reducing 30-day unplanned revisits is a part of the "clinical excellence" perspective, while ensuring each discharge is seen within 30 days is a part of the "operational excellence" perspective. Both perspectives improve health care outcomes and value, and by adding a financial strength perspective, quality care is delivered that keeps in mind that the margin funds the mission.[25]

Other Q&S improvement approaches are widely available and used. These approaches include the Six Sigma DMAIC (define, measure, analyze, improve, and control),[19,26] the Lean method created from the Toyota Production System,[27–29] and the model for improvement by the Institute for Healthcare Improvement.[19] All of these systems overlap with similar attributes and ends–: identify, organize, implement, and reassess processes and outcomes on a continuous basis. For example, the Lean Method focuses on reducing waste from health care processes by reducing activities that do not add value to a process. Lean principles also see the system from the patient's perspective and optimize their experiences. Employees are empowered via a safety-first culture, and there is commitment to "continuous" improvement. Similarly, the Six Sigma method tries to eliminate "defects" in patient care processes systematically. Any of these methodologies will help with Q&S efforts. What is important is not which tool one uses, but that a methodology for process improvement is included in all Q&S efforts.

Variation Versus Standardization

As mentioned earlier, "standardization plus situation awareness leads to quality and safety improvement." The various Q&S methodologies in part advocate improving outcomes by focusing on the standardizations of care. Alternatively speaking, variations in medical care are more likely to lead to adverse outcomes.[10,11,30–34]

Variation can refer to 2 different ideas: –the first concerns the variation in outcomes that naturally occur; for example, operating room turnover times. In this instance, variation or "variance" refers to dispersion from the central tendency. This variation can also be nonrandom, for example, when there is a shortage of postanesthesia care unit nurses. A Q&S initiative to change this variation will look at trend lines in control charts. One would expect changes after the intervention is implemented.

Another critical variation for Q&S is variations in processes that can lead to poor or unreliable outcomes. For example, variations can occur if the components of the surgical time-out were left up to the individual surgeon. Instead, standardizing the surgical time-out leads to better outcomes by ensuring that essential steps (ie, processes) do not get skipped or overlooked.[11]

The surgical checklist is an excellent example of standardization.[34–39] The surgical checklist consists of steps that should be taken with every surgery. Items include elements that address concerns that occur in the preoperative phase, at the time of anesthesia induction, and after completion of the procedure. A prospective observational study of this single intervention was able to reduce all-cause mortality and in-hospital complications at multiple hospitals across different settings.[35] A checklist of processes is one of the simplest ways to standardize care, and their impact has been studied in otolaryngology.

Related to this standard checklist are algorithms and practice guidelines. Algorithms and guidelines can also reduce variations in health care by reminding clinicians of the best practices for a particular problem. For example, how does one manage patients with peritonsillar abscess[40] or obstructive sleep-disordered breathing?[41,42] The otolaryngology literature is ripe with examples of algorithms and practice guidelines. These publications serve as reminders of the power of standardization to reduce variation and improve Q&S.

Toward High-Reliability Organization

Reliability is one of the principal end goals of Q&S efforts. Reliability in health care means having outcomes and processes that are of high quality, that are efficient, and that are safe.[43] High-reliability organizations (HRO), organizations that can perform complex, hazardous, and technically demanding tasks over a long period without significant errors, have become the holy grail of health delivery systems. Models of these organizations include aircraft carriers, nuclear power plants, and commercial airlines. Health care organizations have a similar task as HROs; that is, the work is risky, complicated, and requires expertise.

There are 5 key components of HROs according to Rochlin and colleagues,[44] who described the concept while studying the processes involved in operating an aircraft carrier. Those principles include adherence to and promotion of high-quality standards and procedures with deference to expertise, risk recognition, operations that monitor precarious conditions, communication strategies to mitigate risk, and a rewards system to culturally condition team members toward safe behaviors. Although applying this model on a system-wide level remains elusive for many health care organizations, it has been applied for smaller functional teams,[45] and considering the success of these efforts, otolaryngology is an area that is ripe for such efforts.

One such potential area is pediatric tracheostomy. The care of a child with a tracheostomy requires experts in speech-language pathology, nursing, respiratory therapy, pulmonology, and otolaryngology. The procedure is routinely performed in complex, critically ill children and carries significant catastrophic risk with routine care if errors occur.

An HRO model of tracheostomy care could include a multidisciplinary team of experts who meet regularly to provide care for these children.[24,46,47] This team would defer to the experts within the team on each aspect of the child's care. The team would put the focus on safety and best practices by designing tools and workflows that are used to mitigate risks and common conditions, for example, accidental decannulation, 1-valve utilization, hearing screening, and so forth. Dashboards could be used to monitor essential trends over time, such as accidental decannulation, unplanned emergency department visits, and other critical metrics for process improvement.

Although this model used tracheostomy as the condition, there are numerous other otolaryngology conditions and services whereby the principles of HRO are being utilized: –hearing loss and cochlear implantation, allergy, and head and neck oncology to name a few.

Finally, no discussion of Q&S would be complete without mentioning "the culture of safety." Humans are by nature, rule-bound social creatures and cultural norms often developed naturally via tit-for-tat modes of cooperation.[48] That is, spoken and implied norms permeate individual behavior throughout any organization. Over time, people will voluntarily engage in behaviors that are consistently rewarded and will avoid behaviors that are punished. The culture of safety within an organization therefore tries to align behaviors via rewards that stress the importance of safety.

James Reason[32] developed a popular model of safety culture. He suggested the components consist of a culture of fairness, reporting, support, and learning. Each component works to ensure that emphasis on safety should prioritize rooting out and learning from risky practices. This culture also recognizes that human errors are inherent within any system and acts to mitigate those risks as opposed to blaming the individual for all errors. This practice includes recognizing if someone is engaging in reckless behavior as opposed to the more common risky behavior.

SUMMARY

Dr King argued that the means are the ends in process. He was arguing that just ends cannot be achieved with unjust means. This philosophy holds true for professionalism, quality, and safety as well. That is, the means by which one engages in professional, quality, and safety are what leads to the ends of each in turn. Understanding and implementing these core principles are now as important as understanding the fundamentals of surgical practice and in some respects more so.

REFERENCES

1. ABIM Foundation. American Board of Internal Medicine, ACP-ASIM Foundation. American College of Physicians-American Society of Internal Medicine, European Federation of Internal Medicine. Medical professionalism in the new millennium: a physician charter. Ann Intern Med 2002;136:243–6.
2. Levinson W, Ginsburg S, Hafferty F, et al. Understading medical professionalism. New York: McGraw-Hill Professional; 2015.
3. Goleman D. Emotional intelligence. Why it can matter more than IQ. Learning 1996;24:49–50.
4. Calling a truce on physician-to-physician incivility to avoid burnout. Available at: https://abimfoundation.org/profile/calling-a-truce. Accessed January 20, 2019.
5. Dyrbye LN, Shanafelt TD, Sinsky CA, et al. Burnout among health care professionals: a call to explore and address this underrecognized threat to safe, high-quality care. National Academy of Medicine, Discussion Paper, July 5, 2017.
6. Thom DH. Physician behaviors the predict trust. J Fam Pract 2001;50:323–8.
7. Robert M, Wachter MD. New York Times 2016;1–17.
8. Shanafelt TD, Noseworthy JH. Executive leadership and physician well-being nine organizational strategies to promote engagement and reduce burnout. Mayo Clin Proc 2017;92(1):129–46.
9. Wiggleton C, Petrusa E, Loomin K, et al. Medical students' experiences of moral distress: development of a web-based survey. Acad Med 2010;85:111–7.
10. Kohn LT, Corrigan J, Donaldson MS. To err is human: building a safer health system. Washington, DC: National Academy Press; 2000.
11. Institute of Medicine (U.S.). Committee on Quality of Health Care in America. Crossing the quality chasm : a new health system for the 21st century. Washington, DC: National Academy Press; 2001.
12. Boss EF, Thompson RE. Patient experience in outpatient pediatric otolaryngology. Laryngoscope 2012;122:2304–10.
13. Bowe SN, McCormick ME. Resident and fellow engagement in safety and quality. Otolaryngol Clin North Am 2019;52:55–62.
14. Ishman SL, Hart CK. Improving outcomes and promoting quality in otolaryngology—beyond the national surgical quality improvement program. JAMA Otolaryngol Head Neck Surg 2016;142:247–8.
15. Lavin J, Shah R, Greenlick H, et al. The Global Tracheostomy Collaborative: one institution's experience with a new quality improvement initiative. Int J Pediatr Otorhinolaryngol 2016;80:106–8.
16. Reed G. Why should we care about quality improvement. Quality improvement basics. Dallas (TX): UT Southwestern Medical Center; 2016. p. 1–8.
17. Berwick DM, Nolan TW, Whittington J. The triple aim: care, health, and cost. Health Aff (Millwood) 2008;27:759–69.
18. Taylor MJ, McNicholas C, Nicolay C, et al. Systematic review of the application of the plan-do-study-act method to improve quality in healthcare. BMJ Qual Saf 2014;23:290–8.
19. How to improve. Instiute for healthcare improvement. Available at: http://www.ihi.org/resources/Pages/HowtoImprove/default.aspx. Accessed January 22, 2019.

20. Project charter. Author is Agency for Healthcare Research and Quality (AHRQ). Available at: https://www.ahrq.gov/sites/default/files/wysiwyg/professionals/systems/hospital/qitoolkit/d2-projectcharter.pdf. Accessed January 14, 2019.

21. Kaplan RS, Norton DP. The balanced scorecard: translating strategy into action. Boston: Harvard Business School Press; 1996.

22. Kaplan RS, Norton DP. The strategy-focused organization: how balanced scorecard companies thrive in the new business environment. Boston: Harvard Business School Press; 2001.

23. Kaplan RS, Norton DP. Alignment: using the balanced scorecard to create corporate synergies. Boston: Harvard Business School Press; 2006.

24. Children's health management program. Available at: https://www.childrens.com/specialties-services/specialty-centers-and-programs/ear-nose-and-throat/programsand-services/airway-management-program. Accessed January 20, 2019.

25. Thomas R. Irene Kraus, 74, nun who led big nonprofit hospital chain. The New York Times; 1998.

26. Barry R, Smith AC, Brubaker C. 2nd edition. High-reliability healthcare: improving patient safety and outcomes with Six Sigma. ACHE management series, vol. ix. Chicago: HAP; 2017. p. 270.

27. Kim CS, Spahlinger DA, Kin JM, et al. Lean health care: what can hospitals learn from a world-class automaker? J Hosp Med 2006;1:191–9.

28. Johnson JE, Smith AL, Mastro KA. From Toyota to the bedside: nurses can lead the lean way in health care reform. Nurs Adm Q 2012;36:234–42.

29. Kissoon N. The Toyota way . or not?—new lessons for health care. Physician Exec 2010;36:40–2.

30. Barron CL, Elmaraghy CA, Lemle S, et al. Clinical indices to drive quality improvement in otolaryngology. Otolaryngol Clin North Am 2019;52:123–33.

31. Christianson MK, Sutcliffe KM, Miller MA, et al. Becoming a high reliability organization. Crit Care 2011;15:314.

32. Reason J. Managing RIsk of organization accidents. Aldershot (UK): Ashgate Publishing LImited; 1997.

33. Langley G, Moen R, Nolan KM, et al. The improvement guide: a practical approach to enhancing organizational performance. 2nd edition. San Francisco (CA): Wiley; 2009.

34. Shah RK, Arjmand E, Roberson DW, et al. Variation in surgical time-out and site marking within pediatric otolaryngology. Arch Otolaryngol Head Neck Surg 2011;137:69–73.

35. Helmio P, Blomgren K, Takala A, et al. Towards better patient safety: WHO Surgical Safety Checklist in otorhinolaryngology. Clin Otolaryngol 2011;36:242–7.

36. Kim SW, Maturo S, Dwyer D, et al. Interdisciplinary development and implementation of communication checklist for postoperative management of pediatric airway patients. Otolaryngol Head Neck Surg 2012;146:129–34.

37. Lingard L, Regehr G, Orser B, et al. Evaluation of a preoperative checklist and team briefing among surgeons, nurses, and anesthesiologists to reduce failures in communication. Arch Surg 2008;143:12–7 [discussion: 8].

38. Prager JD, Ruiz AG, Mooney K, et al. Improving operative flow during pediatric airway evaluation: a quality-improvement initiative. JAMA Otolaryngol Head Neck Surg 2015;141:229–35.

39. Soler ZM, Smith TL. Endoscopic sinus surgery checklist. Laryngoscope 2012;122:137–9.

40. Johnson RF. Emergency department visits, hospitalizations, and readmissions of patients with a peritonsillar abscess. Laryngoscope 2017;127(Suppl 5):S1–9.
41. Baugh RF, Archer SM, Mitchell RB, et al. Clinical practice guideline: tonsillectomy in children. Otolaryngol Head Neck Surg 2011;144:S1–30.
42. Roland PS, Rosenfeld RM, Brooks LJ, et al. Clinical practice guideline: polysomnography for sleep-disordered breathing prior to tonsillectomy in children. Otolaryngol Head Neck Surg 2011;145:S1–15.
43. Hendler R. Quality improvement basics. High reliability in health care. Dallas (TX): UT Southwestern Medical Center; 2016.
44. Rochlin GI, La Porte TR, Roberts KH. The self-designing high-reliability organization: aircraft carrier flight operations at sea. Naval War College Review 1987;40: 76–90.
45. Wilson KA, Burke CS, Priest HA, et al. Promoting health care safety through training high reliability teams. Qual Saf Health Care 2005;14:303–9.
46. Baker DP, Day R, Salas E. Teamwork as an essential component of high-reliability organizations. Health Serv Res 2006;41:1576–98.
47. Bedwell JR, Pandian V, Roberson DW, et al. Multidisciplinary tracheostomy care: how collaboratives drive quality improvement. Otolaryngol Clin North Am 2019; 52:135–47.
48. Axelrod R. The evolution of cooperation. New York: Basic Books; 1984.

1. Publication Title	2. Publication Number	3. Filing Date
OTOLARYNGOLOGIC CLINICS OF NORTH AMERICA	466 – 550	9/18/2019

4. Issue Frequency	5. Number of Issues Published Annually	6. Annual Subscription Price
FEB, APR, JUN, AUG, OCT, DEC	6	$412.00

7. Complete Mailing Address of Known Office of Publication (Not printer) (Street, city, county, state, and ZIP+4®)

ELSEVIER INC.
230 Park Avenue, Suite 800
New York, NY 10169

Contact Person
STEPHEN R. BUSHING

Telephone (Include area code)
215-239-3688

8. Complete Mailing Address of Headquarters or General Business Office of Publisher (Not printer)

ELSEVIER INC.
230 Park Avenue, Suite 800
New York, NY 10169

9. Full Names and Complete Mailing Addresses of Publisher, Editor, and Managing Editor (Do not leave blank)

Publisher (Name and complete mailing address)

TAYLOR BALL, ELSEVIER INC.
1600 JOHN F KENNEDY BLVD. SUITE 1800
PHILADELPHIA, PA 19103-2899

Editor (Name and complete mailing address)

JESSICA MCCOOL, ELSEVIER INC.
1600 JOHN F KENNEDY BLVD. SUITE 1800
PHILADELPHIA, PA 19103-2899

Managing Editor (Name and complete mailing address)

PATRICK MANLEY, ELSEVIER INC.
1600 JOHN F KENNEDY BLVD. SUITE 1800
PHILADELPHIA, PA 19103-2899

10. Owner (Do not leave blank. If the publication is owned by a corporation, give the name and address of the corporation immediately followed by the names and addresses of all stockholders owning or holding 1 percent or more of the total amount of stock. If not owned by a corporation, give the names and addresses of the individual owners. If owned by a partnership or other unincorporated firm, give its name and address as well as those of each individual owner. If the publication is published by a nonprofit organization, give its name and address.)

Full Name	Complete Mailing Address
WHOLLY OWNED SUBSIDIARY OF REED/ELSEVIER, US HOLDINGS	1600 JOHN F KENNEDY BLVD. SUITE 1800 PHILADELPHIA, PA 19103-2899

11. Known Bondholders, Mortgagees, and Other Security Holders Owning or Holding 1 Percent or More of Total Amount of Bonds, Mortgages, or Other Securities. If none, check box ► ☐ None

Full Name	Complete Mailing Address
N/A	

12. Tax Status (For completion by nonprofit organizations authorized to mail at nonprofit rates) (Check one)
The purpose, function, and nonprofit status of this organization and the exempt status for federal income tax purposes:
☒ Has Not Changed During Preceding 12 Months
☐ Has Changed During Preceding 12 Months (Publisher must submit explanation of change with this statement)

PS Form **3526**, July 2014 (Page 1 of 4 (see instructions page 4)) PSN 7530-01-000-9931 PRIVACY NOTICE: See our privacy policy on www.usps.com.

13. Publication Title	14. Issue Date for Circulation Data Below
OTOLARYNGOLOGIC CLINICS OF NORTH AMERICA	JUNE 2019

15. Extent and Nature of Circulation			Average No. Copies Each Issue During Preceding 12 Months	No. Copies of Single Issue Published Nearest to Filing Date
a. Total Number of Copies (Net press run)			274	325
b. Paid Circulation (By Mail and Outside the Mail)	(1)	Mailed Outside-County Paid Subscriptions Stated on PS Form 3541 (include paid distribution above nominal rate, advertiser's proof copies, and exchange copies)	116	162
	(2)	Mailed In-County Paid Subscriptions Stated on PS Form 3541 (include paid distribution above nominal rate, advertiser's proof copies, and exchange copies)	0	0
	(3)	Paid Distribution Outside the Mails Including Sales Through Dealers and Carriers, Street Vendors, Counter Sales, and Other Paid Distribution Outside USPS®	87	122
	(4)	Paid Distribution by Other Classes of Mail Through the USPS (e.g. First-Class Mail®)	0	0
c. Total Paid Distribution (Sum of 15b (1), (2), (3), and (4))			203	284
d. Free or Nominal Rate Distribution (By Mail and Outside the Mail)	(1)	Free or Nominal Rate Outside-County Copies included on PS Form 3541	57	21
	(2)	Free or Nominal Rate In-County Copies Included on PS Form 3541	0	0
	(3)	Free or Nominal Rate Copies Mailed at Other Classes Through the USPS (e.g. First-Class Mail)	0	0
	(4)	Free or Nominal Rate Distribution Outside the Mail (Carriers or other means)	0	0
e. Total Free or Nominal Rate Distribution (Sum of 15d (1), (2), (3) and (4))			57	21
f. Total Distribution (Sum of 15c and 15e)			260	305
g. Copies not Distributed (See Instructions to Publishers #4 (page #3))			14	20
h. Total (Sum of 15f and g)			274	325
i. Percent Paid (15c divided by 15f times 100)			78.08%	93.11%

* If you are claiming electronic copies, go to line 16 on page 3. If you are not claiming electronic copies, skip to line 17 on page 3.

16. Electronic Copy Circulation		Average No. Copies Each Issue During Preceding 12 Months	No. Copies of Single Issue Published Nearest to Filing Date
a. Paid Electronic Copies	►		
b. Total Paid Print Copies (Line 15c) + Paid Electronic Copies (Line 16a)	►		
c. Total Print Distribution (Line 15f) + Paid Electronic Copies (Line 16a)	►		
d. Percent Paid (Both Print & Electronic Copies) (16b divided by 16c × 100)	►		

☒ I certify that 50% of all my distributed copies (electronic and print) are paid above a nominal price.

17. Publication of Statement of Ownership

☒ If the publication is a general publication, publication of this statement is required. Will be printed ☐ Publication not required.
in the October 2019 issue of this publication.

18. Signature and Title of Editor, Publisher, Business Manager, or Owner

STEPHEN R. BUSHING - INVENTORY DISTRIBUTION CONTROL MANAGER

Date 9/18/2019

I certify that all information furnished on this form is true and complete. I understand that anyone who furnishes false or misleading information on this form or who omits material or information requested on the form may be subject to criminal sanctions (including fines and imprisonment) and/or civil sanctions (including civil penalties).

PS Form **3526**, July 2014 (Page 3 of 4) PRIVACY NOTICE: See our privacy policy on www.usps.com.

Moving?

Make sure your subscription moves with you!

To notify us of your new address, find your **Clinics Account Number** (located on your mailing label above your name), and contact customer service at:

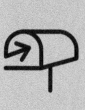

Email: journalscustomerservice-usa@elsevier.com

800-654-2452 (subscribers in the U.S. & Canada)
314-447-8871 (subscribers outside of the U.S. & Canada)

Fax number: 314-447-8029

Elsevier Health Sciences Division
Subscription Customer Service
3251 Riverport Lane
Maryland Heights, MO 63043

*To ensure uninterrupted delivery of your subscription, please notify us at least 4 weeks in advance of move.

ELSEVIER

Printed and bound by CPI Group (UK) Ltd, Croydon, CR0 4YY

03/10/2024

01040404-0001